Health Education

■ ■ ■

The Jones and Bartlett Series in Health Sciences

Health Education

A Cognitive-Behavioral Approach

■ ■ ■

Donald A. Read

Worcester State College

Jones and Bartlett Publishers

Sudbury, Massachusetts

Boston   London   Singapore

Editorial, Sales, and Customer Service Offices
Jones and Bartlett Publishers
40 Tall Pine Drive
Sudbury, MA 01776
1-800-832-0034
508-443-5000
info@jbpub.com
http://www.jbpub.com

Jones and Bartlett Publishers International
Barb House, Barb Mews
London W6 7PA
UK

Library of Congress Cataloging-in-Publication Data
Read, Donald A.
    Health education : a cognitive-behavioral approach / Donald A. Read.
        p.   cm.
    Includes bibliographical references and index.
    ISBN 0-7637-0147-5
    1. Health education.   I. Title.
RA440.5.R39   1997
613—dc20   96-22262
                                                                CIP

Vice President, Editorial: Joseph E. Burns
Senior Production Administrator: Mary Sanger
Manufacturing Manager: Dana L. Cerrito
Design: Susan Gerould, Perspectives
Editorial Production Services: WordCrafters Editorial Services, Inc.
Typesetting: Publishers' Design and Production Services, Inc.
Cover Design: Marshall Henrichs
Printing and Binding: Hamilton Printing Co.
Cover Printing: John P. Pow Company

Printed in the United States of America
00 99 98 97 96   10 9 8 7 6 5 4 3 2 1

To Florence A. Read

Her countenance radiates love. Her expressions of unconditional love for her brother, Robert; my father; my brother, Hugh; our family; my children, Robin and Craig; my daughter's son, Max; her grandson, Kevin; and her countless friends, have all influenced my life. These expressions ultimately have found their way into the words and thoughts of this book.

It is not enough for me to ask the questions; I want to know how to answer the one question that seems to encompass everything I face: What am I here for?

—ABRAHAM HESCHEL

Contents

Introduction

> *Education should, but does not, teach us to make effective use of our bodies and our minds. We are not taught the interrelatedness of movement, sensing, thinking, and feeling functions, or how mind and body interact to determine what we are and what we can do. We are not even taught how to use our bodies efficiently so as to avoid damage to the organism. Nor are we given any inkling of the true range of our human potentials, much less how to use them productively. By suppressing many of our potentials, we develop the personality (and doubtless the brain also) in an imbalanced way. Adequate awareness of the body and of body-mind interactions is basic of self-knowledge, and until these defects are remedied, education will always fail—fundamentally. Whatever is learned and taught by individuals who are thus handicapped by basic self-ignorance cannot be learned or taught as well as it might be.*
>
> —ROBERT MASTERS AND JEAN HOUSTON,
> *LISTENING TO THE BODY*

Building on Masters and Houston's premise, this is a book about the *process* of health education with a focus on the whole person; thus, it will include a comprehensive discussion of the skills and strategies that are of critical importance in this process.

In *Health Education: A Cognitive-Behavioral Approach*, emphasis is placed squarely on you, the reader and health educator. This is because it is my belief that the most effective way to teach health education is through a process by which you are placed in the role of facilitator for change. As Chinese philosopher Lao-tzu said, "If we want things to stay as they are, things will have to change." Health education makes the best vehicle for this change, for it has the potential to direct learning away from the belief that all behaviors are the product of external stimuli alone to an approach that emphasizes the importance of the whole person as a coparticipant in shaping his life and embracing his personal choices.

The first aim of this book is toward *primary prevention*. Here, the focus is on a process that encourages the learner to examine carefully the health choices she is making and how these choices are affecting her present level of personal satisfaction. To achieve this, health education must focus on a behavioral change pattern from how things are, to what they may be, and the changes that need to be made in this process.

At the heart of this book is *secondary prevention*. Here, the focus is on ways of reducing or eliminating negative health behaviors. For lack of a better word, we call this intervention. In this approach, the emphasis is on behavioral changes that can lead to more control over one's health behaviors and thus to a much wider range of personal health choices. In a cognitive-behavioral approach to health education the focus must be placed squarely on identifying unhealthy behaviors and their cognitive supports, and through appropriate health education, such an approach is effective in bringing about change. This often requires a simultaneously multifaceted approach.

The fundamental thesis of this book is simple: *Health education can be more effective if it is not only cognitive and behaviorally understood and practiced, but is also democratic in its approach.* By this I mean that the health educator cannot assume some arbitrary state of mind or skill for the learner, nor can he impose the process of understanding. The process of understanding should not exclude but rather encourage individual thinking and behaving. Health-education goals and objectives can be individualized and collectively involve each individual's thinking, feeling, and acting. Thinking and emotion are at the very heart of health education, because both the subject and the person are so intimately intertwined. The bottom line is health is primarily a matter of choices, however positive or negative, personal or impersonal. And these choices cannot be left to chance but instead to the student's ability to discern what's going on around and within himself; for, as Sartre pointed out, "We are our choices." Health education is in the pivotal position of providing the critical link in what Freire (1973) calls *critical consciousness*—allowing someone to make broad connections between individual experiences and social meanings.

An Overview

Part 1 starts by presenting an overview of what health and health education mean from various perspectives and how these perspectives impact on the future. It also includes a concept of health from a holistic perspective (here the wisdom of the mind/body connection is stressed) and a presentation of the realities that now exist and what health education needs to address as it approaches the twenty-first century. Another focus is to help the reader know and question what has been done and what needs to be done. The section closes with a brief but important introduction to cognitive-behavioral theory.

Part 2 explores the five stages in a cognitive-behavioral approach to health education; namely, the *relationship-building, exploratory, decision-making, working,* and *termination* stages. The final chapter in this section uses AIDS education to bring the five stages together into one suggested model.

Part 3 explores the psychosocial issues of values and self-esteem. Emphasis is placed on both character education and self-esteem, with suggestions as to how using some well-tested theories (including those of humanistic psychology from both Abraham Maslow and Carl Rogers) can lead to both personal empowerment and more positive health choices.

Part 4 explores teaching and learning styles as well as issues and concerns for consideration in health education. Emphasis here is on the fact that we tend to teach the way we learn and the importance of understanding how this impacts our views.

Finally, Part 5 explores the role of the health educator as counselor. Although this may read like a laundromat "wash-and-dry" approach, let it serve as an impetus to further your understanding of this vital aspect of health education.

The purpose of this book is to provide the reader with ways to create response capacity and introduce new ways of looking at and improving personal health choices and satisfaction. By doing this, the health educator can help move the learner from being (or becoming) the victim of her personal health choices toward empowering her to feel good about her choices (based on the premise that these choices are truly adult, informed, and responsible and include the student's personal values). In doing this, the health educator creates an environment conducive to critical thinking, thus helping the learners to flourish intellectually and grow into lifelong, self-directed learners.

A second focus of this book is to present a clear, comprehensive approach to health education that considers the perspective of the learner. I am convinced that real learning takes place when the learner can make sense of the *what* and *why* behind the things he is learning and how they impact his *thoughts, feelings,* and *actions*; as such, a cognitive-behavioral approach is the most logical choice and is the focus of this text. By approaching health education from this perspective, educators are able to adopt a balanced, personal, multifaceted approach.

Health Education: A Cognitive-Behavioral Approach is about forging a bridge between the learner's thoughts, feelings, and actions and a collective set of goals and objectives. Cognitive-behavioral theory provides that bridge by integrating thought and behavior into one synergistic approach to health education that can accommodate the whole person. This encourages the learner to look at and deal with his personal-health behaviors and choices in a much more integrated way, leading to an exciting, process-oriented learning environment in which the individual examines important personal events and considers new behavioral possibilities based on his own thoughts, feelings, and actions. Cognitive techniques, such as lectures, readings, collection of data, and specific planning combined with the behavioral components of emotion and action help in bringing about this synergistic process.

A cautionary note must be mentioned here. In moving toward the above goals, the educator must be aware of the potential risks involved in challenging the learner to consider changing even one—seemingly insignificant—behavior. For example, learned anger toward another person because of the color of her skin or her beliefs may be at the sacrifice of the student's own feelings. These feelings need to be understood by health educators in a way that assumes people are basically good, care about themselves, and are forward moving. And so, if health education is to be true to itself, it must challenge the learner to rethink her personal views, and through this process, help her to become more conscious of how she views herself, others, and the world around her. Through this dynamic process, the health educator can help the learner become more conscious of how she thinks and feels and actively participate in and facilitate holistic learning. By approaching health education in this way, we share in the process of opening doors not only to the learners' knowledge, but to their beliefs and concerns. Existentialists, such as the Danish philosopher Kierkegaard, Sartre, and Heidegger, have presented a view of humankind that gives individuals more responsibility for their actions—to become, in the words of Soren Kierkegaard, "that self thou truly art."

It is important to point out that a new idea becomes self-fulfilling only when someone chooses not only to *take the leap*, but to *make the leap*. To this end—to embrace what we know and have and are happy and secure with, or to take that leap of faith and change our thoughts and actions—is based on one critical factor: the individual. So, what is the role of the health educator? To borrow from the words of Joseph Chilton Pearce in *Evolution's End* (1992), ". . . . to turn scientific ideas into an ingenious and optimistic portrait of human potential." I can't think of a better jumping-off point than that.

Health Promotion for the Whole Person

A person's sense of coherence is crucial to a comprehensive understanding of the choices he makes when it comes to health. Health education provides the critical link through which the individual can create and maintain his way of feeling and behaving rather than being controlled by these behaviors. This sense of coherence includes the whole person—mind, body, personal beliefs, and concerns. In changing his behavior, the learner is often forced to take up new patterns and skills as well as new concerns and meanings. Add to this the fact that most current health literature indicates that someone who practices an unhealthy habit is practicing it on others as well. These changes, if successful, usually cannot just be a layering on of new ideas and behaviors. Old ones need to be altered and, in some cases, dropped altogether. A reorganization of one's life needs to take place, and all or part of this change often requires support within the context of familial as well as social patterns.

Cognitive-behavioral therapies have empirically proven more effective than either cognitive or behavioral therapy alone (Holroyd, Appel, and Andrasik, 1983). The phenomenologist would explain that the combined approach has the advantage of focusing on thinking habits along with feeling and acting. The behavioral approach adds new skills and habits, while the cognitive approach addresses the need and provides the skills for new self-interpretations. In sum, it can be said that a health-education program that is based on a comprehensive cognitive-behavioral approach offers the health educator a much wider range of possible interventions. Since in my view it is assumed that the person is at least a somewhat integrated being, change in any one area will bring about change in others. It is a truism that a change in how one thinks about something or how one understands something will affect how one feels. To get to the very heart of this book, *any change in formal beliefs or in personal meanings will cause a shift in one's emotional outlook, opening up new ways of thinking, feeling, and acting.*

How to Use This Text Effectively

As you move forward, you will be presented with various questions and food for thought in each chapter. These questions are designed to probe your thoughts and feelings. Take some time to respond as you feel. Your response may help in exploring your own feelings and, in some cases, behaviors. I encourage you to question, challenge yourself, and think about what rings true for you.

You can use this text in a number of ways. One is to explore the concept of health from a holistic perspective. Another is to apply this concept to health education. Still another is to think about the concept of health and health education as a theoretical framework including all the phenomena related to human learning and experience that previously have been ignored by traditional academic psychology.

Remember that the central focus of this text is that human beings have vast potentials that are seldom tapped. Health education can tap one of those potentials: it can help the learner to explore the elusive issue of why he behaves the way he does in the context of his health and well-being, and if this behavior is negative, it can help him explore and create alternative ways of thinking, feeling, and behaving.

Acknowledgments

Six years of research and four years in its writing, this text represents the infusion of a great number of people, places, and things. I am ever grateful for the wonderful critiques and creative perspectives that were provided by the reviewers who read and reread various drafts. These people include Rick Barns, East Carolina University; Michael J. Cleary, Slippery Rock University; Myra Edelstein, Worcester State College; Mark J. Kittleson, Southern Illinois University; Larry K. Olsen, the Pennsylvania State University; Gayle Schmidt, Texas A&M University; Margaret M. Smith, Oregon State University; and Walt Stoll, M.D., A.B.E.P., special friend and inner-circle member of my life who read and contributed to the chapters on holistic health and its meanings. I am also grateful to Tom Lyndon for the small miracle of counteracting my genius for not getting the English language quite right. And to Donna Vaillancourt, who edited the final manuscript, much, much thanks. Finally, to Joe Burns, vice president of Jones and Bartlett, thanks for your early and steadfast support.

I remain indebted to my principle mentors whose influence is both explicit and implicit in these pages: Professor William Creswell, my former swimming coach and teacher, who first turned me on to health education at the University of Northern Colorado at Greeley; Dr. Warren Johnson, University of Maryland, who lead me into the arena of health behavior and self-as-agent-for-change during my master's degree years in health education; Dr. Carl Willgoose, who taught me the important concept of commitment to the profession of health education while I was a doctoral student at Boston University; and to Dr. William Darity, former dean of the School of Public Health at the University of Massachusetts at Amherst where I first taught, multiple thanks for helping me sharpen my understanding of the field of public health.

Finally, thanks to Worcester State College for always supporting my work in this vital academic arena and respecting my professional freedom of expression; to Yvonne Chen, M.D., my colleague in the Department of Health Science, who always gifts me with a certain inner peace of mind; to Don Traub, Ph.D., professor of philosophy, for the support and encouragement of my ideas and philosophy during my seminal work in establishing the Department of Health Science at Worcester State College, I shall never forget; and to Patricia A. Houston, my special T.A. at Worcester State, who wrote the interactive scripts for *Philadelphia* and *Forrest Gump* and coauthored the instructor's manual.

I am indebted to the work of such people as Ruth Wylie who, with her book *The Self-Concept* (1961), was the spark for my doctoral dissertation and thus certainly is a part of this book; to the writings and thoughts of John Dewey, whose articulate concept of progressive education led me to a fuller understanding of holistic learning; to Marilyn Ferguson, whose transformational work *The Aquarian Conspiracy* (1980) helped me better understand the mind-body connection as it applied to the changes going on in my own life; to Larry Dossey, M.D., whose book *Beyond Illness: Discovering the Experience of Health* (1984) greatly solidified and reinforced my concept of health; and to Ira Shor, who helped me make the connection between empowerment and education through his book *Empowering Education: Critical Teaching for Social Change* (1992). To Robert Pirsing, fellow biker, for his personal tour through two points in *Zen and the Art of Motorcycle Maintenance* (1975), thanks for the inspiration to continue on. Finally, to Muriel and John James, coauthors of *Passion for Life: Psychology and the Human Spirit* (1991), thanks for helping me recognize the spiritual side of life and health.

Additional acknowledgment is warranted for the writings and work of such people as Fritz Perls, M.D., founder of Gestalt therapy; William Glasser, M.D., founder and creator of reality therapy; Dr. Albert Ellis, whose theory of rational-emotive therapy (RET) is considered part of existential-humanistic psychology; Ashley Montague, anthropologist; Joseph Chilton Pearce, and his special attention to human potential; and Dr. Albert Bandura, a behavioral psychologist who developed an approach to reducing fears and anxieties based on the fact that imitation is one of our basic ways of learning. This belief represents the very infrastructure of this text. Multiple, multiple thanks.

References

Dossey, Larry. *Beyond Illness: Discovering the Experience of Health*. Boulder, CO: New Science Library, 1984.

Ferguson, Marilyn. *The Aquarian Conspiracy: Personal and Social Transformation in the 1980s*. Los Angeles: J.P. Tarcher, 1980.

Freire, Paulo. *Education for Critical Consciousness*. New York: Seabury, 1973.

Holroyd, K.A., M.A. Appel, and F. Andrasik. "A Cognitive-Behavioral Approach to Psychophysiological Disorders." In D. Meichenbaum and M.E. Jaremko (eds.), *Stress Reduction and Prevention*. New York: Plenum, 1983.

James, Muriel, and John James. *Passion for Life: Psychology and the Human Spirit*. New York: Dutton, 1991.

Masters, Robert, and Jean Houston. *Listening to the Body: The Psychophysical Way to Health and Awareness*. New York: Delta Books, 1978.

Pearce, Joseph Chilton. *Evolution's End: Claiming the Potential of Our Intelligence*. New York: HarperCollins, 1992.

Pirsing, Robert M. *Zen and the Art of Motorcycle Maintenance: An Inquiry into Values*. New York: Bantam Books, 1975.

Shor, Ira. *Empowering Education: Critical Teaching for Social Change*. Chicago: University of Chicago Press, 1992.

Wylie, Ruth. *The Self Concept*. Lincoln: University of Nebraska Press, 1961.

The Hows and Whys of Health Education

Underlying Conditions

These introductory chapters examine the relationship between the reality of what is happening today in learning, teaching, and information and the principal targets of this information and teaching—students. What is health education all about? To give students facts? To give them information so they can make healthy choices? To give them a positive sense of self so that they can examine their own beliefs and values? To empower them to change their current negative attitudes and behaviors?

These questions, increasingly asked by health educators, undergird this book, especially these first four chapters. The immense variety of issues faced by young people and adults today requires an approach to teaching that does not fit easily into any one mode. What is needed is an articulation of alternative approaches to health education that are based on the primacy of empowerment and caring. *Empowerment* means health education must become more involved in helping students understand and act on the critical health choices they face from a realistic point of view. *Caring* means emphasizing the connection between information and concerns of the students. Certain teaching techniques will not work unless a basic level of empowerment and caring is in place.

The difference that we need to understand between health education of the past and that of the present is the tendency for past health educators to consider her theories and methods as the only way. Carlos Castaneda said in *Tales of Power* (1974), " . . . the first act of a teacher is to introduce the idea that the world we think we see is only a view, a description of the world." How we as adults view the world is not how students view it; our reality is not necessarily their reality. And so, we must begin by looking inward to what and who we are, how we feel about ourselves, and how we as health educators participate in and take responsibility for our own professional lives.

The overall view of health and health education is of crucial importance in this process. Chapter 1 discusses these issues. Chapter 2 focuses on a much broader concept of health, exploring the fallacy of considering mind and body as separate entities and the significance of holistic health. Chapter 3 offers a reality check by pointing out how society has failed our youth, why this has happened, and what some of the results of this failure are. Chapter 4 delineates the characteristics of a cognitive-behavioral approach and examines the broad theory of cognitive-behavioral teaching.

Part I looks at today's fast-lane, high-tech conditions and how they require a change in the way health education is taught. What follows is the theory and practice that links critical pedagogy to positive health behaviors and personal empowerment.

Reference

Castaneda, Carlos. *Tales of Power.* New York: Simon & Schuster, 1974.

1 Health and Health Education

The questions we should ask of health and health education are both intertwined and manifold. What is health? What are its delimitations? How can we recognize those who have high potential for helping others? Are there valid ways of teaching for positive health potential? What kind of health-education focus do we use? What kind do we need? How can we get from one to the other? Finally, can professional programs in health education help students become critical thinkers, feeling people, and self-motivated health-change agents?

Those in the profession may be left with the conclusion that health education is an enigma. However, if we are concerned enough we can plumb its depths to the extent that we are willing to know ourselves on our own terms.

Whether you are a school- or community-health educator the subject of health is vitally important to all of us. Health is truly a shared phenomenon, with roots extending outside our profession. Cigarette smoking has long been considered a matter of choice, but today we know this choice has serious consequences for those who choose not to smoke. AIDS, drugs, drunk driving, violence, guns, child abuse, and dysfunctional families send a strong message that we are living in an era in which our actions and behavior affect the lives of others. We know that we cannot act in the world without affecting others—extending even to their physiological functioning.

This fact calls for a new, expanded definition of health and illness that involves the whole spectrum of consciousness to include body, mind, and personal meanings and concerns (see Chapter 2). Peper and Kushel (1985) extend this concept to include the individual's local network of relations and belief system. A comprehensive health-education program must evolve, expanding our focus to include the many personal, familial, social environmental, and

Illness is the night-side of life, a more onerous citizenship. Everyone who is born holds dual citizenship, in the kingdom of the well and in the kingdom of the sick. Although we all prefer to use only the good passport, sooner or later each of us is obliged, at least for a spell, to identify ourselves as citizens of that other place.

—SUSAN SONTAG

personal meanings that promote health, prevent illness, and encourage healing. A comprehensive health-education program must also involve the learner in the whole process. This attitude emphasizes the responsibility of the person for his or her own health and the importance of mobilizing the person's own unique health capacities.

Before this chapter moves on to health education, it must define the term *health*. Take a moment to think about how you define health by answering the questions that follow.

Health, Illness, and Disease

Health is not the absence of illness, and illness is not the same as disease (Kleinman, Eisenberg, and Good, 1978). *Illness* is the human experience of loss or dysfunction, whereas *disease* is aberration at the cellular, tissue, or organ level. As Oliver Sacks notes, " . . . animals get disease, but only man falls radically into sickness" (1985).

Since not all illness is caused by disease, illness cannot be reduced to a non-scientific account of disease. Illness has a reality of its own. All objectives of health education must make sense in terms of the human experience. To understand this in a personal sense, we must understand what behavioral psychologist Albert Bandura (1969) says, which is we must *imitate what the model does*—in essence, become, for a moment, the other person, know what they know and feel what they feel. In *Being and Caring* (1984), Daniels and Horowitz describe this further:

Creativity exists when we find new ways of understanding relationships and relating to the world of things. It can occur at the easel, at the kitchen table, or at an insurance executive's desk. Creativity includes perceiving and responding to the world anew, out of the sense of wonder—the ability to enter a situation and see it "as if for the first time." We can begin such exploration by finding out what's already highly developed in us, and what's less so. And therein lies a fascinating tale.

To accomplish this inner state is to unlock some of our latent potentials. How can we learn to use the abilities that may be hidden in our minds? A partial answer may be found in studying people whose unusual abilities have lead to health, love, and joy in their lives.

Health educators must present health as a shared phenomenon, with roots extending outside the individual. The "new" thinking in health education gives us a fresh perspective on the old Delphic precept, "know thyself." Any theory of health education that does not acknowledge this is bound to be, at best, incomplete. So, let's start with some questions:

- What is health?
- What does it mean to me?
- What does it mean for health education?

Toward a Personal Concept of Health

Health is most always measured against a concept of illness. Take for example the often quoted definition given by the World Health Organization:

Health is a state of complete physical, mental, and social well-being and not merely the absence of disease or infirmity.

The question that needs to be addressed is how does one define such words as "state," "complete," "physical," and "mental?" Try this experiment with an unsuspecting friend: Ask him the following questions, and see if you get similar answers:

"What does the word health mean to you?"

"Oh, it's a state of feeling good I guess."

"What's a state of feeling good?"

"It's a kind of feeling I have."

"What's a feeling?"

"Hey, is this a joke?"

You have pushed him into a loss for words. That is because the word *health* defies definition as a measurable quantity. It requires an additional level of *feeling* and *behaving*.

For health educators to help students move closer to a more personal concept of health is to go down the "abstraction ladder," as Hayakawa described in his book *Language in Thought and Action* (1964). He believed we must go to *lower* levels of abstraction where the health educator asks the question, "What does the word health mean to you?" Like peeling an onion, we help the learner get to the very core and content of what health means to her.

For these reasons, it is the contention of the author (along with others) that a definition of health is not operational without including *feelings* and *experiences*. Health includes how one experiences it (as opposed to illness) as well as what and how one feels. Definitions can be found (see Appendix A), but they are limited in their ability to express feelings and experiences: "Many of us have become inured to health. We have lost what we once knew in keen purity, excitement, fulfillment. We are numb to the *experience* of health" (Dossey, 1984). According to Kate Duff (1993), "We have lost the ability to come to terms with pain and suffering, to be changed, informed, and even illuminated by their presence in our lives." These ideas bring to mind the concept of being and nothingness that Sartre (1948, 1957) talked about, in which the person is seen as capable of choosing meanings without regard for past experiences or present understanding.

Which brings me to the point of all of this: In attempting to define health, we tend to lose sight of our feelings and experiences. My suggestion is that we be guided by what Hayakawa (1964) said: "The kind of 'thinking' we must be extremely wary of is that which *never* leaves the higher verbal levels of abstraction, the kind that never points *down* the abstraction ladder to lower levels of abstraction and from there to the extensional world."

In terms of defining the word health, and picking up on the earlier scenario, ask your friend these additional questions:

"What do you mean by feeling?"

"Something inside me."

"What do you mean by inside?"

"Well, I guess I mean a gut feeling, a reaction, a feeling that makes me feel good or not so good, happy or sad."

"Such as?"

"When my brother got killed in a gang fight."

"And that made you feel . . .?"

That health education should never point down to a lower level of abstraction is to deny one's personal concept of health. A personal concept of health means that one's health choices are based not only on one's thinking, but on one's *personal meanings* and *concerns* as well. Health education must provide that vehicle through which the learner can experience all three as one. Paul Lee, in the introduction to Paul Tillich's *The Meaning of Health* (1981), explores this process in his own life:

> *As the son of a doctor, I had decided against medicine and for theology and philosophy as a career. Tillich restored to me the lost unity of these two subject matters, as well, by placing the theme of "healing" and the meaning of health in its old cosmic frame, within the context of salvation and its etymological origins.*

Healing is restored to its religious dignity. Tillich shows this ancient unity of powers and functions before their historical separation. He anticipated the longing for their mutual convergence as currently expressed in the wholistic health movement now sweeping the country in all of its varied forms.

I would like to conclude this discussion on a concept of health with a quote from Donald A. Tubesing (1979): "This book calls for a redefinition of health and illness in the context of a broader view of life, health, and the quality of life in order to include the whole person, and the mental, emotional, and spiritual sides of life as well as the physical. Only a redefinition of health care to include the whole person will begin to lead toward solutions to the problems of the health-care system; only a new way of looking at health and illness will help us to correct some of the ills."

Paul Tillich (1952) with his facility for language and theoretical formulation, picked just the right word to describe his pursuit of the meaning of health and the relation of religion and health: *Thymos*—"the courage to be." If we choose to live, we choose not only joy and love, peace and fulfillment; we must also accept the other side of the package. Since life is not open ended, and since we don't know how long it will last, hadn't we better do some living? Find ways of making the most of the time we do have? Discover the meaning in every single event in our lives, so that we can choose and develop the most significant aspects of them? To give this meaning in terms of health education; *any knowledge that does not change the quality of life is sterile and of questionable value.* Health education is about translating health information into new insights and perceptions, which, in turn, bring about the quality and emotional patterns of life. These new insights can bring about new ways of acting and behaving. Before this is possible, however, a whole new way of being and becoming must be presented that includes the perception that *health is basically a matter of choices.*

Borrowing from Robert Frost, we in health education need to be concerned with helping the learner take "the road less traveled." The end of leniency in the nation's courts for drunk driving and the quest for a smokeless environment are just two examples of the divergent paths taken by those who choose to lead rather than follow. In both examples, a concerted cognitive-behavioral approach is the most critical factor in changing the nation's attitudes and behaviors.

Holistic Health Education: Transforming the Health-Education Paradigm

The role of education in promoting healthy behavior is a fact of life today. Yet, given the broader definition in which health must be defined, there is a greater need to address the development of curriculum, the design of instructional strategies, the creation of assessment mechanisms, and the preparation of health educators for the twenty-first century. How can we educate so that knowledge is not only power, but also insight; so that children and youth not only learn about health but also make health a meaningful part of their lives; so that we guide the development not only of health knowledge but also of character; so that students not only acquire facts but also have enhanced capacity to maintain healthy behaviors?

Together, these questions constitute a challenge to basic health-education assumptions, attitudes, and objectives. They suggest that health education, in its very definition, must reflect the whole of the human condition. To attempt any less guarantees an incomplete education and assures the long-term failure of our efforts.

In keeping with these considerations, a more comprehensive, holistic definition of health, which includes the very personal and often overlooked issues of spirituality and ecology, is included here.

In the past six or seven years, holistic education (as well as holistic medicine) has emerged as a serious critique of modern society and evolved into a truly viable alternative to the mass-production routine of modern learning. This approach has its own journal entitled the *Holistic Education Review*. Holistic education encompasses the revolutionary worldview of so-called new science (quantum physics, and systems and chaos theories), the moral and philosophical teachings of the world's great spiritual traditions, and the new understandings gained by ecologists, neuroscientists, and other researchers about the intricate interconnections between human experience and the natural world.

Holism emphasizes wholeness, interdependence, and meaning in reaction to a culture that has become tremendously fragmented, reductionistic, and crudely materialistic. Holistic thinkers reject Cartesian dualism (the view of the world as split between mind and body), Lockean empiricism (all knowledge comes from experience), and rationalist positivism (any claim that could not be verified in some way is meaningless), which have formed the intellectual underpinnings of modern society. Consequently, holistic educators believe that the "factory" model of schooling, with its behaviorist pedagogy and bureaucratic methods of management and assessment, has outlived its limited usefulness and has become a major source of alienation among today's youth.

In applying its concepts to health education, holism emphasizes integrated and experiential learning, the encouragement of community building, ethical, value-based decision making, and the development of multiple ways of solving problems, including the imaginative and intuitive (e.g., visualization, role playing, and group decision making). These approaches enable students to respond creatively and purposefully to the explosion of information and technology before them and to understand the complex interrelationship between the emotional, physical, spiritual, and ecological. Holistic health education must concern itself with connections in the human experiences of health—connections between mind and body (see Chapter 2), between linear and intuitive ways of thinking, between individual and community, and between mind (how we think) and body (how we feel) (Miller, 1990).

Applying a Holistic Approach to Health Education

Since holistic education involves a radical rethinking of cultural assumptions it is not enough to simply add "curriculum unity" as a subtext of personal beliefs and concerns. This is made very clear in William E. Doll's *A Post-Modern Perspective on Curriculum* (1993), which provides an especially rich and useful overview of the historical development of modern thought. Doll shows how the dominance of scientific, technical rationality has trivialized education by reducing curricula to controlled, measurable fragments. He introduces educators to new possibilities with a postmodern emphasis on process, diversity, flexibility, and creativity:

> *Educationally, we need to be trained in the art of creating and choosing, not just in ordering and following. Much of our curriculum to date has trained us to be passive receivers of preordained "truths," not active creators of knowledge.*

Toward a Comprehensive Community Health-Education Program

As with any health-education program, be it community or school-based, a comprehensive approach must be central to transforming traditional methods into critical and democratic ones. To do this, the health educator must carefully analyze obstacles to and resources for empowering education such that it addresses the economic, political, and personal needs of the learner. To make a holistic health-education program work, the health educator needs to listen carefully to students to draw out the issues and concerns from which critical curricula are built. Student participation provides the raw material for building a curriculum that reflects students' needs in a given situation.

Reflexive teaching, based on a set list of standards constituting a "comprehensive" health-education curriculum, truly negates and violates students' needs and interests and accepts a standard that is not only often remote from what students want, but also violates their right to be heard—and in so doing, denies the richness of their voice and thoughts. The empowering health-education experience opens up the learning experience so all voices can be heard.

With this in focus, it should be acknowledged that the concept of a comprehensive health-education program can be used as a guide only. The content areas established by the American Association for Health Education are

- community health
- consumer health
- family health
- mental and emotional health
- injury prevention and safety
- nutrition
- personal health
- prevention and control of disease
- substance use and abuse

I would now like to give the reader what I see as some assumptions of a traditional cognitive versus a cognitive-behavioral approach to these content areas.

Assumptions of a Cognitive Approach to Health Education	Assumptions of a Cognitive-Behavioral Approach to Health Education
Emphasis on *content*	Emphasis on learning how to learn, how to apply what one is learning to one's feelings and actions
Learning as *protection*	Learning as expansion of one's ability to create new solutions
Emphasis on analytical, linear, left-brain thinking	Emphasis on a holistic approach to *thinking, feeling,* and *acting*
Preoccupation with left-brain performance	Cooperation, personal sense of achievement, and shared goals, with personal values stressed
Getting a good grade stressed	Wrestling with ideas stressed
Bureaucratically determined, resistant to community input	Encourages cooperation and shared sense of personal empowerment
Emphasis on technology	Emphasis on human relationships
Teacher imparts knowledge: one-way street	Teacher is learner, too—learning from students

Adapted from *The Aquarian Conspiracy* by Marilyn Ferguson. Tarcher, 1981.

These issues certainly are important, but the health educator must keep them in perspective for the group or class in which she is working. The key element in the learning environment is that of educating students to be *critical thinkers, feeling thinkers,* and *active thinkers.* The classroom environment should promote democracy and serve all students equitably. A holistic health-education program requires these important equalities.

There are other vital focuses of a comprehensive health-education program, including

- critical decision making
- socialization (Bettelheim, 1990)
- values and ethical decision making
- self-esteem
- empowerment
- critical thinking

In whatever situation you are working, you must always remember that the critical point is to create a learning environment that is problematic enough to inspire students to do intellectual work and that will produce a great deal of cognitive-behavioral learning.

Some hoped-for goals that can be used as guides in this process include:

- open and effective communication with the learner
- an understanding of the values, life-styles, contributions, and history of a pluralistic society
- an ability to recognize and deal with dehumanizing biases and awareness of the impact such biases have on interpersonal relations; an ability to recognize the ways in which dehumanizing biases may be reflected in instructional materials and classroom discussion

- an ability to translate knowledge of human behavior into attitudes, skills, and techniques that result in favorable experiences for the learner
- providing individualized treatment, which requires that he get to know each learner individually
- providing the most knowledgeable and effective information available thoroughly familiar with well-proven alternative methods of health and healing; knowing when to refer the learner to appropriate specialists
- an ability to translate knowledge of human behavior into attitudes, skills, and techniques that will result in positive health habits for the learner
- an ability to relate effectively and positively to all learners regardless of race, sex, ethnic background, religion, or life-style choices
- an ability to maintain a positive classroom environment and assist students with setting healthy boundaries
- being deeply concerned with the aspirations of students and their ability to move toward more positive health behaviors
- an ability to work with students in understanding that multiculturalism is a part of living in a world of diversity
- working with students on ethical issues that will help them in dealing with their own value-based attitudes and behaviors
- an ability to integrate spiritual and ecological issues that relate to health
- providing the total concept of holism: the knowledge that everything students think, feel, and act upon impacts on their health and wellness and that of others
- taking an approach to health education that aims at the concurrent development of the logical and the mystical, the analytical and the intuitive

A basic premise of holistic health education must be focused on the teacher. Holism does not necessarily imply alternative modes of teaching. These methods can often be superficial, nonverifiable, or one-dimensional. Nor does it imply that traditional health education cannot be holistic. What is important is for the practitioner of holistic health education to create an atmosphere where mind and body are seen as interconnected. In this atmosphere, spiritual and ecological dimensions of health and wellness are consistently acknowledged and integrated into the total program of health education.

A holistic health education program needs to ask itself some critical questions:

What is the relationship, if any, between body, mind, spirit, ecology, and human experience?

Why is health important for ourselves, and for humankind?

What is our responsibility for the health of ourselves, others, and humankind?

What is the fundamental meaning and purpose of health education? Is it to increase knowledge, affect attitudes, or affect behaviors?

What are the most appropriate ways of approaching health education: cognitively, behaviorally, or confluently (a combination of both)?

What are the deepest issues we face in the following areas of health education: personal wellness, anatomy and physiology, emotional development and its relation to health, basic nutrition, eating disorders, aging, suicide, death and dying, disease, substance use and abuse, positive personal health, consumerism, sex and sexuality, violence, values and ethics, human relations, ecology, human caring, and global concerns? How can integrate all of these areas into a comprehensive program?

Your Responses

Take a moment to answer the last question about creating an integrated health-education program:

The development of a comprehensive health-education program requires a theoretical framework that includes all the phenomena related to human learning. Freudian, behavioral, and humanistic psychology are useful but incomplete approaches. Holistic education offers a more inclusive vision of human-health potential as well as a new worldview. Using holistic psychology in health education does not require a complete rejection of established health-education approaches but may be used in conjunction with them. Conflict occurs at some points, and agreement occurs at others.

An underlying assumption of holistic health education is that the emotional, physical, spiritual, and ecological mix that makes up what is known as holism is interrelated, and that an optimal health-education curriculum is one that stimulates and nurtures the intuitive as well as the rational, the imaginative as well as the practical, and the creative as well as the receptive functions of each individual. Thus, a holistic health-education program shifts the focus from external to internal awareness. As the students become aware of their inner states, they begin to recognize important conditions that affect their wellness, not because they are *told* that health is important, but because they *feel* it is important.

Qualities of Caring

In a book by Ram Dass and Paul Gorman (1985) entitled *How Can I Help?*, the authors say,

> Caring for one another, we sometimes glimpse an essential quality of our being. We may be sitting alone, lost in self-doubt or self-pity, when the phone rings with a call from a friend who's really depressed. Instinctively, we come out of ourselves, just to be there with her and say a few reassuring words. When we're done, and a little comfort's been shared, we put down the phone and feel a little

more at home with ourselves. We're reminded of who we really are and what we have to offer one another. . . . When the experience of helping seems so natural, it's not surprising we find ourselves wishing or wondering if things could be like that more or even most of the time.

Implicit in caring is motive. Why do you want to care for others? To answer this, you must step outside yourself, look at your motives, and then answer the question, "Why do I want to help?" Before you respond, think about the question. What is it asking? What are you seeking for yourself? How much time and energy will it take?

Your Responses

See if you can isolate the personal reasons from the professional reasons you come up with to answer these questions on caring.

Personal:

Professional:

To follow are some qualities for working in the helping professions drawn from the works of Noddings (1984), Mayeroff (1971), Rogers (1961), and Carkhuff (1983).

- **Effective health education involves a process of interpersonal influence.** How you present yourself depends to a great extent on how you feel about yourself. To help another, you must have a high degree of self-esteem, because helping requires a great deal of focus outside yourself. Statements about the goals of helping often include terms such as self-actualization, an increased ability to respond and cope, an ability to love and work, reaching out to others, and being yourself. If health education is a process of positive change, the process of interpersonal influence is primary to that change.
- **Act on the desire to care for others.** Nell Noddings, in her book *Caring* (1984), states "Everywhere we hear the complaint 'Nobody cares!' and our increasing immersion in bureaucratic procedures and regulations leads us to predict that the complaint will continue to be heard. As human beings, we want to care and to be cared for. *Caring* is important in itself." Caring for others requires " . . . helping another grow and actualize himself . . .[it] is a process, a

way of relating to someone that involves development, in the same way that friendship can only emerge in time through mutual trust and a deepening and qualitative transformation of the relationship" (Mayeroff, 1971). Someone once remarked, a friend is a person who leaves you with all your freedom intact but obliges you to be fully what you are. In that spirit of being *authentic,* you do not want to intrude on another's authenticity but are willing to give a great deal of warmth and caring. In this vein, Carl Rogers (1961) describes an attitude of "unconditional positive regard," which he defines as an atmosphere demonstrating "I care," not "I care *if* you behave thus and so." This kind of caring and acceptance is not easy. It takes hard work to set aside your goals for another—what you want for them and what you think is best for them. But the potential outcome is well worth it.

- **Establish certain conceptual frameworks and theories of health education.** Expanding your cognitive-response repertoire for helping is not enough; it is also necessary to examine your conceptual framework or worldview. Put in simplest terms, how do you think health education works? If you have not thought about this before, think about a friend you have tried to help in some way. What did you do to help? How did you approach her? What did you say? Did you help? How do you know? Did you follow up? The manner in which you view and answer these questions provides a small picture of how you view the world. It is out of this worldview that you make a decision on how to act. Your worldview and theories determine how you relate to others and probably shaped what you said to your friend.

- **Initiate trusting.** This means developing the ability to reach out unselfconsciously to those who are in need. To help another, you must begin by becoming involved with him. Involving him means engaging him, informing him of your availability, and encouraging him to use your help (Carkhuff, 1983). While someone may be less able to reach out to you, you need to be able and willing to transcend that boundary, to recognize his need through his initial inability to trust. It allows you, as helper, to move forward without permission, trusting your own initiative, which you *must* do if you hope to meet others halfway.

- **Believe that people are capable of change.** Your theoretical orientation and your basic assumptions about the nature of human beings will largely determine your beliefs regarding the degree of change possible for any individual you are working with. Health educators may hold distinct and varied opinions on the kinds of changes they believe are possible, but all health educators must hold to the assumption that *individuals are capable of and want to change.* Further, all health educators must communicate this belief by their actions and attitudes and not depend on verbal communication alone. The use of words such as "I believe in you; you can do it" will not, by and of itself, persuade the individual of your belief. Other communication channels, such as body gestures, facial expressions, voice tone, and role modeling are more subtle yet more powerful ways of communicating your attitudes and beliefs.

- **Know how individuals function.** Health educators need to understand the psychological principles that guide human behavior and be aware of the environmental factors that influence this behavior. This knowledge is ordinarily

Respond to the following questions as simply as you can:

1. If I were absolutely free to choose my occupation, my choice would be

2. When I consider my future career prospects, I become

3. The thing that most excites me about becoming a helping person is

4. The most challenging aspect of my career is

5. The most rewarding aspect of my career is

6. I think I could find more meaning in my career if I

7. The most significant effect my career choice will have on the rest of my life is

Look over your answers to see whether there is a significant pattern in your responses. What can you say about your attitudes and values as they relate to selecting your career?

gained through advanced study in psychology. Knowledge of how individuals function is essential to the entire health-education process. It is important, when you are trying to build trust for a working relationship, that you explore and understand the factors delimiting a person's behaviors. Then you can decide on a particular teaching strategy and employ an intervention strategy in a sound and appropriate manner.

- **Be willing to become involved.** The bottom line in any successful health-education program is the willingness to become involved in the interpersonal process called health education. This commitment to share yourself goes beyond merely giving the time and energy required to assist another person. It includes bringing as much of yourself as is necessary into the helping relationship and communicating to those you are working with that nothing is more important at that moment than what they are and what they have to say. Health educators who have good feelings of self-worth, adequacy, and self-discipline transcend their own limitations and are free to give the necessary attention to those they are working with and to focus on ways of assisting them.

- **Know yourself.** Effective health educators must have self-esteem and feel secure within themselves. Be aware of your own feelings, attitudes, values, and motivations when working with others. You will need to know your own skills and to acknowledge your limitations willingly. Be open to self-improvement and growth through additional learning and experience, and acknowledge that all persons, including yourself, have a range of talents and limitations. Effective health educators realize they cannot help everyone with every issue and must acknowledge that people sometimes require specialized knowledge in an area of expertise they may not possess. Become sensitive to those areas and exercise appropriate discretion and judgment in making referrals. The process of self-knowledge and facing up to your limitations has two important influences for health education. First, the better you understand and appreciate your own feelings, thoughts, and behaviors, the better you understand those of others. Second, health educators who are comfortable with themselves communicate an attitude of genuineness to those they are working with. The learner, sensing that sincerity, develops a sense of trust in the helping relationship and thus will unfold more deeply his or her internal frame of reference, moving the health-education process along.

Synthesis

In this chapter, I have explained the essential concepts of health, holism, and health education. In all of this, the most important single ingredient in helping people to maintain and increase their health potential, is the health educator. Some simple guiding principles in helping students achieve these goals are

- learn to appreciate and enjoy yourself, your life, and other people rather than deprecating and judging

- live in a self-determined, authentic way based on who you are rather than on what others want you to be
- develop the neglected sides of who you are to become a more fully integrated person
- increase your freedom and power by accepting responsibility for your behavior
- sharpen your awareness of events both within and outside yourself
- learn to teach not only from the head but also from the heart
- believe not only in the factual but also in the spiritual dimension of what you are teaching
- lead students to discover and understand their own best path to personal-health realization
- never stop believing in yourself as a positive force in the lives of those you are working with

If we truly believe in health education and what it is all about, then we will be armed against the four horsemen—war, pestilence, famine, and death. We will master the process of teaching for transformation—a process of bringing out insights in students and helping them reconstruct experience so they see things in a new and life-changing way. This type of health education assumes that the learner brings to the educational task certain experiences and concepts that can be used for growth. It realizes that each learner is different. Health education in this context is a process of unfolding rather than a program of indoctrination. It is open-ended and always open to that "teachable moment" when something clicks in the mind of the learner and transformation occurs.

References

Bandura, Albert. *Principles of Behavior Modification.* New York: Holt, Rinehart, and Winston, 1969.

Carkhuff, Robert R. *The Art of Helping.* Amherst, MA: Human Resource Development Press, 1983.

Daniels, Victor, and Laurence J. Horowitz. *Being and Caring: A Psychology for Living.* Palo Alto, CA: Mayfield, 1984.

Dass, Ram, and Paul Gorman. *How Can I Help?* New York: Knopf, 1985.

Doll, William E. *A Post-Modern Perspective on Curriculum.* New York: Teachers College Press, 1993.

Dossey, Larry. *Beyond Illness: Discovering the Experience of Health.* Boulder, CO: New Science Library, 1984.

Duff, Kate. "The Alchemy of Illness." *Common Boundary,* May/June 1993.

Ferguson, Marilyn. *The Aquarian Conspiracy.* Los Angeles: J.P. Tarcher, 1980.

Freire, Paulo. *Education for Critical Consciousness.* New York: Seabury, 1973.

____.Interview. *Omni,* April 1990.

Hayakawa, S.I. *Language in Thought and Action.* New York: Harcourt, Brace, 1964.

Kleinman, A., L. Eisenberg, and B. Good. "Culture, Illness, and Care: Clinical Lessons from Anthropologic and Cross-cultural Research." *Annals of Internal Medicine,* February 1978.

Mayeroff, Milton. *On Caring*. New York: Perennial Library, 1971.

Noddings, Nell. *Caring: A Feminine Approach to Ethics and Moral Education*. Berkeley, CA: University of California Press, 1984.

Peper, Erik, and Casi Kushel. "A Holistic Merger of Biofeedback and Family Therapy," in Dora Kunz (ed.), *Spiritual Aspects of the Healing Arts*. Wheaton, IL: Theosophical Publishing House, 1985.

Sacks, Oliver. *The Man Who Mistook His Wife for a Hat and Other Clinical Tales*. New York: Simon & Schuster, 1985.

Sartre, Jean-Paul. *Existentialism and Humanism*. P. Mairet, trans. London: Methuen, 1948.

___. *The Transcendence of the Ego*. Williams and R. Kirkpatrick, trans. New York: Noonday, 1957.

Sontag, Susan. *Illness as Metaphor and AIDS as Its Metaphors*. New York: Anchor Books, 1989.

Tillich, Paul. *The Courage to Be*. Hartford: Yale University Press, 1952.

___. *The Meaning of Health*. Richmond, CA: North Atlantic Books, 1981.

Tubesing, Donald A. *Wholistic Health: A Whole-Person Approach to Primary Health Care*. New York: Human Sciences Press, 1979.

Additional Resources

Breckon, Donald J., John R. Harvey, and R. Brick Lancaster. *Community Health Education: Settings, Roles, and Skills for the 21st Century*. Gaithersburg, MD: Aspen, 1994.

Corey, Gerald, et al. *Issues and Ethics in the Helping Professions*. Pacific Grove, CA: Brooks/Cole, 1993.

Cortese, Peter, and Kathleen Middleton (eds.). *The Comprehensive School Health Challenge: Promoting Health through Education*, vols. 1 & 2. Santa Cruz, CA: ETR Associates, 1994.

"CSHE: Comprehensive School Health Education." *Journal of Health Education*, March/April 1995.

Daniels, Victor, and Laurence J. Horowitz. *Being and Caring: A Psychology for Living*. Palo Alto: Mayfield, 1984.

Ilardo, Joseph. *Risk-Taking for Personal Growth*. Oakland, CA: New Harbinger, 1992.

James, Muriel, and John James. *Passion for Life: Psychology and Human Spirit*. New York: Penguin, 1991.

Parsley, Bonnie K. *The Choice Is Yours: A Teenager's Guide to Self-Discovery, Relationships, Values, and Spiritual Growth*. New York: Fireside, 1992.

Reynolds, David K. *Constructive Living*. Three audiocassettes for gaining insight into one's feelings of self and seeing one's life more clearly. Available from Sounds True, Dept. FC8, 735 Walnut Street, Boulder, CO 80302.

Shor, Ira. *Empowering Education: Critical Teaching for Social Change*. Chicago: The University of Chicago Press, 1992.

2 Toward a Holistic Concept of Health

Practitioners of the modern concepts of health feel compelled to choose between the "scientific" and the "unscientific," between the objective and the subjective, between the precise and the vague, and between the measurable and the nonquantifiable. This is one of the great agonies of the profession. This selection process is certainly an integral part of our profession, for it is at the very center of what we do and what our goals are all about. And thus, these questions arise:

- Must we choose between a scientific and an unscientific definition of health, or can the two coexist (Dossey, 1984)?
- How are mind and body connected? Is mind part of the soul, and if so, can it exist apart from the body (Kunz, 1985)?
- How do we know how healthy we are? Are our perceptions built into our minds, or do we develop them from our external perceptions and experiences (Sontag, 1979)?
- How does perception work? Are our impressions of health and illness true representations of what we are? How can someone know whether or not she is healthy (Frank, 1974)?
- Which is the right road to true health—pure knowledge from the outside, data gathered from the inside, or a combination of both (Oyle, 1979)?
- Does the mind rule the body, or vice versa? Do they play an equal role (Bishop, 1994)?
- Can we present not only the analytical and logical but also the intuitive in health education (Goleman, 1995)?

As you move forward in this chapter, the answers to these questions should become evident. Before reading further, please write down your initial responses to them. They are important to our profession and the way in which we approach it.

Healthy people are healthy because of what's going on in their heads, not what's going on in their bodies.

—BERNIE SIEGEL

Early Holistic Thinking

In 1898, William James, the Harvard-trained physician who has been called the father of American psychology, successfully testified before the legislators of Massachusetts in opposition to a bill that would have outlawed "mental" healing by nondoctors. "If medicine were a finished science," James said, "such a bill might be possible. But the whole face of medicine changes unexpectedly from one generation to another, in consequences of widening experience." He deplored the unwillingness of his colleagues to investigate the practices they were so quick to condemn, like homeopathy (like cures like) and mind cures. He sympathized with the wish to protect the public from quackery but believed the only answer was education. He urged his medical peers to fight "not for license and monopoly, but for freedom and conciliation. . . . There is too much that we do not understand" (Hunt, 1993).

Albert Schweitzer (1961) was more forward about his thoughts concerning the internal healing power of the human. He often talked about this potential of the human body to heal itself. Among his favorite examples was a story he liked to share with visitors to his famous African jungle clinic. When Schweitzer first started his clinic, he found himself in competition with the local witch doctor. What surprised Schweitzer was that the witch doctor was able to heal patients. Not only that, but the witch doctor was able to heal patients whom Schweitzer himself had given up on.

Schweitzer discovered that, simply by using rituals to make the healing process elaborate and believable, the witch doctor had helped his patients tap into their own internal healing power. This led him to predict that western medicine would eventually come to realize the human body itself holds the ultimate secret prescription for healing.

A Broader Definition

Our widening experience with holistic health from the late 1980s onward demonstrates the durable truth of James's argument. Widening experience has shown us that acupuncture triggers the release of powerful brain chemicals, the existence of which was not even suspected a decade ago. We can indeed "die of a broken heart" (Frankl, 1963), because grief sabotages the immune system. Hostility has been correlated to everything from the common cold to serious illness. The mind has been shown to cure through biofeedback and other technologies (Oyle, 1979).

The word *health* comes from the same root as the words *hale* and *whole*. Its etymology suggests the way our development should be measured. Body, mind, feelings, and spirit are all part of one whole. They do not act on one another as subject and object—like billiard balls striking each other from first one and then another direction. They are inextricably interwoven, a fabric of interactions. To treat them separately and sequentially as agents of stimulus and response is to reduce the human being to a mechanical model composed of interchangeable, independent parts. We may isolate a physical or mental function; we may alter a person's behavior with drugs or through surgery; but we cannot pretend that in so doing we are dealing with the whole person. René Dubois, in *Man Adapting* (1965), puts the matter this way:

> The components of the body-machine react with the environment, but living man responds to his environment. In fact, man's responses are not necessarily aimed at coping with his environment. They often correspond rather to an expressive behavior and involve using the environment for self-actualization. Health in the case of human beings means more than a state in which the organism has become physically suited to the surrounding physico-chemical conditions through passive mechanism; it demands that the personality be able to express itself creatively.

The creative expression of personality is another way of describing the process of becoming a whole person. This expression of the personality is the function of the private and public actions in accord with the values and goals of our personal natures. Whole health, then, is using what we have in *all* of our human systems to express those values.

New-Age Thinking and Holistic Health

The concept of holism was first introduced by the South African philosopher Jan Christian Smuts in 1926. To Smuts, holism was an antidote to the analytic reductionism of the prevailing sciences. It was a way of comprehending whole organisms and systems as entities greater than and different from the sum of their parts (Smuts, 1926).

In the last several years, holistic (sometimes spelled "wholistic") medicine has come to denote both the relationship of the whole person and his environment to the healing process and a variety of health-promoting approaches to health education. These approaches to wellness, encompassing and at times indistinguishable from humanistic-behavioral approaches, include an appreciation of learners as emotional, social, and spiritual as well as physical beings. Holistic teaching respects their capacity for healing themselves and regards them as active partners in, rather than passive recipients of, health education.

This important holistic connection can be found in Kenneth R. Pelletier's *Mind As Healer, Mind As Slayer;* Joan Borysenko's *Minding the Body, Mending the Mind;* Larry Dossey's *Meaning and Medicine: A Doctor's Tales of Breakthrough and Healing;* Deepak Chopra's *Unconditional Life;* and the PBS television series, "Healing and the Mind" with Bill Moyers. What all of these people are saying is that we can better control our own lives (and health) by gaining greater control of the mind.

The major thesis of Deepak Chopra's book *Unconditional Life* (1991) is that our perceptions create our experience, so the outside world can be radically altered by changing the world within. Chopra, who has emerged as one of the most powerful writers in the field of mind-body medicine, is one of the holistic medical thinkers who explores the perils of self-generated illness. Others are Larry Dossey, Joan Borysenko, and Bernie Siegel. All of these writers believe that the universe, human life, and health are participatory and consciousness-dependent; in short, unconditional health can be in our hands if we accept responsibility for our well-being.

Dossey, who practices internal medicine with the Dallas Diagnostic Association, feels that the most prominent possibility in the field of health is finding meaning in the experience of illness. Allopathy (conventional western medicine) long ago outlawed meaning in pathology; after all, if the human body is a machine, then illness is simply a loose screw or burned-out motor. Allopathy disregards the individual's interpretation of the significance of an illness as bad science and irrelevant to its cause, contending that the mind and body are independent systems. For Dossey, the way a patient perceives the meaning of his or her illness is crucial to its outcome; "patient attitudes are actually the most reliable predictors of how an illness will be resolved, whether the outcome is recovery or death" (1991).

Is there an atom of meaning in illness? Is disease a biological code trying to say something to us? Emphatically yes, according to Dossey. He makes the case that our own perceptions enter the body and actually change it on the molecular level. The pioneers of psychoneuroimmunology (the study of the relationship between the mind and the body) first established this connection. Dossey gathered up their data and commentaries to create a wider net of meaning. For many, illness is often the first pivotal experience in which life's meaning involves the dramatic interaction of mind and matter. Understanding this interaction must go beyond science to a fundamental shift in consciousness. Meaning is being, Dossey argues; healing requires "a fundamental change in our own being."

In an earlier book, *Beyond Illness: Discovering the Experience of Health* (1984), Dossey argued that the problem of viewing health is a matter of pure experience; until we make a painful reassessment of who we are, we will not be able to experience a state of health. This emotional experience alone can lead us to the physical reality; conscious awareness and insight are required to become totally healthy. Health is difficult to achieve through external intervention alone.

Chopra's concern is not just for our physical and emotional health. He wants to promote healing in the metaphysical foundations of our existence—to heal our "hurt awareness." If we make our own reality, then we can make it better. For most of us, reality is a highly subjective, personalized realm of experience. Chopra says

> the forces that shape our personal reality are beliefs, attitudes, perceptions, and the boundaries of subjective conditioning—what the ancient Indian sages called "mistakes of the intellect." Disease is not the way to solve the core issues of life. People have to be transformed before the crisis (1991).

To put this into perspective, for most people illness is an opportunity for learning; that is, we learn from the experience. Chopra suggests that we must act *before* the crisis, for most of us do not learn from negative experiences.

Joan Borysenko is former director of the Mind-Body Clinic at New England Deaconess Hospital and instructor in medicine at Harvard Medical School. In her latest book, *Fire in the Soul: A New Psychology of Spiritual Optimism* (1993), she develops the following themes in understanding the dynamics of healing, medicine must not overlook the role of the spirit. Her explorations of seemingly miraculous healings, near-death experiences, the power of prayer, and other often dismissed topics have added resonance coming from a scientist trained as a cell biologist and psychologist who has taught at Harvard Medical School. Borysenko goes beyond psychology as currently practiced and taps a deeper vein of healing. She reveals the power of spiritual optimism, a philosophy that views life crises as opportunities for personal growth and spiritual homecoming.

On Mind, Body, and Spirituality

Under the direction of Herbert Benson, M.D., Harvard Medical School and the Mind-Body Medical Institute at Deaconess Hospital, a conference on spirituality and healing in medicine was presented in Boston in 1995. That a prestigious medical school and world-renowned institute would cosponsor such a workshop is a testament to the fact that the connection between spirituality and health has become a serious field of study ("Spirituality and Healing in Medicine," 1995).

The objective of the three-day workshop was to provide participants with an understanding of the following aspects of health promotion:

- the relationship between spirituality and healing from the perspective of major world religions
- the scientific evidence for the effects of spirituality on healing
- the physiologic and neuralgic effects of spirituality on healing
- the relationship between healing, spirituality, and mind-body effects

For more than twenty-five years, laboratories at Harvard Medical School have systematically studied the benefits of mind-body interactions. The research established that when a person engages in a repetitive prayer, word, sound, or phrase, and when intrusive thoughts are passively disregarded, a specific set of physiologic changes occur. Metabolism, heart rate, and rate of breathing decrease, and brain waves become distinctly slower. These changes are the opposite of those induced by stress and are an effective therapy in a number of diseases including hypertension, cardiac-rhythm irregularities, chronic pain, insomnia, infertility, the symptoms of cancer and AIDS, premenstrual syndrome, anxiety, and mild to moderate depression. In fact, to the extent that any disease is caused or made worse by stress, this physiologic state is an effective therapy.

The work at Harvard led to consideration of the healing effects of spirituality, because later research established that people felt increasingly spiritual when eliciting this state regardless of whether or not they used a religious focus. Spirituality was defined as experiencing the presence of a power, force, or energy or was perceived of as God, whose presence was close to the person. This sense of spirituality was associated with fewer medical symptoms.

Bernie Siegel, M.D., who has been deeply involved in humanizing medical education and making the medical profession and patients aware of the mind-body connection, is a firm believer in giving ourselves healing messages through techniques of meditation, visualization, relaxation, and peace of mind, as expressed in his book *Peace, Love, and Healing* (1989). In his earlier book *Love, Medicine, and Miracles* (1986), he discusses the importance of self-love in health and healing:

The fundamental problem most patients face is an inability to love themselves, having been unloved by others during some crucial part of their lives. This period is almost always childhood, when our relations with our parents establish our characteristic ways of reacting to stress. As adults we repeat these reactions and make ourselves vulnerable to illness, and our personalities often determine the specific nature of the illnesses. The ability to love oneself, combined with the ability to love life, fully accepting that it won't last forever, enables one to improve the quality of life. My role as a surgeon is to buy people time during which they can heal themselves. I try to help them get well, and at the same time, to understand why they became sick. Then they can go on to true healing, not merely a reversal of one particular disease.

Dr. Siegel's basic premise is that we need to understand the extreme importance of the mind-body connection and be receptive to the messages our minds give our bodies.

Attitudes and Health

"The brain is a health-care system," psychologist Gary Schwartz said at a conference sponsored by the Holmes Center in Los Angeles (1991). Schwartz and his colleagues at Yale University have undertaken a number of experiments demonstrating the role of the mind in regulating health—or producing the "disregulation" that leads to disease.

When looking at emotions and health, we should consider the following points (*Brain-Mind Bulletin Collections,* 1991).

- Emotions and health are closely related. It has been known for many years that negative emotions and experiences can have a deleterious effect on health and can complicate medical treatment. Not as well-known is the connection between positive attitudes and the possible enhancement of the body's healing system. This relationship is now the subject of study at a number of medical-research centers.
- It is likely that numerous emotional and physical factors, many of them yet to be delineated, influence health and disease, probably in different ways for different individuals. There is no single, simple factor that causes or cures cancer and other major illnesses.
- Even though positive attitudes and a good mental outlook cannot influence the physical outcome, they can and do affect the quality of life. Few things are more important in the care of seriously ill patients than their mental state and the general environment in which they have to be treated. Unfortunately, human beings are not able to exercise control over all of their biological and disease processes. Therefore, they should not be encouraged to believe that positive attitudes are a substitute for competent medical attention.
- Feelings of panic are not uncommon among patients on learning that they have cancer. Panic is itself destructive and can interfere with effective treat-

ment. The wise physician, therefore, is mindful of the need to combat feelings of panic and emotional devastation.

The reciprocal mind-body relationship is complex. We must be aware of both the potential and the limitations of attitudes and their effects on health and disease.

What Does It All Mean?

The creative expression of personality is just another way of describing the process of becoming a whole person. A soundly functioning body is one aspect of that expression, but it is not the entire expression. A healthy human being may be someone confined to a wheelchair who uses what she has in the way of a sound body to express her authentic purpose, working for what she believes to be true and important for her. (In this vein, it is not surprising that the term "physically challenged" has replaced "physically disabled.") Therefore, we need to challenge the traditional norms regarding health. What is health for one may be very different for another, *but both are equally healthy.*

Physical health is the most palpable evidence we have of the state of the organism. Our bodies are the outward structure of our public natures, the surfaces exposed to the world. In the body is the brain we use to formulate the language of thought and feeling. The gift we call life is given originally to those bodies, and we share with everything else in the living kingdom the biology of life forces. Being material, the human body is our primary connection with the world of matter.

The direction of influence between illness and disease goes both ways. Illness, the human experience, affects disease through a climate of hopefulness, fear, despair, and denial; disease, in turn, can alter the illness experience through direct impact on neuroendocrine and other bodily functions and states (e.g., hunger, fatigue, thirst, muscle weakness, or paralysis). This can never be a simple story of mind over matter or physical determinism (body over mind), because the mind and body are not dual realities, as the Cartesian tradition of a mind-body split portrays. The mind both constitutes and is constituted by the body. The influence between mind and body is synergistic and mutual. Thus, since health education deals with both health and illness, growth and loss, the mind and body must be considered in theory and practice and within its own reality.

Implications for Health Education

Placing Chopra's concept of illness as subjective conditioning and personal reality in the context of health education and, more specifically, in the transformation taking place in health and health education, requires a totally different approach to the field in the future. We need to incorporate the following concepts:

- the mind-body connection does exist, and we must take this connection into consideration in our teaching
- mind-body approaches to teaching include such areas as biofeedback, visualization, meditation, self-esteem, and self-empowerment

- Understanding the mind-body connection includes explaining how psychological and social-support systems can lead to better health; exploring the role of the mind in unhealthy life-styles; and emphasizing the need to take full responsibility for managing our physical, emotional, and spiritual well-being.

An approach to health education that focuses on life-style stresses all of these concepts. It says "I am not a victim; I choose—on some level—whatever happens to me." What we as health educators need to talk about is cause and effect.

We have deadly germs in our bodies now. Why don't they take over? This has been a medical conundrum for years. Some say it has to do with our mental state. We need to study correlatives between attitudes and physical well-being. We experience illness, but we find that the mind is the central control system; as such, we need to better understand what is going on in our minds as well as our bodies. As Robert Ornstein and David Sobel state in their book *Healthy Pleasures* (1989),

> *Hundreds of scientific studies on thousands of people now report that individuals who expect the best, who are hopeful and optimistic, and who regularly enjoy sexual pleasures are, in general, healthier and live longer. While the results of any single study could always be debated or challenged, the collective weight of the evidence strongly points to how positive moods influence resistance to and recovery from disease. The opposite is true as well: negative moods, depression, hostility, and the lack of pleasure all seem to contribute to poor health. There appears to be a physiology of happiness which communicates to our heart, our immune system, our entire body.*

Imagine telling a class that feelings are chemicals; that how we feel about ourselves may be the single most useful rule in our well-being; that three hugs a day are healthier for us than taking a vitamin pill; that expressions of hostility are unhealthy for both mind and body; that health is a state of mind more than body; that our unhealthy behaviors—such as drug abuse, unsafe sex, and low self-esteem—are not the product of our external environment but of our internal feelings.

A Specific Application

Holistic applications to learning situations are part of an emerging point of view that allows greater freedom and flexibility in education. Insights gained from meditation, biofeedback, mental imagery, eastern thought, and altered states of consciousness are finding their ways into the classroom. Stripped of their jargon, these fields of study are accelerating and improving conventional learning and have been most applicable in the field of health education. They offer immense opportunities to expand the effectiveness of the learning environment in health education and offer powerful tools and possibilities for the health educator. Students are excited when they find that a holistic approach is not limited to subject matter but can be extensively applied to their personal lives and wellness.

A specific application of the mind-body approach to health and health education can be found in the work of Herbert Benson, M.D. Dr. Benson, who is an associate professor of medicine at Harvard Medical School, coined the term *relaxation response,* a stress-management technique. From meditation to biofeedback, the aim is to induce a positive parasympathetic state. Benson believes these techniques increase self-esteem, lower blood pressure, reduce stress and anxiety, and refocus the individual from external to internal demands and needs (Benson, 1987, 1993).

Dorchester High School, an inner-city school in Boston, is using the relaxation-response technique in the classroom to help students cope with stress by helping them develop their own inner resources. The object is to show students that, although they may be influenced by external forces, they control their internal powers. This allows students to gain better control over their emotions and response patterns and is empowering for them.

Jon Kabat-Zinn, director of the Stress Reduction Clinic at the University of Massachusetts Medical Center, uses what he calls "mindfulness meditation" to induce deep states of relaxation that can often directly improve physical symptoms of stress, pain, and chronic illness. In follow-up studies, he found patients in his program had shown a sharp drop in the number of medical symptoms reported as well as in such psychological problems as anxiety, depression, and hostility (1993). These findings have profound implications for health education, for it seems clear that our current educational efforts are aimed primarily at the left side of the brain, thereby leaving an entire model of consciousness to chance development.

Synthesis

In the last decade or two, emphasis seems to have swung from a technocentric culture that barely acknowledged the possibility of a mind-body connection to the somewhat focused assumption that everything that goes wrong in our bodies is caused by our minds. But, as Carl Jung observed, "Psyche cannot be totally different from matter, for how otherwise could it move matter? And matter cannot be alien to psyche, for how else could matter produce psyche? . . . If research could only advance far enough . . . we should arrive at an ultimate agreement between physical and psychological concepts" (1971).

It is the premise of the author that if health educators combined what is knowable about inner nature and psychological process with what we have learned about the outer process of wellness, we could resolve a number of problems that have long concerned traditional health education: *If our minds contain the stuff for determining our behavior, there is every reason to believe that our mental processes reflect and extend the basic laws guiding our personal health choices.* Current and future health educators must, therefore, respond to the question, What is the process through which health education can focus to present both aspects as one?

There is an old Zen saying, "If you do not find it within yourself, where will you go to get it?" Among some traditional American Indian peoples, mind-body separation does not exist. This is largely due to a learning process that includes mind, body, and spirit (Neihardt, 1972). The old Native languages have no separate word for mind—anything you call "body" is the total being, implying a different kind of relationship than what we have traditionally been taught.

Health education is a process. The health educator is the central figure in applying techniques that most support the concept of health not just as an event in the mind but as shaping and affecting one's *whole being*.

Time Out for Personal Thoughts

Science is beginning to reveal the psychological mechanisms that allow mind to affect the body. Thus, mind-body, life-style approaches to teaching health hold real value. Take a moment to think about that value. How do you see it working?

Take a moment to think about how you have treated yourself up to this point—both physically and emotionally—and respond briefly to the following questions.

1. If your body could speak to you, what would it tell you about how it is being treated?

2. Which emotion(s) is easiest for you to express?

3. Which emotion(s) is the most difficult for you to express?

4. What are three things you think you could do to get in touch with your body?

Terminology in Alternative Medicine

Like their conventional counterparts, alternative-medical practitioners have black bags overflowing with treatments. The treatments they offer, however, can be anything from acupuncture, dancing by the ocean, or massage, to taking vitamins, drinking cocktails of fresh vegetable juices, or adopting a new, spirit-reviving vocation. The following are definitions of treatment options (Baar, 1994).

Acupuncture: The insertion of fine sterile needles into the body at points (called acupoints) along the meridians through which the *qi,* or vital energy, is said to flow. The needles help restore the normal flow of this energy, but this restoration can also be achieved by other means, such as moxibustion, which involves the placing of burning herbs over acupuncture points, or, by recent invention, with electronic devices.

Alexander technique: Re-educating the body to correct faulty posture and thus restore function and coordination.

Aromatherapy: The use of scents made from essential oils of herbs to boost energy, relieve stress, or alleviate the symptoms of disease.

Biofeedback: The use of electronic devices to monitor subtle changes in muscle tension, body temperature, heart rate, or other physiological responses. Once the patient has become aware of these reactions, she can use guided relaxation techniques like meditation and visualization to control them.

Bodywork: The broad heading of bodywork includes numerous hands-on therapies. They are designed, variously, to stimulate the nervous and lymphatic systems, to stretch and relax muscles, and to improve circulation. Bodywork therapies include:

- *Craniosacral therapy:* The manipulation of the bones of the skull to enhance the functioning of the central nervous system and treat a host of ailments including headache, chronic pain, temporomandibular joint syndrome, ear infections, and strokes.
- *Reflexology:* Application of deep pressure to specific locations on the hands and/or soles of the feet that are believed to correspond to various organs, and the consequent stimulation of energy to those organs.
- *Rolfing:* Formally called Structural Integration, the use of thumbs, fingers, knuckles, and elbows to manipulate connective tissue and reestablish the proper alignment of the body.
- *Shiatsu:* A therapy closely related in principle to acupuncture in which pressure is applied with thumbs, fingers, elbows, and sometimes feet to specific points on the body's meridians of energy to improve and balance the flow of the life force. Acupressure is an American version of shiatsu.
- *Therapeutic massage:* The systematic application of strokes and pressure to muscles, tendons, and joints to promote circulatory and lymphatic movement and to relax and stretch muscles.

Chiropractic: A major system of healthcare in which musculoskeletal structures of the body, primarily the spinal column, are manipulated to bring them into their proper relationship with the nervous system which chiropractic doctors maintain is the key to ensuring health throughout the body.

Feldenkrais method: Movement exercises designed to release habitual patterns of tension brought about by everyday posture and movement.

Guided imagery: Trained concentration on specific mental images with the goal of reducing pain, inducing relaxation, and boosting the immune system's ability to fight disease.

Herbal medicine: The use of botanical medicines to treat or prevent a wide array of ailments.

Hydrotherapy: The therapeutic use of water, including compresses, saunas, enemas, baths, and steam treatments.

Hypnotherapy: The induction of a state of consciousness in which normal critical powers are suspended and the mind becomes highly suggestable and able to consciously influence the body.

Magnetic field therapy: The use of magnets or electromagnetic-generating devices to stimulate energetic responses that help relieve pain, aid the healing of broken bones, and diagnose and treat disease.

Meditation: Trained focusing and freeing of the mind—achieved by such means as the repetition of a sound, concentration on an image, or close observation of the breath—in order to induce calm, control pain, and reduce anxiety and stress.

Qigong: A system of exercise that incorporates breathing, meditation, and movement to restore the free flow of vital energy and boost the body's natural healing abilities.

Tai Chi: A form of meditation through movement in which slow-motion exercises are combined with mental concentration and coordinated breathing to quiet the mind, increase relaxation, and improve the flow of vital energy through the body.

Yoga: A body of disciplines that include, in addition to such practices as meditation and dietary prescriptions, an extensive series of postures that stretch, condition, and improve organs. Special attention is placed on proper breathing.

Excerpted with permission from "Alternative Medicine's Pharmacopia" by Karen Baar, *Natural Health,* November/December 1994. For a trial issue of *Natural Health,* call 1-800-526-8440.

References

Baar, Karen. "Alternative Medicine's Pharmacopoeia." *Natural Health,* November/December 1994.

Benson, Herbert. *Your Maximum Mind.* New York: Times Books, 1987.

Bishop, George D. *Health Psychology: Integrating Mind and Body.* Boston: Allyn and Bacon, 1994.

Borysenko, Joan. *Minding the Body, Mending the Mind.* New York: Bantam Books, 1988.

___. *Guilt Is the Teacher, Love Is the Lesson: A Book to Heal You, Heart and Soul.* New York: Warner Books, 1990.

___. *Fire in the Soul: A New Psychology of Spiritual Optimism*. New York: Warner Books, 1993.

Borysenko, Joan, and Miroslav Borysenko. *The Power of the Mind to Heal*. Carson, CA: Hay House, 1994.

Chopra, Deepak. *Unconditional Life: Mastering the Forces that Shape Personal Reality*. New York: Bantam Books, 1991.

"Cousins, Cassileth Agree: Mind Can Alter Illness." *Brain/Mind Bulletin Collections* 11:1G, 1991.

Dossey, Larry. *Beyond Illness: Discovering the Experience of Health*. Boulder, CO: Shambhala, 1984.

___. *Meaning and Medicine: A Doctor's Tales of Breakthrough and Healing*. New York: Bantam, 1991.

Dubois, René. *Man Adapting*. New Haven, CT: Yale University Press, 1965.

Frank, Jerome D. *Persuasion and Healing*. New York: Schocken Books, 1974.

Frankl, Victor. *Man's Search for Meaning*. New York: Washington Square Press, 1963.

Goleman, Daniel. *Emotional Intelligence: Why It Can Matter More than IQ*. New York: Bantam Books, 1995.

Hunt, Morton. *The Story of Psychology*. New York: Doubleday, 1993.

Jung, Carl. In Joseph Campbell (ed.), *The Portable Jung*. New York: Viking Press, 1971.

Kabat-Zinn, Jon. "Mindfulness Meditation: Health Benefits of an Ancient Buddhist Practice," in Daniel Goleman and Joel Gurin (eds.), *Mind/Body Medicine*. Yonkers, NY: Consumer Reports Books, 1993.

Kunz, Dora (ed.). *Spiritual Aspects of the Healing Arts*. Wheaton, IL: Theosophical Publishing House, 1985.

Moyers, Bill. "Healing and the Mind" (1993). Available on videocassette from Parabola, 656 Broadway, Dept. H1, New York, NY 10012.

Neihardt, John. *Black Elk Speaks*. New York: Pocket Books, 1972.

Ornstein, Robert, and David Sobel. *Healthy Pleasures*. Reading, MA: Addison-Wesley, 1989.

Oyle, David. *The Healing Mind*. Berkeley, CA: Celestial Arts, 1979.

Pelletier, Kenneth R. *Mind as Healer, Mind as Slayer*. New York: Delacorte, 1977.

Schwartz, Gary. "Brain as Health Care System." *Yale Journal of Biology and Medicine* 52: 1991.

Schweitzer, Albert. *Out of My Life and Thought* (trans. by C.P. Campion). New York: Holt, Rinehart, and Winston, 1961.

Siegel, Bernie. *Love, Medicine and Miracles*. New York: Harper & Row, 1986.

___. *Peace, Love and Healing: Body-Mind Communication and the Path to Self-Healing*. New York: Harper & Row, 1989.

___. "Beyond Medicine and Miracles." *New Age Journal,* March-April 1993.

Smuts, Jan Christian. *Holism and Evolution*. New York: Macmillan, 1926.

Sontag, Susan. *Illness as Metaphor*. New York: Vintage Books, 1979.

"Spirituality in Healing and Medicine." Conference sponsored by the Harvard Medical School and the Mind-Body Institute at Deaconess Hospital. Boston: December 3–5, 1995.

Additional Resources

Aceves, Carlos. "Mythic Pedagogy: An Approach." *Holistic Education Review.* Summer, 1992.

Campbell, Joseph. "The Power of Myth." Available on videocassette from Parabola, 656 Broadway, Dept. H1, New York, NY 10012

Chopra, Deepak. *Perfect Health: The Complete Mind-Body Guide.* New York: Harmony Books, 1991.

Cousins, Norman. *Anatomy of an Illness as Perceived by the Patient: Reflections on Healing and Regeneration.* New York: Bantam Books, 1981.

Dennis, Gregory. "What's Deepak's Secret?" *New Age,* February 1994.

Epstein, Alice Hooper. *Mind, Fantasy, and Healing: One Woman's Journey from Conflict and Illness to Wholeness and Health.* New York: Delacorte, 1989.

"Exploring the Mystery of Spiritual Healing." *New Age Journal,* February 1996.

Ferrucci, Piero. *What We May Be: Techniques for Psychological and Spiritual Growth.* Los Angeles: J.P. Tarcher, 1982.

Fox, Matthew, "Toward a Spiritual Renaissance." *Common Boundary,* July/August 1990.

James, Muriel, and John James. *Passion for Life: Psychology and the Human Spirit.* New York: Dutton, 1991.

Kirby, Joan. "Poverty, Spirit, and Education." *Holistic Education Review,* Spring 1993.

Masters, Robert, and Jean Houston. *Listening to the Body: The Psychophysical Way to Health and Awareness.* New York: Delta Books, 1978.

Metzger, William. "Prayer, Healing, and Traditional Medicine: An Interview with Dr. Larry Dossey." *The Quest,* Winter 1992.

Moss, Richard. *The I that Is We: Awakening to Higher Energies through Unconditional Love.* Millbrae, CA: Celestial Arts, 1981.

Moyers, Bill. "Healing and the Mind." Available on videocassette from Parabola, 656 Broadway, Dept. H1, New York, NY 10012.

Occhiogrosso, Peter. "What Is Spirituality?" *MindField,* Winter 1992.

Ornstein, Robert, and David Sobel. *Healthy Pleasures.* Reading, MA: Addison-Wesley, 1989.

Robbins, Jim. "Wired for Miracles." *New Age Journal,* April 1996.

Sanford, John. "Building Soul." *Common Boundary,* July/August, 1990.

Schwartz, Tony. "Uncovering the Essential Self." *New Age Journal,* May-June 1995.

Shapiro, Debbie. *The Bodymind Workbook: Exploring How the Mind and the Body Work Together.* Rockport, MA: Element, 1990.

Thomashow, Cynthia. "Seeking the Sacred in Everyday Life." *Holistic Education Review,* Autumn 1993.

Wakefield, Dan. "In Search of Miracles." *New Age Journal,* May-June 1995.

"When The Body Speaks, Who Listens?" *Psychology Today,* January-February 1995.

3 The Initial Reality

The struggle to make the educational process one in which students learn to respect, love, and value themselves and thus choose positive life-styles ranks as one of the most important goals of health education. To understand and act on this important concept of personal empowerment tomorrow, health educators must be willing to move beyond what is happening today. As the great psychiatrist Carl Jung said in *Modern Man in Search of a Soul* (1963), "Any knowledge that does not change the quality of life is sterile and of questionable value." This cuts to the heart of what health education needs to be all about in the twenty-first century: *if the quality and emotional patterns of life are to be changed, the change must be traceable to some new insight or perception that translates into a behavioral change.*

This invites the proposition that individual attitudes and behaviors are programmed not only by our genes but also by our internal needs and wants. Theories to explain this process of attitudinal and behavioral learning are plentiful, but scientifically verifiable explanations have been elusive. Until the past two decades, nothing could be said with scientific authority about any dimension of the learning process, let alone about how specific aspects of positive health behaviors could be taught. Today, the multitude of voices can be confusing to health educators who must make decisions about how to transmit health information.

What do learners need to *feel* to believe that the world of people is a positive and healthy place and that they have value? What experiences can we provide so they feel confident in their ability to make wise and healthy choices, to value and love themselves, to develop healthy peer relationships, to rebound from adversity, and to resist negative peer pressure? What sort of an environment can we cre-

The field cannot well be seen from within the field.

—RALPH WALDO EMERSON

ate to best serve their emotional needs? All these questions are of huge theoretical and practical interest.

Because of deep cuts in government financing of schools and other programs for youth, the diminished role of the family has become a critical factor for educators. Children spend too little time engaged in structured activities with positive role models and too much time at loose ends and susceptible to negative role models. Today—with mothers and fathers working longer hours and thus spending less time at home; with families falling apart and being reshaped in new and sometimes confusing combinations; with debates raging over the emotional needs of children and the advantages and disadvantages of day care; with teenagers concerned about crime, drugs, suicide, sexual abuse, parental drug problems and abandonment, and whether the world will be around long enough for them to grow up—children are being systematically destroyed (see Jonathan Kozol's *Savage Inequalities,* 1991).

A report by the Center for the Study of Social Policy called the *Kids Count Data Book* (1991) gives us some interesting facts about changes in the lives of young people between 1985 and 1990.

- The number of teenagers finishing high school in four years declined to 69 percent in 1990 from 72 percent in 1985. Seventy-five percent of whites, 61 percent of blacks, and 42 percent of Hispanics graduated on time.
- Juvenile violent-crime arrest rates increased by 48 percent, from 314 per 100,000 in 1986 to 466 per 100,000 in 1991. For whites, this was an increase of 58 percent; for blacks, 29 percent. For girls, the increase was 57 percent; for boys, 46 percent.
- Teen deaths from accidents, homicides, or suicides grew by 13 percent, from 62.8 per 100,000 in 1985 to 70.9 per 100,000 in 1990. For blacks, the figure was up 78 percent; for whites, 10 percent.
- Births to single teenagers grew by 16 percent, from 7.5 percent of all births in 1985 to 8.7 percent in 1990. For whites, this was an increase of 26 percent; the rate was unchanged for blacks.
- The child-poverty rate inched down from 21 percent to 20 percent between 1985 and 1990 but is still higher than in 1979.
- According to the American Psychological Association, the average child has watched 8,000 murders and 100,000 acts of violence simulated on television before she finishes elementary school.
- Statistics by the Centers for Disease Control found that, in 1988, 26 percent of girls aged fifteen reported being sexually active compared with only 5 percent in 1970.

In addition to these sobering facts, nearly fifty-thousand children and teenagers were killed by guns between 1979 and 1991—a total roughly equal to the number of battle deaths in the Vietnam War, according to the Children's Defense Fund. Arrests from 1982 to 1991 for murder and non-negligent manslaughter rose 11 percent for adults, while the number of juveniles arrested for those crimes rose 93 percent. There was also a 79-percent increase during the 1980s in the number of ten- to seventeen-year-olds who used firearms to commit murder (Dixon, 1994).

The Reality

According to *Handgun Control,* in 1992 handguns killed

- **13,220 people in the United States**
- **33 people in Great Britain**
- **36 people in Sweden**
- **13 people in Australia**
- **128 people in Canada**

Except for the United States, all of these countries have stringent gun-control laws.

In his book *Tales out of School* (1993), Joseph Fernandez, former chancellor of the New York City school system, points out that schools have been dealing with the problem of neglected and disaffected students since the 1950s.

Where [have the] people been? More important, where were their eyes and hearts? In New York, at this pivotal moment in time, we are faced with some frightening realities: that as many as 80 percent of our teenagers are sexually active, and that 10 percent of the nation's full-blown AIDS cases reported among adolescents live in New York City. . . . But the larger issue [has been] missed again, as it is missed almost every time. The teaching of values isn't the problem. The problem is drugs, and crime, and violence, and truancy, and broken dreams, and hopelessness, and despair. The problem is two-thirds of black children in America are born out of wedlock and more than half grow up with only one parent, often below the poverty level, and in an environment ravaged by crime and drugs. The problem is that the ills and sins of the society are visited on the schools of America.

No matter how punitive we become, no matter how strong a message we send to the streets, teenagers who are self-destructive will always turn a deaf ear to deterrence. The national trend toward trying juveniles as adults so they are incarcerated longer may address the need for justice and retribution, but it does nothing to dissuade teenagers from the negative pressures that confront them.

Health Educators in the Middle

As an example of what health educators face, a recent nationwide opinion poll found that nearly nine out of ten beginning teachers believed many of their pupils were too overwhelmed by family and other outside problems to succeed in class. Seventy-five percent of the teachers agreed that a number of children came to school with so many problems it was difficult for them to be good students. After these same teachers taught for one year, 89 percent held this view.

That young people caught in these circumstances resort to negative and unhealthy behaviors should surprise no one. The development of loyalties and values within peer groups and gangs can put them permanently beyond the constructive reach of most health educators and society at large. It is a myth that we can reverse unhealthy, socially unacceptable behavior with simple facts. For some of these youths, the savagery and contempt are so deep-rooted that the chance for redemptory caring and connecting is negligible (*Reaching the Hip-Hop Generation*, 1992). These often insecure youths have difficulty finding positive role models because the strategies they have adopted to get along in the world tend to alienate them from the very people who might be able to help. The behavior of insecure individuals—whether aggressive or passive, puffed up or easily deflated—tries the patience of peers and adults alike, which reinforces the individual's distorted view of the world—"People will never love me, they treat me like an irritation, they don't trust me," and so on. Harold Hodgkinson (1991) points out that "one-third of preschool children are destined for school failure because of poverty, neglect, sickness, handicapping conditions, and lack of adult protection and nurturing."

About Hope and Caring

There is hope for young people today, and this hope is based on the need for compassion and commitment on the part of those who are in a position to form a positive, helping relationship with at-risk kids. It calls on us as health educators to devote energy and enthusiasm to a method of teaching that has personal meaning. It calls on us to be more than we are and to do more than we are doing. We must focus our attention on early-childhood health-education programs, because young children are more impressionable and we have a better chance of instilling good-health values and behaviors that will carry over into the teen years and adulthood. We must also reinvest in our youth and strive to make healthy life-styles more attractive than unhealthy life-styles. This will take both creative teaching and positive reinforcement of prosocial behavior to outweigh negative reinforcement for antisocial behavior.

All health-education specialists, whether working in the community or in school, must shift their focus so the objective is not just increasing cognitive knowledge but also changing attitudes and behaviors. Gilbert J. Botvin writes in *Strengthening Health Education for the 1990s* (1990),

> *The challenge facing health educators has been to demonstrate that preventive interventions can be developed which really work—i.e., which reduce tobacco, alcohol, and drug-use behavior. Considerable research has been conducted in the past decade testing a variety of strategies hypothesized to prevent drug abuse. Most of these approaches targeted the various psychosocial factors believed to promote substance abuse among adolescents (Botvin, 1983). The approaches tested differ from previous tobacco, alcohol, and drug-abuse pre-*

vention approaches in several important ways. These approaches 1) are based on a more complete understanding of the causes of health-compromising behavior; 2) are grounded in theory; 3) use well-tested, cognitive-behavioral intervention techniques; and perhaps most important, 4) they have been tested using rigorous evaluation designs.

This body of research has been summarized in a number of review papers (Botvin, 1987; Flay, 1985). Botvin also argued that broad-based health-education programs, which include the teaching of personal and social skills, are successful prevention strategies because they provide students with the know-how to resist social pressure to use tobacco, alcohol, and other drugs and reduce the motivation to use these substances. Teaching refusal skills can increase students' ability to resist the social influences that promote substance use. At the same time, they improve students' personal and social competence, thus reducing their motivation to use drugs (1990).

Inroads in HIV Education

In a review of school-based AIDS-prevention programs, Kirby and DiClemente (1994) provide several key elements to enhance program effectiveness:

1. Use social-learning theories as a foundation for program development (e.g., cognitive-behavioral theory or social-influence theory).
2. Maintain a narrow focus on reducing sexual risk-taking behaviors.
3. Use active-learning methods of instruction.
4. Include activities that address social or media influences and pressures to have sex.
5. Focus on and reinforce clear and appropriate values against sexual risk-taking (e.g., postponing sex, avoiding unprotected intercourse, or avoiding high-risk partners).
6. Provide modeling and practice of communication skills.

Furthermore, to maximize effectiveness, AIDS-prevention programs must also be tailored so they are developmentally appropriate and culturally relevant. Stryker et al. (1995) put HIV-infection prevention in this context.

[One] misconception is that knowledge alone is sufficient to inoculate individuals against risk-taking. The sexual behavior changes noted among middle-class gay men in the 1980s may represent the most profound behavior changes ever observed in the literature on health-behavior change. For some, these dramatic changes are evidence that efforts should be directed toward other problems or groups at risk of HIV. Yet, as is evident from other areas of health promotion, intellectual appreciation of risk does not necessarily translate into sustained behavior change, particularly for activities as inherently pleasurable as sexual intercourse.

Whatever aspect of health education we focus on, developing a program that really works is the primary focus of this text. This process must include theories that balance cognitive and behavioral learning, and must draw from research not only in health education but also in the related fields of counseling, psychology, and sociology.

A Focus on Positive Goals

Although the facts and figures may suggest that health educators are facing an impossible fight against insurmountable odds, the reality is we are not. Although the statistics suggest a rise in negative behaviors, our approach needs to remain positive.

One beauty of health education is its focus on meaning through health; this implies a strong faith in humankind, in opportunities for personal growth, and in the infinite possibilities of experience. As Albert Camus said, "The meaning of life is the most urgent of questions" (1955). What greater meaning than the search for positive health?

Goals 2000

On March 31, 1994, President Clinton signed the Goals 2000 school-reform bill into law. Under the goals set by the law, by the year 2000

- *all children in America will start school ready to learn*
- *the high-school graduation rate will increase to at least 90 percent*
- *students will leave grades 4, 8, and 12 having demonstrated competence over challenging subject matter*
- *teachers will have access to programs for the continued improvement of their professional skills and the opportunity to acquire the knowledge and skills needed*
- *American students will be first in the world in mathematics and science achievement*
- *every adult American will be literate and possess the skills necessary to compete in a global economy and exercise the rights and responsibilities of citizenship*
- *every school in the United States will be free of drugs, firearms, alcohol, and violence and will offer a disciplined environment conducive to learning*
- *every school will promote partnerships that will increase parental participation in promoting the social, emotional, and academic growth of children*

Healthy People 2000

The nation's health goals for the year 2000 were set forth with the release of *Healthy People 2000* (1991), which reviewed the principal health challenges for Americans and identified in measurable terms the opportunities for health gains during the 1990s. *Healthy People 2000* presented three broad goals for the health of the nation: (1) to increase the life span, (2) to reduce health disparities among Americans, and (3) to achieve access to preventive services. To accomplish these goals, the U.S. Department of Public Health (1991) also set forth three-hundred measurable objectives for the year 2000 in twenty-two areas of priority involving health promotion, health protection, and clinical preventive services (Table 3–1):

Health promotion

  Physical activity and fitness

  Nutrition

  Tobacco

  Alcohol and other drugs

  Family planning

  Mental health and mental disorders

  Violent and abusive behavior

  Educational and community-based programs

Health protection

  Unintentional injuries

  Occupational safety and health

  Environmental health

  Food and drug safety

  Oral health

Preventive services

  Maternal and infant health

  Heart disease and stroke

  Cancer

  Diabetes and chronic disabling conditions

  Human immunodeficiency virus infection

  Sexually transmitted diseases

  Immunization and infectious diseases

  Clinical preventive services

Surveillance and data systems

  The *health-promotion priorities* have a prominent behavioral component, requiring strategies to address the social contexts that shape personal attitudes and choices. The *health-protection priorities* emphasize population-wide interventions to protect entire communities. *Preventive-services priorities* are the counseling, screening, immunization, and chemoprophylactic interventions that are best provided through clinical settings. Objectives specific to people in certain age, ethnic, or socioeconomic groups are found in each of the priority areas. In addi-

Table 3–1

Quantitative goals of *Healthy People 2000*

Objective	Change Targeted, %	Baseline, %*†‡	Update, %†§	Year 2000 Targets, %†‡	Right Direction||
Health Promotion					
Physical activity					
More people exercising regularly	36↑¶	22#	24**	30	Yes
Fewer people never exercising	38↓	24#	24**	15	No change
Nutrition					
Fewer people overweight	23↓	26††	34###	20	No
Lower-fat diets	17↓	36††	34###	30	Yes
Tobacco					
Fewer people smoking cigarettes	48↓	29	25	15	Yes
Fewer youth beginning to smoke	50↓	30	27	15	Yes
Alcohol and other drugs					
Fewer alcohol-related automobile deaths	13↓	9.8/100 000‡‡	6.8/100 000‡‡	8.5/100 00‡‡	Yes
Less alcohol use among youth aged 12 to 17 y	50↓	25.2¶¶	18.0	12.6	Yes
Less marijuana use among youth aged 12 to 17 y	50↓	6.4¶¶	4.9	3.2	Yes
Family planning					
Fewer teen pregnancies	30↓	71.1/1000#§§	74.3/1000||||§§	50.0/1000§§	No
Fewer unintended pregnancies	46↓	56¶¶	NA##	30	No data
Mental health and mental disorders					
Fewer suicides	10↓	11.7/100 000‡‡	11.2/100 000‡‡	10.5/100 000‡‡	Yes
Fewer people reporting stress-related problems	21↓	44.2#	39.2	35	Yes
Violent and abusive behavior					
Fewer homicides	15↓	8.5/100 000‡‡	10.3/100 000‡‡†††	7.2/100 000‡‡	No
Fewer assault injuries	10↓	9.7/100 000‡‡***	9.9/100 000‡‡†††	8.7/100 000‡‡	No
Educational and community-based programs					
More schools with comprehensive school health education	NA	NA	NA	75	No data
More workplaces with health promotion programs	31↑	65#	81†††	85	Yes
Health Protection					
Unintentional injuries					
Fewer unintentional injury deaths	16↓	34.7/100 000‡‡	29.6/100 000‡‡	29.3/100 000‡‡	Yes
More people using automobile safety restraints	102↑	42¶¶	67‡‡‡	85	Yes

Occupational safety and health					
Fewer work-related deaths	33↓	6/100 000‡‡§§§	5/100 000‡‡	4/100 000‡‡	Yes
Fewer work-related injuries	22↓	7.7/100 000‡‡§§§	7.9/100 000‡‡	6.0/100 000‡‡	No
Environmental health					
No children with blood lead level > 1.21 μmol/L (>25 μg/dL)	100↓	234 000|||||¶¶¶	93 000|||||###	0|||||	Yes
More people with clean air in their communities	71↑	49.7¶¶	76.5	85	Yes
More people in radon-tested houses	700↑	5****	11.4	40	Yes
Food and drug safety					
Fewer salmonella outbreaks	68↓	77*****††††	63††††	25†††	Yes
Oral health					
Fewer children with dental caries	34↓	53	NA	35	No data
Fewer older people without teeth	44↓	36***	30	20	Yes
Maternal and infant health					
Fewer newborns with low weight	28↓	6.9	7.1†††	5	No
More mothers with first-trimester care	18↑	76	77.7†††	90	Yes
Heart disease and stroke					
Fewer coronary heart disease deaths	26↓	135/100 000‡‡	114/100 000‡‡†††	100/100 000‡‡	Yes
Fewer stroke deaths	34↓	30.4/100 000‡‡	26.4/100 000‡‡	20.0/100 000‡‡	Yes
Better control of high blood pressure	355↑	11††	21###	50	Yes
Lower cholesterol levels	6↓	5.51 (213)††‡‡‡	5.30 (205)######‡‡‡	5.17 (200)‡‡‡	Yes
Cancer					
Decrease in cancer deaths	3↓	134/100 000‡‡	133/100 000‡‡	130/100 000‡‡	Yes
Increase screening for breast cancer (age > 50 y)	140↑	25	55	60	Yes
Increase screening for cervical center (age > 18 y)	8↑	88	95	95	Yes
Increase fecal occult blood testing (age > 50 y)	85↑	27	30†††	50	Yes
Diabetes and chronic disabling conditions					
Fewer people disabled by chronic conditions	15↓	9.4	10.6	8	No
Fewer diabetes-related deaths	11↓	38/100 000‡‡***	38/100 000‡‡††††	34/100 000‡‡	No change
Human immunodeficiency virus (HIV) infection					
Slower increase in HIV infection	In revision§§§§	400/100 000‡‡*****	NA	In revision§§§	No data

Continued

Table 3–1 (Continued)

Objective	Change Targeted, %	Baseline, %*†‡	Update, %‡§	Year 2000 Targets, %‡	Right Direction‖
Sexually transmitted diseases					
Fewer gonorrhea infections	25↓	300/100 000‡‡*****	172/100 000‡‡	225/100 000‡‡	Yes
Fewer syphillis infections	45↓	18.1/100 000‡‡*****	10.4/100 000‡‡	10.0/100 000‡‡	Yes
Immunization and infectious diseases					
No measles cases	100↓	3058¶‖‖‖‖‖‖	312‖‖‖‖‖	0	Yes
Fewer pneumonia and influenza deaths	63↓	19.9/100 000‡‡¶¶¶¶	23.1/100 000‡‡###¶	7.3/100 00‡‡	No
Higher immunization levels (ages 19-35 mo)	53↑	54–64	67	90	Yes
Clinical preventive services					
No financial barrier to recommended preventive services	100↓	16****	17	0	No
Surveillance and Data Systems					
Common and comparable health status indicators in use across states		0*****	48*****	40*****	Yes

*From US Public Health Service. *Healthy People 2000: Midcourse Review and 1995 Revisions.* In press.

†1987 unless otherwise noted.
‡Data are expressed in percentages unless otherwise indicated.
§1993 unless otherwise noted.
‖A total of 32 objectives were progressing in the right direction; nine, in the wrong direction; two, no change; four, no data.
¶Arrows indicate whether trend was increasing (up arrow) or decreasing (down arrow).
#1985.
**1991.
††1976–1980.
‡‡Data are expressed as rate per 100 000 population.
§§Data are expressed as rate per 1000 population
‖‖1990.
¶¶1988.
##NA indicates not available.

***1986.
†††1992.
‡‡‡1994.
§§§1983–1987.
‖‖‖Data are expressed as number of children.
¶¶¶1984.
###1988–1991.
****1989.
††††Data are expressed as number of salmonella outbreaks.
‡‡‡‡Data are reported in mmol/L (mg/dL).
§§§§Targeted percentage change and year 2000 targets in revision (1995) (see text).
‖‖‖‖Data are expressed as number of measles cases.
¶¶¶¶1979–1980 through 1986–1987 influenza seasons.
####1987–1988 through 1989-1990 influenza seasons.
*****Data are expressed as number of states.

tion, goals for improving surveillance and data systems at the national, state, and local level were established to help target interventions to areas of greatest need.

Community health needs. At the community level, *Healthy People 2000* has provided a framework for local health initiatives. To assist communities in planning and implementing prevention agendas, the American Public Health Association and the Centers for Disease Control (CDC) jointly developed *Healthy Communities 2000: Model Standards, Guidelines for Community Attainment of Year 2000 National Health Objectives* (1991).

Objectives into Theory

What is to be done with these goals for the decade? First, we must look at them as a challenge due to the magnitude of the problems that exist, the shortfalls with respect to our aspirations, and the changes necessary to rebuild the eroding infrastructure supporting our youth. We must shift the focus of health education from external to internal awareness. As students become aware of their own inner states, they can begin to recognize important conditions that affect their learning ability.

We must also recognize that people are whole beings, with cognitive, social, emotional, and spiritual potential. A cognitive-behavioral approach to health education *is* education for the whole person, and the educational setting is a place where this wholeness can be supported and encouraged. To accomplish this, we must address issues raised by Robert Ornstein (1972). From his research on the brain, he surmised that there were two modes of consciousness at work in human beings: one, a rational, logical, and active mode associated with the left side of the brain; the other, a mystical, intuitive, and receptive mode associated with the right side of the brain. Thus, a strictly cognitive approach to health education simply will not work in the long term. We need to take a multifaceted approach that includes not only the learner's *thinking* (cognitive) level, but their *feeling* and *acting* (behavioral) level as well.

Philosophers and psychologists of education, as well as teachers, curriculum planners, textbook writers, and material makers, can learn from Ornstein's research that the linear, verbal-intellectual mode of imparting knowledge is not the only mode available to the teacher. The field is wide open for reconceptualizing what it means to teach and to learn, for creative classroom innovations, for research on new teaching styles, and for the development of new topics of study and supporting materials.

Learning to understand and control our own consciousness includes learning to pay attention to what we want instead of being at the mercy of a roaming, untrained mind. Learning how to relax, concentrate, be in control, feel empowered, and freely associate are skills we seldom teach, but compelling evidence suggests they can improve current instruction.

Theory into Action

A Cognitive-Behavioral Approach

A cognitive-behavioral approach to health education that focuses on positive behavioral responses requires the educator to teach students *how* to be aware of their thoughts, feelings, and actions. The cognitive (thought-based) technique is based on the underlying assumption that the way people interpret their experiences determines how they feel and behave (Beck and Weishaar, 1989; Burns, 1980). For students to truly connect feelings with behavior, some kind of cognitive work is essential. No one disputes that knowledge leads to empowerment, but changing power into action means abandoning old, disabling teaching methods in favor of new ones that support feeling and acting. One such method is to educate for positive self-esteem, which might involve the following experiences:

- letting students talk about themselves
- taking notes on what students say and then telling them what you have heard
- starting each learning experience by talking about things that students have said in past classes
- offering constructive solutions to issues based on student input
- using students' work and ideas as the basis for future teaching themes
- inviting students to suggest future teaching themes

Self-Esteem

Low self-esteem often leads to self-destructive behavior including drug abuse, unhealthy risk-taking, and unprotected sex. Conversely, when people feel positive about themselves they react differently. When people have high self-esteem, they approach negative feelings by exercising one of several options:

- *they accept the feelings*
- *they express the feelings in a respectful way*
- *they act on the feelings in a constructive way*

In essence, people with high self-esteem change their feelings by changing their negative thoughts.

A great deal of emphasis has been placed on helping the learner to identify and express his or her feelings. Every moment of our lives has a feeling attached to it, and these feelings are most often centered on our perception of ourselves. Love, self-esteem, acceptance, sensuality, vulnerability, and attractiveness all have emotional components that color most of our hours and days.

What this means to us in health education is that when we improve the way someone *thinks* about something, we also change the way they *feel* about it and the way they *behave* toward it. Thus, when we change the way students feel about something, we alter the way they think and act. Thinking and feeling are vital components in the cognitive-behavioral process, but bringing about action is essential if the goal in our teaching is behavioral change. Students can spend countless hours talking about health issues and how to identify and change certain behaviors, but it remains nothing more than an academic exercise. We as health educators must implement an action-oriented program for change. We do this by applying feelings and thoughts to real-life situations ("reality" education). There is considerable merit in a health-education focus that is reality based. Begin by asking students these questions:

- What are you doing with yourself, healthwise?
- What do you see for yourself now and in the future?
- Does your present health behavior have a reasonable chance of getting you what you want now, and will it take you in the direction you want to go?

If the focus of the teacher is on what learners are doing, there is a greater chance that they will be able to change the learner's thoughts and feelings (Glasser, 1986).

In closing, a basic underlying premise in any self-esteem program is that self-esteem as an end in itself is futile (Baumeister et al. 1996). Self-esteem *must* be rooted in achievement and in acquiring of new ways of feeling and acting. In health education, this would translate into new thoughts and actions that lead to more positive health choices.

Closing the Gap

Cultural, economic, and ethnic issues, as well as the realities of single parenthood, guns, and violence, have been around for awhile. That they dictate relationships between teachers, students, and community-health educators should not be a surprise to those whose careers give them firsthand experience with what is going on in our schools and communities today. The reputation of urban schools and community health centers suggests that there is a need to change the way health educators prepare for working in inner city schools. Teachers are not often fully prepared to work with the growing number of urban students who live in poverty and come to class tired, scared, hungry, distressed, and thus less able to learn than their suburban counterparts. Training should expose new teachers to multicultural issues and make them aware of the preconceptions, expectations, and values that damage children and youth. The bottom line is, a new type of education is taking place today that is really about the teacher's approach, and this approach must be more reality focused.

Reality-Based Education

Reality-based education is about tailoring the educational environment to the specific needs of those we are working with. Urban education certainly has a different flavor from other arenas because we are dealing with children and youth with unique needs.

We must start by building relationships between the teacher and the students. (See Chapter 8 for further discussion.) If a student senses that you care about her, she won't care if you are black, blue, or green. She will simply respond to your caring (see Chapter 12). The major focus in reality education is on what is real to students—how they feel, function, and behave, as well as their environment.

A Reality-Based Program for Health Education

"I think, therefore I am," said Descartes. I would add, "I also feel, therefore I am fuller and more complete in my being." If we were only physical, we would simply react, as an amoeba does when touched with a probe under a microscope. By combining emotional and cognitive skills, we can *respond,* which is far more than just reacting—an unconscious, automatic response. People can modify their behavior, mull things over, and experience events more fully when they bring together all aspects of their selfhood.

Health education stands at the threshold of a new reality. This reality includes establishing an educational process that encompasses the following principles (Figure 3–1):

- **A health education program must be democratic.** It must promote fairness, compassion, and community rather than maintaining a morally blind focus on a single concept of health. It needs to celebrate the wonderful variety of human expression and talent rather than homogenizing the concept of good health or giving undue status to an established avenue for its attainment. It invites all learners to become active participants in the process of building a multiethnic, multi-age, gender-specific concept of health.
- **A health education program must be learner-centered.** It is appropriate to the audience it is working with rather than to a given curriculum or other worn out teaching concept that has little or no meaning for the learner. The real lives, experiences, and interests of human beings must have priority over abstract ideologies or a technocratic interest in standardization, classification, and control.
- **Health education must be reality-based rather than abstract.** It should focus the curriculum on the student's reality (i.e., his age, sex, and culture). It seeks to engage the learner with his own experience of life.
- **A health-education program should be holistic.** It needs to recognize the complexity of human life in its physical, emotional, cultural, and spiritual dimensions. It should also acknowledge that human existence is a quest for meaning, and that meaning arises only through connections to the natural world, to culture and community, and to archetypal layers of experience.

Integrating these four principles into a new curriculum calls for changes in the way health education is presented. But changes may pose tricky problems for some health educators. Developing alternative models of teaching is just as diffi-

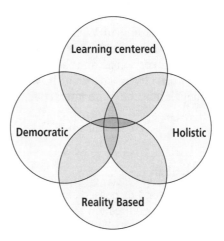

Figure 3–1

The four principles of a reality-based program in health education.

cult as abandoning the old health-education model of cognitive knowledge for one of behavioral response. Getting students more involved in their own learning can bump up against well-entrenched traditions. It's fine to set up a well-functioning learning environment in which students take charge of their own education, but learning does not exist in a vacuum. It is part of a process including the learner and an outside environment that is not always friendly to those who set out to do things differently. Health-education subject matter is often like a loaded gun: it can kill even those with the best intentions. Educating students on condom use and distribution and alternative life-styles can become a professional death sentence, even if you back yourself up with solid facts and a sound educational rationale for their discussion. And so, in endorsing a health-education program that is both cognitively and behaviorally oriented, a knowledgeable understanding of the value and need for such an approach is vital to its success.

The proper synthesis of these principles may not be easy to define and certainly will not be easy to achieve. However, the goal should be to encourage a lifestyle that includes a balance of emotional reactivity and rationality. Carl Rogers (1961) described the fully functioning person in these terms:

> *Psychological adjustment exists when the concept of self is such that all the sensory and visceral experiences of the organism are, or may be, assimilated on a symbolic level into a consistent relationship with the concept of self.*

This means that any experience, whether emotional, perceptual, or rational, should be consistent and congruent with the person's concept of who she is.

Recognizing the dual nature of human beings, the interplay between the cognitive and the behavioral, should excite every health educator's interest. We may have made a mistake in our philosophical approach to health education in the past. The prevalent assumption has been that knowing precedes doing, but this is not the case according to William Glasser (1965), among others. He believed that reflection always occurs after an event. To illustrate, talk to anyone who has had a near-death experience, and they will tell you about the major changes they have made in their lives. The point is, we *must* rethink our philosophical approach to teaching; it must be more interactive, more behaviorally focused, and more reality based.

Synthesis

In this chapter, I discussed some of the issues that we face in health education as well as teacher education today. One issue that needs to be addressed is incorporating the reality of the lives many young people face into the curriculum. Their fear and their perception of their lives as meaningless and irrelevant can have a devastating affect on their ability to learn.

To help young people gain a sense of selfhood when they have not yet learned to deal logically with the world or to take responsibility for their decisions, the teacher must enter the student's frame of reference, understand and

---

Time Out for Personal Thoughts

The purpose of this chapter was to challenge you to examine your thoughts and feelings about making the learning experience more meaningful for students. It's easy to lash out at or write off those who lack motivation, are slow learners, or come from less than desirable backgrounds. It's more difficult—and more honest—to look at yourself and ask, "When I teach a class of high achievers, do I get fully involved and become excited about my teaching?" or, "When I am in a class of perceived slow learners, do I become passive and bored and expect less of them?" Even if your own educational experiences taught you to be a passive learner and to fear taking risks in your teaching, becoming aware of this influence gives you the power to change your style.

In this chapter, I presented some bleak statistics on young people and suggested alternative models for dealing with students who live with these realities. Now it's your turn. List some of the ideas in this chapter that had the greatest impact on you. Write them down, whether they reflect your own experience or you disagree with them:

Exercises

1. Go to an inner-city school and observe a classroom (ideally, in health education) for one day. Write down what you observe. Ask yourself the following questions?

   - Would I teach in this school?
   - What aspects of the classroom experience bothered me the most?
   - What things could be done to make the learning experience more meaningful for the students?
   - What was the most meaningful experience for me?
   - What did I learn?
   - How has it affected me?

2. Interview a person you do not know who is in failing health. Some questions you might want to ask are:

   - How can I help?
   - What do you see as the major problem within the health-care system?
   - What do you see as the major cause of your illness?
   - What can you teach me?

3. If you are considering a particular job in the health field, seek out a person who is actively engaged in that type of work and arrange to talk with her. Ask questions concerning the chances of gaining employment, the experience necessary, the satisfactions and drawbacks of the position, and so on. In this way, your perception of the job will be more realistic, thus avoiding disappointment if your expectations don't match reality.

4. Think back to your own high-school learning experience and list the top-ten most negative aspects of it. Now ask yourself how you would change it. Make a top-ten positive list.

appreciate the uniqueness of each student's experience, and use this experience to affirm a student's right, desire, and ability to change. According to Robert Carkhuff and Richard Pierce, in their beautifully simple book *Teacher as Person* (1976), this process "requires developing the skills of truly hearing what students are saying, acknowledging our understanding by providing meaningful responses, and developing educational activities based on the individual needs of the student. These interpersonal skills are the first building blocks for increasing one's effectiveness in the classroom."

The learner needs your emotional availability and responsiveness! Health educators don't need to be popular or smart or talented or funny; they just need to be *there,* in both senses of the word. To a student in need, none of the rest matters, except insofar as it enables the health educator to give of himself.

Finally, although the focus was on youth, their reality is also the reality of adults. The youth of today become the adults of tomorrow. Thus, we cannot let our efforts stop at the school-age person; we must follow through onto adulthood.

References

American Public Health Association. *Healthy Communities 2000: Model Standards, Guidelines for Community Attainment of Year 2000 National Objectives* (3rd ed.). Washington, DC: U.S. Government Printing Office, 1991.

Baumeister, Roy F., Laura Smart, and Joseph M. Boden. "Relation of Threatened Egotism to Violence and Aggression: The Dark Side of High Self-Esteem." *Psychological Review,* January 1996.

Beck, A.T., and M.E. Weishaar. "Cognitive Therapy," in R.J. Corsini and D. Wedding (eds.), *Current Psychotherapies.* Itasca, IL: F.E. Peacock, 1989.

Botvin, Gilbert J. "Substance Abuse Prevention Research: Recent Developments and Future Directions." *Journal of School Health,* November 1983.

____. *Drug Abuse and Drug Abuse Research: Second Triennial Report to Congress* (DHHS Publication No. ADM 87–1486). Washington, DC: U.S. Government Printing Office, 1987.

____. "Personal and Social Skills Training: Applications for Substance Prevention," in *Strengthening Health Education for the 1990s.* Reston, VA: Association for the Advancement of Health Education, 1990.

Burns, D. *Feeling Good: The New Mood Therapy.* New York: Morrow, 1980.

Carkhuff, Robert, and Richard Pierce. *Teacher as Person.* Washington, DC: National Education Association, 1976.

Dixon, Jennifer. "Report Details Toll of Guns on Youths." *Boston Globe,* 21 January 1994.

Emerson, Ralph Waldo. *Emerson: A Modern Anthology.* Alfred Kazin and Daniel Aaron (eds.). Boston: Houghton Mifflin, 1959.

Fernandez, Joseph A. *Tales out of School.* Boston: Little, Brown, 1993.

Flay, B.R. "Psychosocial Approaches to Smoking Prevention: A Review of Findings." *Health Psychology,* 4:5, 1985.

Glasser, William. *Reality Therapy: A New Approach to Psychiatry.* New York: Harper & Row, 1965.

____. *Control Theory in the Classroom.* New York: Harper & Row, 1986.

Hodgkinson, Harold. "Reform versus Reality." *Phi Delta Kappan,* September 1991.

Jung, Carl. *Modern Man in Search of a Soul.* New York: Harcourt Brace Jovanovich, 1963.

Kids Count Data Book. Washington, DC: Center for the Study of Social Policy, 1991.

Kirby, D., and R.J. DiClemente. "School-based Behavioral Interventions to Prevent Unprotected Sex and HIV among Adolescents," in R.J. DiClemente and

J.L. Peterson (eds.), *Preventing AIDS: Theories and Methods of Behavioral Interventions.* New York: Plenum, 1994.

Kozol, Jonathan. *Savage Inequalities: Children in America's Schools.* New York: Crown, 1991.

Ornstein, Robert E. "The Education of the Intuitive Mode," in *The Psychology of Consciousness.* San Francisco: W.H. Freeman, 1972.

Reaching the Hip-Hop Generation. Philadelphia, PA: West Philadelphia Enterprise Center, 1992.

Rogers, Carl. *On Becoming a Person: A Therapist's View of Psychotherapy.* Boston: Houghton Mifflin, 1961.

Stryker, Jeff, et al. "Prevention of HIV Infection: Looking Back, Looking Ahead." *Journal of the American Medical Association,* 12 April 1995.

U.S. Dept. of Public Health. *Healthy People 2000: National Health Promotion and Disease Prevention Objectives.* Washington, DC: U.S. Government Printing Office, 1991.

Additional Resources

Anspaugh, David, and Gene Ezell. *Teaching Today's Health.* Boston: Allyn & Bacon, 1995.

Carnegie Council on Adolescent Development. *A Matter of Time: Risk and Opportunity in the Out-of-School Hours.* Carnegie Corporation, July 1994.

Comer, James P., and Alvin F. Poussaint. *Raising Black Children.* New York: Plume, 1992.

Cortese, Peter, and Kathleen Middleton. *The Comprehensive School Health Challenge: Promoting Health through Education.* Santa Cruz, CA: ETR Associates, 1994.

Currie, Elliott. *Reckoning: Drugs, the Cities, and the American Future.* New York: Hill and Wang, 1993.

Devine, Joel A., and James D. Wright. *The Greatest of Evils.* Hawthorne, NY: Aldine de Gruyter, 1993.

Elam, Stanley M., Lowell C. Rose, and Alec M. Gallup. "The 24th Annual GALLUP/Phi Delta Kappa Poll of the Public's Attitudes toward the Public Schools." *Phi Delta Kappan,* September 1992.

Goodman, Berney. "When the Body Speaks, Who Listens?" *Psychology Today,* January-February 1995.

Hendricks, Gay, and James Fadiman. *Transpersonal Education: A Curriculum for Feeling and Being.* Englewood Cliffs, NJ: Prentice-Hall, 1976.

Johnson, Lenora. "Beyond Knowledge and Practice: A Challenge in Health Education." *Journal of Health Education,* January-February 1991.

Morrison, Toni. *The Bluest Eye.* NY: Pocket Books, 1970.

Naylor, Thomas H., et al. *The Search for Meaning.* Nashville: Abingdon Press, 1994.

Nickerson, Carl J. "Getting in Touch with Realities of the Classroom and Community Service Agencies." *Journal of Health Education,* May-June 1991.

Page, Randy M., and Tana S. Page. *Fostering Emotional Well-Being in the Classroom.* Boston: Jones and Bartlett Publishers, 1993.

Pollock, Marion B., and Kathleen Middleton. *School Health Instruction: The Elementary and Middle School Years.* St. Louis: Mosby, 1994.

Sheley, Joseph F., and James D. Wright. *In the Line of Fire: Youth, Guns, and Violence in Urban America.* Hawthorne, NY: Aldine de Gruyter, 1995.

Wallerstein, Nina, and Michael Hammes. "Problem-Posing: A Teaching Strategy for Improving the Decision-Making Process." *Journal of Health Education,* July-August 1991.

4 Steps toward a General Theory

Which teaching approach, under what conditions, and for what purpose? We will explore these questions, increasingly asked by health educators, in this chapter. The immense variety of health issues and the people dealing with and affected by them do not fit easily into theoretical pigeonholes. One group may respond well to a given approach, while another may resist the same techniques. Evidence is mounting that teaching health requires more than a single set of methodological and theoretical approaches if we are to meet the needs of an increasingly diverse clientele. Thus, the road we travel must have a sure objective.

General theory (as opposed to specific theory) is concerned with the search for connections and underlying unity among the differing cognitive and behavioral approaches to teaching. Because general theory is only in the initial stages of development, the ideas presented here should be considered only a beginning. As you study the concepts presented in this chapter, you will want to start making your own connections and developing your own general theory for your work as a health educator. Keep these important questions in mind as you go along: What are *your* reactions to the ideas presented here? What methods and techniques make most sense to *you?* What do you want to bring to the lives of those you are working with? How will you go about developing your own general theory of educating for healthy behaviors?

Specifically, this book is concerned with producing health educators who can alter helping behaviors to any given situation, who can provide several alternative helping models to respond to individual needs, and who can apply these responses to assist others in reaching long-term behavioral goals. Thus, the focus of the health educator must be to *increase his response capacity and his ability to support and maintain healthy feelings and behaviors in the learner.*

> **When you don't know where you are going, any road will take you there.**
>
> —UNKNOWN

Early Thinking on General Theory

Nearly two-thousand years ago, the philosopher Epictetus anticipated the theory behind a major form of current psychotherapy: "People are disturbed not by things but by the view which they take of them" (Crossley, 1937). Some may find this observation shallow or pat, but its validity is shown by the effectiveness of cognitive psychotherapy. Albert Ellis, one of the originators of this form of therapy, summed it up similarly: "You largely feel the way you think, and you can change your thinking and thereby change your feeling" (Ellis, 1991).

Cognitive psychotherapy is often called cognitive-behavior therapy, since it incorporates elements of behavior therapy. But although the two forms overlap, they have a somewhat different focus. Behavior therapy often treats the person as an unthinking being whose behavior and reactions can be shaped by desensitization and other forms of conditioning. Cognitive therapy seeks to modify the person's feelings and behavior by modifying his or her conscious thoughts.

The cognitive approach to treating mental disorders emerged in the early years of the cognitive revolution in psychology. In the 1940s and early 1950s, several psychologists theorized that flawed cognitive processes rather than unconscious conflicts were responsible for many neurotic conditions. One of the therapists was Julian Rotter, whose work on internal and external locus of control has been used in health-education research for years. Both an academic and a therapist, he devised *social-learning* therapy, a method of getting the patient to rethink his or her faulty expectations and values (Burke, 1989).

As a result of an intensive search for better ways of teaching conducted between 1957 and 1967, schools today in every major city and most outlying areas are trying nongrading, team teaching, reality education, flexible scheduling, and other interesting and creative ways of teaching. Questions about how people learn best and organize knowledge cut across the established disciplines of psychology, counseling, philosophy, and sociology. Counseling techniques have been incorporated into teaching subjects that deal with human behavior. No other subject area qualifies to use these techniques more clearly than health education. It is unique in the field of teaching and learning because it covers cognitive knowledge, affective attitudes and behaviors, and the psychosocial issues of health and self-esteem.

The study of health is more than a matter of learning about cause and effect. It is understanding the nature of human behavior and how knowledge of cause and effect influences behavior. It is virtually impossible to sharply differentiate the study of health education from the study of human behavior in general. For example, today's researchers view knowledge as what we perceive. Consequently, knowledge does not merely accumulate but is recast again and again in fresh theoretical structures based on our perception of reality. This reality is based on our sense of who we are, our environment, our knowledge of the world around us, and our values, perceptions, and feelings. Facts become facts only when they fall within the perspective of the viewer. For instance, talking about safe sex will not affect a teenage girl who wants to get pregnant because of self-directed inner thoughts and feelings (e.g., to have and hold something she can love and be loved by). Understanding the nature of learning and designing approaches to teaching health are complicated by the uniqueness of the subject matter and the powerful forces that drive individuals to accept the risk at all costs (as evidenced by cigarette smoking, unprotected sex, drinking and driving, etc.) while they remain unwilling to accept responsibility for their behaviors.

To recognize that all these factors play a part in health education is a good beginning, but debate has tended to languish within each category. There are competing schools of thought over a single focus such as "teaching techniques," power struggles over current definitions of health education, and conflict over which basic concepts of health should be starting points for education. The differences among these opposing views are often so slight that they are overshadowed by other factors, such as the sobering statistics discussed in Chapter 4. In the words of the former surgeon general Joycelyn Elders, schools teach drivers' education, "but when we come to health education, which includes sexuality education, we refuse to teach them that. . . . A major cause of children dying is really related to many of the social problems impacting their health, so I really feel we need to have a comprehensive health-education program in our schools from kindergarten through twelfth grade. This is the equalizer."

According to Elders, health education must cover the entire spectrum of social issues including drugs, alcohol, sex, and violence. "It's not going in there and giving them a plumbing lesson. I feel that's a waste of time." Only 5 percent of public schools now have comprehensive programs in health education.

Elders, the former top health official in Arkansas who has been outspoken on the need to provide condoms to sexually active teenagers, said that while contraceptives should be made available, "if you don't have the education, I could go out and throw condoms up in the air and let them rain" ("This Week with David Brinkley," July, 1994).

Clearly, statements of this kind have profound implications for health education, for they support the position that we are truly the *first line of defense against unhealthy behaviors.*

Some Specific Theories Explored

In reading over the professional literature, we would have to conclude that there are almost as many approaches to health education as there are health educators. However, most health-education approaches owe some allegiance to three major theoretical influences—psychodynamic, behavioral, and existential-humanistic. Historically, the psychodynamic approach came first. Freud's work was seminal as he was the first to discover that human behavior follows certain consistent patterns. Behaviorism was the second major force. John Watson, B.F. Skinner, and many others demonstrated that we do not need to uncover unconscious forces to produce change and growth in people. More recently, existential-humanistic approaches have developed, at least partially as a reaction against the pessimism and mechanism of the first two theories. Works by existentialists such as Kierkegaard, Sartre, and Heidegger present a view of humankind that gives individuals more responsibility for their actions. Carl Rogers looms large in the humanistic point of view with his dignified view of humankind coupled with a thoughtful methodology of counseling and teaching. However, as we view the three major theories today, there is an increasing search for commonalties and similarities among them.

Psychodynamic Theory

What does Freud's research offer us today? First, his extensive writings organize human functioning and conceptualize the emotional and irrational feelings underlying behavior. Second, his many disciples provide a constant impetus for change in psychotherapy through additions to and modifications of his concepts. Those theorists with a Freudian perspective include close followers such as Ernest Jones and revisionists and neo-Freudians such as Alfred Adler, Eric Erikson, Erich Fromm, Karen Horney, Carl Jung, Wilheim Reich, and Harry Stack Sullivan. The Freudian worldview has been summarized as follows:

> . . . *essentially pessimistic, deterministic, mechanistic, and reductionistic. According to Freud, human beings are determined by irrational forces, unconscious motivations, biological and instinctual needs and drives, and psychosexual events that occurred during the first five years of life (Corey, 1977).*

In short, this theory tends to a paternalistic view that encourages the individual to accept things as they are and then cope with them. Those with strictly Freudian views often see their job as repairing human beings damaged by their own internal destructive forces or by the competitive, destructive aspects of society through the "medical model" of diagnosis and redemption.

Learned Personality: Behaviorism

Behaviorist theory, unlike psychodynamic theory or trait theory, sees personality as nothing but a set of learned (conditioned) responses to stimuli. Psychodynamic and trait theories, in their different ways, see personality as inherent qualities of the individual that determine behavior.

In the 1940s, Yale scientist John Dollard and psychologist Neal Miller jointly worked out a theory of *social learning* as an expansion of behaviorism. These researchers found that much learning is social and takes place through high-level cognitive processes as well as through the drives and needs that underlie motivation (Dollard and Miller, 1950). To put this into proper context, it is a fairly well accepted fact that the staying power of teen smoking despite the hazards is really about social bonding.

From the 1950s on, a number of other behaviorists developed further social-learning theories, particularly the cognitive aspects. Central to all versions of the theory is the concept that human personality and behavior are shaped not only by rewards but by the individuals' expectations based on what they have observed. Although this view is much more cognitive than strictly behaviorist, it differs from both trait theory and psychoanalytic theory in that it still sees experiences and situations—external influences—as the major determinants of personality and behavior.

A trait-like modification of the social-learning view of personality was made by Julian Rotter (1954). Rotter found that often his patients' basic attitudes toward life had been formed by critical experiences, some good and others bad. Recasting this in behavioral terms, he theorized that when particular acts are either rewarded or not rewarded, people develop "generalized expectancies" about which kinds of circumstances and behaviors will or will not be rewarding (1954).

Rotter (1972) went on to conduct research that led to the major discovery of his career: the *locus of control* test. The test includes twenty-nine items comprised of two statements; the person taking the test says which of each pair of statements seems more true to him or her.

The concept of locus of control and the I–E scale struck a responsive chord among personality psychologists. Since the scale appeared in 1966, some two-thousand studies have been published that use it. It has long been one of the most popular personality tests (Singer, 1984).

Many research studies have shown how locus-of-control expectations affect behavior. For instance, elementary school students who scored as "internals" got higher grades on average than "externals"; helpless children ("externals") did worse after failing a test containing difficult problems, while mastery-oriented children ("internals") tried harder and did better. In experiments where volunteers were confronted with a dilemma, "internals" were more likely to seek useful information; "externals" relied on others to help them. Among people hospitalized with TB, "internals" knew more about their illness and asked more questions of their doctors than "externals." Internals brushed and flossed their teeth more, and were more likely to use seat belts, get preventive shots, engage in physical-fitness activities, and practice effective birth control (Singer, 1984; Mischel, 1990; Baron, Byrne, and Kantowitz, 1980).

Social-learning and locus-of-control research led to some notable developments in personality theory and clinical psychology. One was a growing recognition that conscious attitudes and ideas, not just unconscious ones, account in considerable part for an individual's traits and actions. What psychologist George Kelly called *personal constructs*—conscious ideas about our abilities and character, what other people expect of us in various situations, how others behave in response to us, and how we interpret what they say—are important determinants of personality and behavior (Kelly, 1955).

The Existential-Humanistic Approach

As discussed earlier, Freudian psychology is concerned with the unconscious and hidden meanings. Behaviorism takes the polar position with emphasis on observed behavior, stimulus-response patterns, and concrete action. The existential-humanistic approach focuses on people as empowered to act on the world and determine their own destinies. The existential-humanistic view in health education is positive and forward-moving and holistic in definition and behavioral outcomes.

While the roots of the existential-humanistic tradition rest in philosophy, Carl Rogers (1961) and his client-centered approach to therapy were most influential in popularizing this point of view and making it relevant. French existentialists Camus and Sartre, among others, provided a solid theoretical basis for the existential-humanistic position. In most cases, the existential, client-centered framework has become part of the health-education milieu. It emphasizes the fact that people are essentially good, forward moving, and able to master their health behavior. Basic to existential-humanistic health education is a consistent effort to understand and experience the uniqueness in each person we work with. The importance of these ideas cannot be overstated.

Perhaps more than anyone else, Carl Rogers was able to listen empathically and carefully to other human beings. As he came to understand them, he consistently found positive, self-actualizing forces in even the most troubled individuals. As such, health educators must always believe that each individual, even if in a very hidden part of himself, holds some small promise for changing his negative health behaviors.

A Cognitive-Behavioral Approach to Teaching

There are many variations on the cognitive-behavioral approach that can be used in the classroom, all with the same set of goals—the reinforcement of healthy behaviors and positive behavioral change. The thinking-feeling-acting (TFA) model (Hutchins, 1979, 1982, 1984) is particularly suited to classroom use because it integrates the three major cognitive-behavioral approaches into the learning environment. This model draws from a combination of resources including counseling, group dynamics, crisis intervention, and the well-recognized PRECEDE-PROCEED model often used in health education (Green and Kreuter, 1991).

The TFA technique is based on the underlying assumption that the way people mentally frame experiences determines how they feel and behave (Beck and Weishaar, 1989; Burns, 1980). For students to truly connect feelings with behavior, some kind of cognitive work is essential; it is, in fact, the backbone of the feeling and acting processes (see Chapter 3). To approach students on a cognitive-behavioral level, we need to ask them the following questions:

- In what ways are you damaging your current state of health?
- In what ways are you maintaining or improving your health?
- Will your present health behavior help you get what you want out of life?
- What changes do you need to make to achieve your goals?
- When and how do you intend to improve your health behavior?

The cognitive-behavioral approach to teaching health education differs sharply from the strictly cognitive approach, which emphasizes subject matter. Cognitive teaching relies solely on talking between the teacher and student, on the student's comprehension of textbook material, and on verbal interaction among the students. Its purpose is to provide the learner with knowledge and teach him to make judgments and decisions based on that knowledge. The strictly cognitive approach to teaching is usually considered the "scientific" method, whereas the behavioral approach is often considered "anti-intellectual," or "irrational."

Cognitive methodology may provide the student with needed knowledge, but it does not offer (although it could) alternative concepts of intellect and reason—concepts that are broader, more spiritual, and potentially more liberating and empowering. Cognitive-behavioral approaches, conversely, dissolve the traditional dichotomy between mind and body, spirit and matter. The central tenet of health education must include a holistic emphasis on the integration of the inner life with the outer physical and social world. Health education as a holistic science is essentially ecological—no phenomenon, physical, mental or spiritual, can be adequately studied apart from its whole context.

Cognitive-behavioral education also focuses on learning by doing. The health educator must be an organizer who selects problems of interest to students, helps them plan an attack on the problems, and provides suitable materials and guidance to enable them to make positive changes in their health behavior. For instance, a smoker who's worried about her health may choose one of four courses of thinking and acting about her smoking:

- she may smoke because her girlfriends do (social bonding)
- she may stop because of the health risks
- she may deny to herself that it is really dangerous
- she may compromise by changing to a low-tar brand
- she may exercise, eat better, etc.

Horowitz (1966) demonstrated that behavior change can lead to attitude change and that we infer our attitudes from our behavior. Based on what we perceive ourselves doing, we attribute certain attitudes about our health to ourselves.

Research by Leon Festinger (1957) stressed two kinds of situations. The first situation required decision making: whenever we freely decide between two or more alternatives and commit ourselves to one of them dissonance occurs, because there is always *something* desirable about the option foregone and *something* negative about the choice we have made. The urge to reduce that dissonance can lead to a reappraisal that makes us feel more positive toward our chosen alternative and more negative toward the other option.

For example, Knox and Inkster (1968) found that gamblers at a racetrack were more confident their horse would win after placing their bets, than just before they placed them. And Brehm and Cohen (1962) found that after children chose one of two toys they had rated as equally attractive, their liking for the toy they selected went up and their liking for the other one went down.

This research tells us something about an individual's health choices as well as how to teach positive health choices. It suggests that we can reduce postdecision dissonance through *selective exposure to information*. A person who purchases a certain cold remedy from an array of choices rereads the parts of the cold-remedy description that induced him or her to make that choice in the first place, and pays less, if any, attention to the directions, warnings, and cautions.

Cognitive-dissonance studies describe situations where we do something inconsistent with our beliefs or self-image *when minimal justification* convinces us to. People given barely enough incentive to do something—in one study it was eating grasshoppers—developed more positive attitudes toward the action than those who were given much larger incentives; i.e., "Eating grasshoppers must be okay because I chose to eat them." By contrast, if there was a big return for eating grasshoppers, subjects figured they did it for the payoff.

These and other studies suggest that a cognitive-behavioral approach to health education is the best possible choice to turn around some of the most critical health trends we are facing today.

Time Out for Personal Thoughts

1. What three things have you learned from this discussion?

2. How would you apply this knowledge in teaching high-school students about smoking?

3. If you could apply only one approach to teaching (cognitive or behavioral), which would you choose? Why?

Health educators should keep in mind that, although they may be highly skilled in their field, they may not be experts on the cultural issues that exist within the age group they teach. Whatever you have been taught about health education in your undergraduate or graduate programs, it is *not* the reality of the students' world in which you are working. In addition, many schools and other community-health programs may have an unrealistic, subject-centered curriculum unrelated to student needs and interests; thus, you will have to transform it into a cognitive-behavioral curriculum. To do this, start with your learning environment. What do they want to know? What do they know? How do you find this out?

Ask them. Much educational-curriculum development is based on what adults think about what young people need rather than what the young people want. We need a combination of the two. Essentially, a health educator who uses a cognitive-behavioral approach stays in touch with her students, listens to them, incorporates their views into her teaching, and gains their acceptance and respect.

Advantages of a Cognitive-Behavioral Approach

One of the great benefits of the cognitive-behavioral approach to health education is that it employs a wide range of teaching strategies—cooperative learning, lectures, role playing, media, group work, problem solving, assertiveness training, comprehensive-values education, self-esteem building, and much more. Many of these strategies will be explored further on in this book, but a few will be briefly covered here.

One example of teaching strategy would be *cognitive restructuring,* where the teacher seeks to help students find alternative ways of thinking to combat, for example, early sexual behavior (including intercourse) and behavioral disorders (including drug abuse). Dysfunctional or distorted patterns of thinking are identified, and students are taught methods of challenging and changing negative thoughts and actions and replacing them with more rational responses.

Restructuring involves getting students to ask, "How else can I think about this activity and why I'm doing it?" Instead of telling themselves the same story day in and day out, they can think of a new one that not only casts things in a different light but may be more plausible than the old one.

Variations of this process have evolved under several names. Albert Ellis (1975) developed his well-known rational-emotive therapy (RET). Behavioral psychologist Arnold Lazarus (1971) coined the term *cognitive restructuring,* which is used within this book as a general term for RET and all the cognitive-behavioral methods. **Assertiveness training** empowers students to use more effective interpersonal functioning. It has a behavioral emphasis that builds on the cognitive knowledge and skills developed by the student absorbing positive health information. The **problem-solving** approach teaches students how to tackle issues that might lead to cognitive or behavioral problems. It is a reality-based approach to dealing with problems such as peer pressure, unprotected sex, drug abuse, and violence.

All of these cognitive-behavioral approaches to health education are about getting people to take responsibility for their lives, teaching them that they can change, empowering them to act, and helping them make appropriate changes that *they* deem are necessary and positive.

Carl Rogers, who pioneered client-centered psychotherapy and was perhaps the leading figure in human-potential theory, was an important influence on the humanistic-education movement, especially with his book *Freedom to Learn* (1969). Rogers expressed the central themes of holistic education: that true learning involves the whole person (including feelings, personal concerns, and creativity); that human beings aspire to growth and integration but need an emotionally supportive environment that encourages exploration and self-discovery; that every student and every teacher ought to be respected as a unique and precious person and not be forced into role-bound behavior by rigid, extrinsic goals. These themes were extensions of Roger's central principles of client-centered therapy—trust, unconditional acceptance, emphatic understanding, and personal authenticity and integrity (1951). He confirmed that, ultimately, the holistic approach represented a very positive approach to teaching.

It would be most unlikely that one could hold the . . . attitudes I have described, or could commit himself to being a facilitator of learning, unless he has come to have a profound trust in the human organism and its potentialities. If I distrust the human being, then I must cram him with information of my own choosing, lest he go his own mistaken way (Rogers, 1969).

Some Perceived Goals of Health Education

The outcome of effective health education is twofold: first, it helps to reinforce feelings of self-worth (which then translates into positive health behaviors), and it helps bring about positive behavioral change in those whose feelings of low self-worth affect their health behavior. Since the way we think influences the way we act (Clark, 1988), we must first change the way we perceive things.

One of the great illusions of the information age is that the way to affect people's thinking is to feed them facts. Most literature and research seems to indicate that information by itself may help but may not be enough to affect our perceptions, because it is the mind-set that shapes perception and behavior. For example, to affect the mind-set of a generation raised in an environment of sexual division and sexist attitudes, we need a new way of thinking about the relationship between women and men.

If we are to reconceptualize the meaning of health education, we must step back and look at some of the traditional ways of thinking and teaching in health. Perhaps a way to start is by thinking about "context" as an appropriate synonym

Time Out for Personal Thoughts

1. A cognitive-behavioral approach to health education can make a change in the personal behavior of students. How could you use it in your field of study?

2. What do you see as the three most important aspects of affecting behavioral change in the learner?

3. What specific personal qualities do you feel you bring to the teaching profession? Be specific:

for "health." Just as effective health education should result in positive health behaviors, it is contextual. As such, health education should provide integrative framework within which any subject can be understood more completely. In this sense, health education is about the "big picture"—giving meaning and relevance to ideas via the five stages of cognitive-behavioral teaching we will now discuss.

Stages in the Cognitive-Behavioral Process

Tuckman (1972) reviewed the literature on small-group settings, including therapy groups, T-groups, natural groups, and laboratory-task groups. Based on his rather extensive analysis, he concluded that, although the fit was not perfect, four stages of development could be defined. (He acknowledged that some experts described fewer or more than four stages.) Those who concurred with the four stages described them somewhat differently, yet there was great commonality. Tuckman labeled these four stages as (1) forming, (2) storming, (3) norming, and (4) performing. He observed that this four-stage developmental sequence held up under widely varied conditions of group composition, duration, and task.

Other approaches to these stages have been described. Gazda (1971) described four stages of counseling as (1) exploration, (2) transition, (3) action, and (4) termination. These stages are similar to Tuckman's, but Tuckman did not include a termination stage as such. Gazda's stages also have been related to Carkhuff's (1969) model for helping.

I choose to present a five-stage cognitive-behavioral model for health education:

- *relationship-building:* developing the foundation for a sound collaborative teaching-learning environment
- *exploratory:* examining and understanding each learner and his frame of reference
- *decision making:* formulating a health-education goal and an intervention-oriented teaching focus
- *working:* expanding efforts to present an effective cognitive-behavioral approach to the learning environment
- *termination:* concluding the learning unit

The stages of a cognitive-behavioral approach to health education have been explored and defined by a number of researchers such as Botvin et al. (1984, 1990a, 1990b), Clark et al. (1992), Coates (1990), Kennedy et al. (1991), Petosa and Jackson (1991), and Zimmerman and Connor (1989). Their research indicates that, even though there is no agreement on the number, names, or characteristics of each stage, there is a consensus that the learning process moves in a sequential, orderly progression. This writer sees the five stages in the cognitive-behavioral process as developmental in nature and therefore transitional, overlapping, and continuous rather than rigid and discrete (Figure 4–1). This transitional concept implies that, while each of these stages has its own theme and developmental tasks, elements of any stage may be evident at another stage.

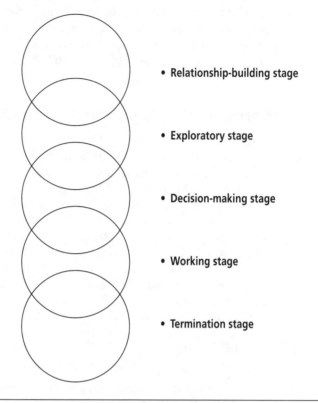

- Relationship-building stage

- Exploratory stage

- Decision-making stage

- Working stage

- Termination stage

Figure 4–1

The five stages of cognitive-behavioral teaching.

The particular stage you are teaching can be discerned by the dominant activities of that time span. Furthermore, the major theme of each stage must be accomplished to a minimal degree before the learning process can progress to the next stage. Until each task is adequately performed, the teaching-learning process will be somewhat constrained and limited. At any point, however, the teacher may go back and focus on the developmental tasks of an earlier stage to enrich the process or overcome any difficulties or blockages. This concept is similar to the structured-stage concepts outlined by other developmental-stage theorists (Lerner, 1986; Turiel, 1969). When a particular concern of the student has been resolved, the process may be repeated to focus on another unresolved issue.

Health education often does not progress on a steady, predictable course. The subject matter is very often personal and requires flexibility. Health is not a constant state. Consequently, the character, duration, and intensity of each stage also varies. Occasionally, all five stages may occur in one teaching session. Normally, they take a minimum of several sessions and often take many sessions. Some health issues require considerable time on one or two stages and little time on other stages; others require considerable time on all stages.

The tasks outlined in each of these five stages are pantheoretical. All approaches to health education, regardless of the methodology of the health issue, should progress through these stages. The specific tasks associated with each stage are outlined in Part II.

Synthesis

The development of a comprehensive educational psychology requires a theoretical framework that includes all the phenomena related to human learning; it must, therefore, include areas of human experience that previously have been ignored by traditional teaching. A cognitive-behavioral approach to teaching offers a more inclusive vision of human potential, suggesting both a new image of the learner and a new worldview. Using a cognitive-behavioral approach does not require a complete rejection of established educational psychologies but may be used in conjunction with them. Conflicts occur at some points, and agreements occur at others.

An underlying assumption of cognitive-behavioral theory is that physical, emotional, intellectual, and spiritual growth are interrelated. The optimal educational environment stimulates and nurtures the intuitive as well as the rational, the imaginative as well as the practical, and the creative as well as the receptive functions of each individual. A cognitive-behavioral approach focuses attention on the human capacity for self-transcendence and self-realization and is concerned with the optimal development of the person.

Time Out for Personal Thoughts

Suppose you were teaching a class in which the subject was drug use among teens. You have been informed that drug use in the high school you are teaching in is moderately high. You have two weeks to present your teaching-learning unit. How would you proceed? Be specific.

References

Baron, Robert A., Donn Byrne, and Barry H. Kantowitz. *Psychology: Understanding Behavior.* New York: Holt, Rinehart and Winston, 1980.

Beck, A.T., and M.E. Weishaar. "Cognitive Therapy," in R.J. Corsini and D. Wedding (eds.), *Current Psychotherapies.* Itasca, IL: Peacock, 1989.

Botvin, G.J., E. Baker, N. Renick, A.D. Filazzola, and E.M. Botvin. "A Cognitive-Behavioral Approach to Substance Abuse Prevention." *Addictive Behavior, 9,* 1984.

Botvin, G.J., E. Baker, L. Dusenbury, S. Tortu, and E.M. Botvin. "Preventing Adolescent Drug Abuse Through a Multimodal Cognitive-Behavioral Approach: Results of a Three-Year Study." *Journal of Consulting and Clinical Psychology,* 58:4, 1990a.

Botvin, G.J., E. Baker, A.D. Filazzola, and E.M. Botvin. "A Cognitive-Behavioral Approach to Substance Abuse Prevention: A One-Year Follow Up." *Addictive Behaviors,* 15, 1990b.

Brehm, Jack, and Arthur R. Cohen. *Explorations in Cognitive Dissonance.* New York: Wiley, 1962.

Burke, Joseph F. *Contemporary Approaches to Psychotherapy and Counseling: The Self-Regulation and Maturity Model.* Pacific Grove, CA: Brooks/Cole, 1989.

Burns, D. *Feeling Good: The New Mood Therapy.* New York: Morrow, 1980.

Carkhuff, R.R. *Helping and Human Relations: A Primer for Lay and Professional Helpers: Vol. 2, Practice and Research.* New York: Holt, Rinehart and Winston, 1969.

Clark, Edward T. "The Role of Mindset in Global and Peace Education." *Holistic Education Review,* Winter 1988.

Clark, Noreen M., Nancy K. Janz, Julia A. Dodge, and Patricia A. Sharpe. "Self-Regulation of Health Behavior: The 'Take PRIDE' Program," *Health Education Quarterly,* Fall 1992.

Coates, T.J. "Strategies for Modifying Sexual Behavior for Primary and Secondary Prevention of HIV Disease." *Journal of Consulting and Clinical Psychology,* June 1990.

Corey, G. *Theory and Practice of Counseling and Psychotherapy.* Monterey, CA: Brooks/Cole, 1977.

Crossley, Hastings (ed.). *The Golden Sayings of Epictetus.* New York: Collier, 1937.

Dollard, John, and Neil E. Miller. *Personality and Psychotherapy.* New York: McGraw-Hill, 1950.

Elders, Joycelyn. Interview with David Brinkley on ABC's "This Week with David Brinkley," July 1994.

Ellis, Albert. "Using RET Effectively," in M.E. Bernart (ed.), *Using Rational-Emotive Therapy Effectively.* New York: Plenum, 1991.

Ellis, Albert, and R.A. Harper. *A New Guide to Rational Living.* Englewood Cliffs, NJ: Prentice-Hall, 1975.

Festinger, Leon. *A Theory of Cognitive Dissonance.* Stanford, CA: Stanford University Press, 1957.

Gazda, G.M. *Group Counseling: A Developmental Approach.* Boston: Allyn and Bacon, 1971.

Green, Lawrence, and Marshall W. Kreuter. *Health Promotion and Planning.* Mountain View, CA: Mayfield, 1991.

Horowitz, Laurence J. "Parental Intervention and Behavior Modification of Underachievers." Unpublished doctoral dissertation. Stanford, CA: Stanford University, 1966.

Hutchins, David E. "Systematic Counseling: The T-F-A Model for Counselor Intervention." *Personal and Guidance Journal,* February 1979.

___. "Ranking Major Counseling Strategies With The TFA-Matrix System." *Personal and Guidance Journal,* March 1982.

___. "Improving the Counseling Relationship." *Personal and Guidance Journal,* June 1984.

Kelly, George A. *The Psychology of Personal Constructs.* New York: W.W. Norton, 1955.

Kennedy, Cassondra J., Claudia K. Probart, and Steve M. Dorman. "The Relationship between Random Knowledge, Concern, and Behavior and Health Values, Health Locus of Control, and Preventive Health Behaviors." *Health Education Quarterly,* Fall 1991.

Knox, R.E., and J.A. Inkster. "Postdecision Dissonance at Post Time." *Journal of Personality and Social Psychology,* June 1968.

Lazarus, Arnold A. *Behavior Therapy and Beyond.* New York: McGraw-Hill, 1971.

Lerner, R.M. *Concepts and Theories of Human Development* (2nd ed.). New York: McGraw-Hill, 1986.

Mischel, Walter. "Personality Dispositions Revisited and Revised: A Review after Three Decades," In Lawrence A. Pervin (ed.), *Handbook of Personality.* New York: Guilford Press, 1990.

Petosa, Rick, and Kirby Jackson. "Using the Health Belief Model to Predict Safer Sex Intentions among Adolescents." *Health Education Quarterly,* Winter 1991.

Rogers, Carl. *Freedom to Learn.* Columbus, OH: Merrill, 1969.

___. *On Becoming a Person.* Boston: Houghton Mifflin, 1961.

Rotter, Julian *Social Learning and Clinical Psychology.* Englewood Cliffs, NJ: Prentice-Hall, 1954.

___. "Generalized Expectancies for Internal versus External Control of Reinforcement," in J.B. Rotter et al. (eds.), *Applications of a Social Learning Theory of Personality.* New York: Holt, Rinehart and Winston, 1972.

Singer, Jerome L. *The Human Personality.* San Diego: Harcourt Brace Jovanovich, 1984.

Tuckman, B.W. "Developmental Sequence in Small Groups," in R.C. Diedrich and H.A. Dye (eds.), *Group Procedures: Purpose, Process, and Outcomes—Selected Readings for the Counselor.* Boston: Houghton Mifflin, 1972.

Turiel, E. "Developmental Processes in the Child's Moral Thinking," in R.H. Mussen, J. Langer, and M. Covington (eds.), *Trends and Issues in Developmental Psychology.* New York: Holt, Rinehart & Winston, 1969.

Zimmerman, Rick S., and Catherine Connor. "Health Promotion in Context: The Effects of Significant Others on Health Behavior Change." *Health Education Quarterly,* Spring 1989.

Additional Resources

Basen-Engquist, Karen, and Guy S. Parcel. "Attitudes, Norms, and Self-Efficacy: A Model of Adolescents' HIV-Related Sexual Risk Behavior." *Health Education Quarterly,* Summer 1992.

Bernstein, Ira H., and Judith B. Keith. "Reexamination of Eisen, Zellman, and McAlster's Health Belief Model Questionnaire." *Health Education Quarterly,* Summer 1991.

Kaplan, Joseph S., and Barbara Drainville. *Beyond Behavior Modification: A Cognitive-Behavioral Approach to Behavior Management in the School.* Austin, TX: Pro-Ed, 1991.

Soloman, Michael R. *Consumer Behavior.* Englewood Cliffs, NJ: Prentice-Hall, 1996.

Sternberg, Robert J. *Mechanisms of Cognitive Development.* Prospect Heights, IL: Waverland Press, 1984.

Wechsler, Henry, et al. "Health and Behavioral Consequences of Binge Drinking in College." *Journal of the American Medical Association,* 7 December 1994.

Cognitive-Behavioral Theory into Action

This unit presents the five important cognitive-behavioral stages in the teaching-learning process and describes the distinctive activities that occur in each of them. It includes a discussion of the characteristics of each stage, outlining some of the ways to implement them in the classroom.

The five stages, which were introduced in Chapter 4, outline some critical components for effective teaching. The *relationship-building stage* (Chapters 5 and 6) is based on the fact that the health educator must establish an environment of caring and acceptance. This is critical to the success of cognitive-behavioral teaching. Students need to feel a sense of trust, genuineness, and respect. As a health educator, you must take responsibility for providing the conditions that will facilitate open, honest, and complete communication. Learners need to be at ease with you and feel accepted by you, and believe that they are understood in appropriate ways. You need to communicate a positive regard for those you are working with and an understanding and respect for their thoughts, feelings and behaviors.

The *exploratory stage* (Chapter 7) defines the scope of the topic under discussion and also lets you gain an understanding of each student's knowledge, attitudes, and behaviors, along with their internal strengths and external resources. Here, you attempt to answer the question, "am I teaching what students want to know?"

In the *decision-making stage* (Chapter 8), emphasis is placed on your goals for your student and how these goals can be achieved. The bottom line is that the right kind of health education consists of understanding the learner as she is without imposing on her an ideal of what you think she should be.

Chapter 9 deals with the *working stage,* which involves the application of an appropriate cognitive-behavioral strategy. The major task at this stage is helping those you are working with resolve their concerns and learn to function more healthfully. This may require you to provide emotional support, encouragement, and reinforcement of newly gained insights.

Finally, Chapter 10 explores the *termination stage,* an extremely important period in which you need to focus on accomplishing three interrelated tasks: first, progress made should be summarized and evaluated; second, other issues that require attention should be brought forward; and third, methods to foster student growth should be handled effectively. The health education process is then successfully completed. If these tasks are not dealt with, the process is truncated and the important progress that might have occurred is curtailed.

In addition to outlining the characteristics of the cognitive-behavioral process through the five-stage developmental process, these chapters also provide some important concepts for working with resistant students. Throughout all of these chapters, keep in mind the overriding message: *The highest function of health education is to bring about an integrated individual who is capable of dealing with thoughts, feelings, and actions as a whole.*

5 The Self in Health Education

The late Joseph Campbell said, "The privilege of a lifetime is being who you are" (Osbon, 1991). This privilege extends to your choice to become a health educator. It is my belief that when you choose to teach in this field the most important factor is *who* you are rather than what you are. According to research, your personality, values, and approach have a profound influence on your effectiveness (Combs, 1967). This belief serves as the framework for this chapter.

Facing the Self First

In a sense, the self is like a tool kit that contains all the necessary tools to work effectively with life. The ability to make the choices about which tools to use is based on a deep understanding of your own personal center. The ability to make choices that truly reflect your personal values is indeed your best resource in the helping professions, and in health education specifically. Thus, the decision to become a health educator was, hopefully, a matter of personal choice, a way of defining yourself. As such, your most important task as a teacher is to help *others* define the role of the self in choosing.

A Student's World: Learning from the Inside Out

The major premise of control theory (Glasser, 1986) is that all human behavior is generated by what goes on *inside* the person. Thus, a young person stops abusing drugs not because the teacher tells her that drugs kill (a premise of the stimulus-response theory, which believes that human behavior is caused by external events) but because that person says, "I want to stay alive." In Glasser's words, "All that we

Everybody can be great . . . because anybody can serve. You don't have to have a college degree to serve. You don't have to make your subject and verb agree to serve. You only need a heart full of grace. A soul generated by love.

—MARTIN LUTHER KING, JR.

get from the outside world is information. We then choose to act on that information in the way we believe is best for us" (1987).

Reality *is* the classroom for many students, for it is the place where they often find love, friendship, consistency, support, guidance, and the acceptance they may not be receiving in the outside world. Students leave school with a more open awareness of the world. The *process* of learning has been experienced first-hand. Teachers exist as facilitators to aid in the development of their students' special gifts and talents. A shared process of learning among parents, students, and teachers builds trust. Responsibility is shared, but consequences are experienced by the student who makes the choices. Students can never learn all they need to know from a class on health education, but they can learn *how* to learn. Health education should be a lifelong learning process.

Carl Rogers, in his article "The Interpersonal Relationship in the Facilitation of Learning" (1967), states:

> *We are, in my view, faced with an entirely new situation in education where the goal of education, if we are to survive, is the facilitation of change and learning. The only man who is educated is the man who has learned how to learn; the man who has learned how to adapt and change; the man who has realized that no knowledge is secure, that only the process of seeking knowledge gives a basis for security. Changingness, a reliance on process rather than upon static knowledge, is the only thing that makes any sense as a goal for education in the modern world.*
>
> *So now with some relief I turn to an activity, a purpose, which really warms me—facilitation of learning. When I have been able to transform a group—and here I mean all the members of a group, myself included—into a community of learners, then the excitement has been almost beyond belief. To free curiosity; to permit individuals to go charging off in new directions dictated by their own interests; to unleash curiosity; to open everything to questioning and exploration; to recognize that everything is in process of change—here is an experience I can never forget.*

When the health educator views himself more as a facilitator of learning rather than a teacher, then authoritarian practices are replaced by dialogue, cooperation, friendship, and mutual respect. Time-honored educational goals such as discipline, order, and academic excellence often mask more authoritarian interests on the part of teachers, such as "I have all the answers," "I control the learning environment," and "I am the authority." In facilitated learning, students are valued for their individuality, not for their conformity to authoritative standards; they are valued for their input into the learning environment.

Facilitation of Learning

Basic to control theory is the concept that our genes instruct us to survive, to love and belong, and to struggle for power, fun, and freedom (Glasser, 1985). If what we offer in school and how we offer it is not seen by students as related to these built-in needs, they will struggle against or withdraw from the curriculum.

Without expanding on existing resources, we can use this theory to make some lasting improvements in the classroom. As Glasser stated in his article "Discipline Is Not the Problem" (1985), any school can provide warmth and human care. To the extent that it does, there are immediate payoffs. Warmth and care are done *with* those we are working with, not to or for them. Additional skills in the facilitation of learning include:

Empathy. "Walking a mile in another person's shoes" is a phrase often used to describe empathy. Empathy is a necessary and basic skill in understanding a student and where he or she is coming from. In an important paper on the counseling process entitled "The Necessary and Sufficient Conditions of Therapeutic Personality Change," Carl Rogers made a strong case for empathy and related concepts as being all that is needed to produce change in a client. According to Rogers, helping another person grow requires (1) an integrated, congruent relationship with the client; (2) unconditional, positive regard for the client; and (3) communication of empathy from the counselor to the client. "No other conditions are necessary" (1957).

Respect, warmth, and caring. Cold, distant teachers may be professional and competent, but underlying the professionalism may be conscious or unconscious hostility and dislike for students and teaching in general. Teachers should respect students, be warm and caring toward them, and communicate these feelings verbally and nonverbally. Respect, warmth, and caring are necessary aspects of true, self-motivated learning on the part of the student.

Active listening. Active listening is hearing not only what is being said but what is *meant*. When an individual is truly heard—not just his words but their meaning—he is moved, released, and grateful. As Carl Rogers states in *A Way of Being,* "Almost always, when a person realizes he has been deeply heard, his eyes moisten. It is as though he were saying, 'Thank God, somebody heard me. Someone knows what it's like to be me.'" Too often he is like a prisoner, "day after day tapping out a Morse code message: 'Does anybody hear me? Is anybody there?' And finally one day he hears some faint tapping that spell out 'yes.' By that one simple response he is released from his loneliness; he has become a human being again" (1980). Examples of active listening include such things as

- positive eye contact with the person speaking
- repeating back part of what the person has said
- giving the person a response that is directly related to what he said
- telling that person that you appreciate his participation
- using his first name in follow-up questions

Positive regard. If you want to help people grow and change, you must truly believe they *can*. In its most simple form, positive regard may be defined as selective attention to positive aspects of student verbalization and behavior. A health educator who truly cares for her students operates on the assumption that they are good, can change, and want to change. Glasser (1965) noted that in schools, mental hospitals, jails, and juvenile homes we often imprison people in their pasts. We expect people to act as their case histories state. Caught in those expectations, a person is indeed likely to act that way. Glasser refused to read case histories in areas where a person showed strength and promise. My experience is that most of the information that has been compiled about a person tells me almost nothing about his or her capacity to grow and change. In the words of Gandhi, "What I said yesterday, you can't go by. It's what I say today" (Fisher, 1962).

Congruence, genuineness, and authenticity. Carl Rogers defined the concepts of congruence, genuineness, and authenticity when he stated that the therapist in a counseling relationship should be "a congruent, integrated person" (1951). For educators, it means that you are freely and deeply yourself, and your actions accurately represented your awareness of yourself. It is the opposite of presenting a facade, either knowingly or unknowingly. Using this theory, you need to ask yourself the questions, "How much room do I have to be myself in this situation?" "How much room do I use?" The closer you are to being yourself, the better you get along with yourself and with others. If you are in a relationship with another person, you will find that the more authentic you are, the closer you'll get. At the same time, you find that you do not need to limit the other person from being himself.

Cultural-environmental focus. "That sounds like a problem girls would talk about," is a common sexist statement some teachers make. What this produces is women who blame themselves for perceived failures when the educational system is the real villain. In health education, we continually deal with gender, culture, religion, and other issues. While teaching in health education is mainly about building positive health behaviors, it is also about the environmental factors (cultural, societal, institutional, religious, and ethnic) that undergird personal and behavioral development. Fully effective health education demands that multicultural and life-style issues be attended to.

Self-disclosure. Self-disclosure occurs when the teacher shares his feelings, thoughts, experiences, and life with the class. This allows the teacher to be a real person to the class. Self-disclosure in teaching can be demonstrated by the use of the personal pronoun "I"; the inclusion of an expression of feeling about one's own experience; and using the past, present, or future tense to describe one's own experience. Self-disclosure builds teacher-student rapport and adds to the mutuality of the relationship. It gives a feeling of sharing and can serve as a model of interpersonal openness. It can also serve as a facilitator for student sharing and self-exploration.

Limits on Disclosure

Sidney Jourard, a seminal thinker in the area of self-disclosure, stated that "only a fool discloses everything" (1968). In essence, teachers should be careful about what they share for they may intimidate students in the class. In an interesting study of a work group, one of the two least liked and most maladjusted members was the most secretive and undisclosing person in the group, while the other was the highest discloser (Jourard, 1971). Those who were better liked and more effective had the ability to anticipate how much disclosure was appropriate to a given situation.

In *The Transparent Self,* Jourard discussed the importance of the counselor's sharing himself genuinely in an interview. Jourard believed that the counselor's courage to be known as a person is critical in counseling success. Authenticity and genuineness as a person are best achieved by sharing what we are.

> *[M]any recollections came rushing to me of patients who had begged me to tell them what I thought, only to be met by cool, faultless reflection or interpretation of their question, or else by a downright lie; e.g., "Yes, I like you," when in fact I found them boring or unlikable. Also, there came to me recollections of instances where I had violated what I thought were technical rules, for example, holding a weeping patient's hand or bursting out laughing at something the patient had said, and of patients telling me that when I had done things, I [had] somehow become human, a person, and that these were significant moments for the patients in the course of their therapy (Jourard, 1971).*

This interview illustrates one type of self-disclosure, in which the counselor and the client honestly confront a difficult point and share their experience of each other in the moment. Such sharing can be close and warm, or it can be more distant. What is critical is honest sharing.

Common Errors in Interpersonal Communication

The following is a list of common errors people make when communicating with others (Weinhold, 1976):

- Making an evasive statement instead of asking for what you want or need: "I wish you were going into town"
- Asking a question instead of making a statement: "Don't you think that . . ."
- Saying "I feel" when you mean "I think": "I feel that you are rude"
- Referring to others when expressing your point of view: "People are afraid to . . ."
- In a group, talking *about* a person rather than *to* him: "I like her idea"
- Using "I can't" to mean "I don't" or "I don't want to": "I can't go with you because I'm too tired"
- Using "have to'" and "should" when you mean "choose to": "I have to go to the school play tonight"
- Not answering a question directly: responding to "How do you feel today?" with "Why do you want to know?"
- Using words like "I guess," "I think," and "maybe" when you are sure.
- Using "try" instead of "do": I'll try to do that today," instead of "I'll do that today"
- Blaming your feelings on someone else: "You made me angry," instead of "I am angry"

- Confusing inference and observation: "John is a poor sport," instead of "John hit Jimmy with the ball (observation), and I think he is a poor sport" (inference)
- Interrupting someone when he is speaking: this usually means you aren't listening
- Changing the subject, or "chaining"—listening to just enough of what someone says to change the subject to something you know more about or want to talk about: responding to "I watched the Monday night football game and it was really exciting," with "We have tickets to see the Colorado–Nebraska football game next week"
- Using statements like "always" or "never" to support your point of view

Synthesis

Facilitated learning focuses on actually *doing* rather than talking about what needs to be done. Insight, self-actualization, positive self-esteem, and realizing potential may be lofty, useful goals in health education, but the reality-based teacher is concerned with what can be done to help students *now* in their daily lives.

This view, which is now commonplace in counseling and psychotherapy, is reinforced by the writings of Carl Rogers, who stressed that the individual can take charge of her life, can make decisions, and can act on the world. Underlying this is a worldview that believes people are positive, forward-moving, basically good, and capable of self-actualization. Health may ultimately be defined as experiencing full "humanness" in all its dimensions, without limits or goals. As William Glasser (1990) stated,

> . . . we search for ways to satisfy our needs for love, belonging, caring, sharing, and cooperation. If a student feels no sense of belonging in school, no sense of being involved in caring and concern, that child will pay little attention to academic subjects. Instead, he or she will engage in a desperate search for friendship, for acceptance. The child may become a behavioral problem, in the hope of attracting attention.

Students are trying to live as best they can. If you feel a tendency to devalue them for something, look at yourself: Are you willing to give the time to show them a better way, without judgment, so they will be able to hear and feel that you care?

References

Combs, A.W. "Florida Studies in the Helping Profession." *University of Florida Social Science Monograph No. 37,* 1967.

Dass, Ram, and Paul Gorman. *How Can I Help?* New York: Knopf, 1985.

Fisher, Louis (ed.). *The Essential Gandhi: An Anthology.* New York: Random House, 1962.

Glasser, William. *Reality Therapy: A New Approach to Psychiatry.* New York: Harper & Row, 1965.

___. "Discipline Is Not the Problem: Control Theory in the Classroom." *Theory Into Practice,* Autumn 1985.

___. *Control Theory in the Classroom.* New York: Perennial Library, 1986.

___. "The Key to Improving Schools: An Interview with William Glasser." *Phi Delta Kappan,* May 1987.

___. *The Quality School: Managing Students without Coercion.* New York: Harper & Row, 1990.

Jourard, Sidney. *Disclosing Man to Himself.* New York: Van Nostrand, 1968.

___. *Self-Disclosure: An Experimental Analysis of the Transparent Self.* New York: Wiley Interscience, 1971a.

___. *The Transparent Self.* New York: Van Nostrand, 1971b.

King, Martin Luther. *Strength to Love.* New York: Pocket Books, 1964.

Osbon, Diane K. (ed.). *Reflections on the Art of Living: A Joseph Campbell Companion.* New York: HarperCollins, 1991.

Rogers, Carl. *Client-Centered Therapy: Its Current Practice, Implications, and Theory.* Boston: Houghton Mifflin, 1951.

___. "The Necessary and Sufficient Conditions of Therapeutic Change." *Journal of Consulting Psychology* 21, 1957.

___. "The Interpersonal Relationship in the Facilitation of Learning," in Robert R. Leeper (ed.), *Humanizing Education: The Person in the Process.* Washington, DC: Association for Supervision and Curriculum Development, 1967.

___. *A Way of Being*. Boston: Houghton Mifflin, 1980.

Weinhold, Barry K. "Transpersonal Communication in the Classroom," in Gay Hendricks and James Fadiman (eds.), *Transpersonal Education: A Curriculum for Feeling and Being*. Englewood Cliffs, NJ: Prentice-Hall, 1976.

Additional Resources

Benner, Patricia, and Judith Wrubel. *The Primacy of Caring*. Reading, MA: Addison-Wesley, 1989.

Borysenko, Joan. *Guilt Is the Teacher, Love Is the Lesson*. New York: Warner Books, 1990.

James, Muriel, and John James. *Passion for Life: Psychology and the Human Spirit*. New York: Dutton, 1991.

Naylor, Thomas A., William H. Willimon, and Magdalena R. Naylor. *The Search for Meaning*. Nashville, TN: Abingdon Press, 1994.

Powell, John. *Why Am I Afraid to Tell You Who I Am?* Allen, TX: Tabor Publishers, 1969.

Viscott, David. *The Language of Feelings*. New York: Pocket Books, 1976.

6 Creating Understanding and Cooperation

No one, of course, can ever climb into another's skin and see this construct we call the self. But there are a number of ways you can get to know those with whom you are working, so let's explore a few. Be aware that it is extremely important to let those you are working with get to know you as well.

Community Building

Recent research in classroom learning demonstrates that informal patterns of friendship and influence and a feeling of group cohesiveness play an important role in motivating students toward the goals of the group. Far from being a waste of time, the effort spent in establishing a sense of community invariably pays off in the ability of the class to pursue common goals and in the positive attitudes of the members of the class toward those goals. Even in cases where a group has been working together for some time, the leader should not assume that there is an established community. All of the activities that follow will be more effective if there is a feeling of positive regard and support among the members of the group.

A Beginning

Part of a student's environment are other students. A member of your class might look around and say, Who are they? Where are they from? Why do they look different from me? All these questions are valid. Remember, your class is truly a home away from home for some students and also the most stable, consistent, accepting, and safe environment they may currently have in their lives. It is important that the teacher attempt to provide such an environment.

"First of all," he said, "if you can learn a simple trick, Scout, you'll get along a lot better with all kinds of folks. You never really understand a person until you consider things from his point of view—"

"Sir?"

"—until you climb into his skin and walk around in it."

—HARPER LEE, *TO KILL A MOCKINGBIRD*

One way to achieve it is to have an introduction process, in which students have a chance to introduce themselves to the other members of the class before they have to deal with the academic issues that must be faced. It is a process of getting to know their neighbors before getting to know the subject matter. This introduction can include

- their names
- where they are from
- their favorite thing to do
- what they do best
- who their best friend is

One of the interesting things about adults is that they tend to seek information about students from other adults (for example, through interviews with parents or other observers). They rarely seek this information from children themselves (Garbarino et al., 1992). In the classroom-introduction process, you receive priceless information because you give students the opportunity to share their feelings and history without adult interpretation or control.

You can do introductions in a number of ways: Have all students in your class sit in a circle and introduce themselves one at a time, stating a few things about themselves that are unique, something about their future goals and what they want to be, etc. A variation on this is to have students choose someone they don't know well and have them sit facing each other. (If you have an unequal number of students, you can have one group of three.) Ask each pair to label themselves as A and B (or A, B, and C in a group of three). Now give A one minute to share with B her life history (you time it). Tell B not to interrupt A during this sharing. When the minute is up, allow B an opportunity to clarify anything that A has shared. Now

A Note on Community-Building Activities

1. For activities that involve individuals forming pairs and then sharing, it is important for the leader to specify a definite time limit and adhere to it. This reduces the risk involved in opening up to a person that one does not know very well.

2. The physical arrangement of the room is important at all times, but especially during community-building activities. For class discussions and activities, the seats should be arranged in a full circle rather than in rows or in a horseshoe. The leader should also try to avoid taking a position traditionally associated with power, such as behind a big desk or in front of the blackboard. If students are working in small groups, the leader should be sure that no member is left on the outside of a group because of the positions of the desks or chairs. If necessary, she should go from group to group arranging positions so that everyone has an equal opportunity to participate.

reverse the process. When both are done, have the class sit in a circle, and let each member of a pair introduce the other; A introducing B first, then B introducing A.

A third variation that can help students get acquainted with one another is to hand out the following exercise. The first student to fill his or her list with names for each category could be the winner if you choose to end it this way.

Exercise: Getting Acquainted

Have participants walk around the room collecting signatures of fellow classmates based on statements that help define who they are. Students may only sign once for each person who approaches them, but they may sign each list differently, since many characteristics and hobbies may apply to them. Have the students introduce themselves as they carry out the exercise.

I am someone who: **Signature:**

- has never smoked   _____
- has quit smoking   _____
- is into exercise   _____
- loves to read   _____
- would like to be a professional athlete   _____
- plays a sport   _____
- plays a musical instrument   _____
- wants to be:
  a lawyer   _____
  a doctor   _____
  a teacher   _____
  a police officer   _____
- spends his extra time helping others   _____
- prefers jeeps over other cars   _____
- has lived in another state or country   _____

Name Tags

This is what William Glasser (1990) had to say about the use of name tags in the educational setting:

> *An effort should be made to increase the number of people in the school who know each other by name. People who call each other by name work together much better and become friends much faster. To accomplish this, the faculty might agree that they, and all adults in the school on school business, will wear name tags. This would set an example and encourage students to do the same. The name tags could be creative, standard, or both. . . . While it should not be compulsory to wear a name tag, every effort should be made to persuade all to do so. No teacher would then have to talk to a student without knowing his or*

her name. This simple procedure, more than anything else that can be done, would reduce discipline problems.

Name tags can be a very positive aspect of the classroom environment, and every teacher should consider them. All students should be allowed to design their own name tags and they should include elements that say who they are—ethnic origin, family origin, personal values, etc. The bottom line is that you are promoting pride by allowing students to say, "I am someone who . . . !" I also feel strongly that the teacher should participate in this process of designing and wearing a personal name tag.

You want to start by providing students with a 5 × 8-inch card. Ask them to write their first name in the very center (large enough so that other class members can see it from across the room). Then, have them begin to personalize the card.

One method of personalizing name tags is to ask students certain questions and have them write down their response on their name tags. Example: "In the upper righthand corner of your tag, write down the names of the three most important people in your life. In the upper middle of your tag, write down your favorite color. In the upper lefthand corner of your tag, write down three things about yourself that you are most proud of. In the bottom lefthand corner of your tag, write down two things you want to accomplish before you die. In the bottom middle, write the name of your best friend. In the lower righthand corner, list three things you feel you do well."

Here are some additional questions you can have students respond to:

- What do you value most in a relationship?
- Write down the first name of the person you most trust.
- Given the choice of anyone in the world, living or dead, who you would like to talk to, who would it be?
- What are the two greatest accomplishments you have achieved in your life?
- If you could live anywhere in the world for one year, where would you choose?
- Name one event that changed your life.
- If you could become proficient in one thing, what would it be?
- If you had an unlimited amount of money, what would you do first?
- Name someone you are especially close to.
- If you could go back in time for one day, where would you go?

Allow Students to Know You

I am a firm believer in equality. This extends to the belief that, if students are asked to share things about themselves, they should have the opportunity to find out those same things about the teacher. Ask students, independent of each other, to come up with two questions they would like to ask you. These questions can be of their own making, but the first should be of a professional nature and the second of a personal nature. Tell them that they will be asking their questions aloud, not turning them in. Let them know you have the right to pass on any question for whatever reason you choose, but stress that they have this right also. This should be a full classroom experience, just as the getting-acquainted exercise was.

Establishing Classroom Rules

The primary way to bring ethics and character back into schools is to create a positive moral environment in schools. The ethos of a school, not its course offerings, is the decisive factor in forming character. The first thing we must change is the moral climate of the schools themselves. What we seem to have forgotten in all our concern with individual development is that schools are social institutions. Their first function is to socialize. Quite frankly, many of them have forgotten how to do that (Kilpatrick, 1992).

Classroom behavior is something all teachers face, and it can make or break a learning environment. However creative or innovative you are as a teacher, you will not be effective if you do not have control of the class. So, how do you get this control?

In some neighborhoods around the country, residents have established what is known as a "Neighborhood Watch." People gather together to establish certain rules about how they want their neighborhood to be and how they should police themselves to achieve it. In short, they look after each other. This dynamic is what you want to establish in the classroom.

Ask the class to nominate a group of students who will establish a "code of classroom conduct" to spell out

- what classroom behavior(s) will or will not be tolerated
- what measures will be taken to see that these guidelines are met
- what punishment will be administered to those who do not adhere to the agreed-on standards
- what rewards will be given to those students who stay within the guidelines
- who will be in charge of overseeing the administration of these rules

Such a committee should be voted on and put into action in every classroom. The bottom line is that students must be allowed to determine what classroom conditions they want to be involved in and learn in.

Conflict Resolution

A second part of guiding conduct in the classroom is conflict resolution. One program to address this issue was started in 1984 by Annette Townley, executive director of the National Association for Mediation in Education. This Amherst, Massachusetts–based group represents just a handful of conflict resolution programs.

Conflict-resolution techniques, which go by a variety of names, essentially help young people learn to stop a fight before it starts by thinking of the consequences first. In some cases, students themselves become peer tutors or mediators that step in and resolve problems. Teachers help young people practice skills like empathy, appropriate social behavior, and anger management.

Curbing Youth Violence

Another approach to youth violence substitutes constructive behavior for violent acting out. At the Harvard School of Public Health, associate dean Jay Winsten directed a campaign to popularize the street expression "squash it," meaning to walk away from a fight. Researchers discovered the term in focus groups of Mission Hill teenagers and later learned it was part of the lingo in New York, Los Angeles, and Chicago. Now, using sports and entertainment heroes, Winsten hopes to spread both the phrase and its hand-signal: a clenched fist rapped once on top by the opposite hand, a kind of time-out signal. He wants to promote the idea that it's cool and smart to stop a fight before it starts. "The hopeful news," Winsten says, "is that social expectations are subject to change" (Drexler, 1994).

In essence, conflict resolution is a process in which children learn the skills to respond creatively to conflict in the context of a supportive, caring community (Kreidler, 1984). To choose a conflict-resolution technique, Kreidler suggests considering these four things:

1. *Who's involved?* How many, how old, how mature, and how angry are they? What are their needs?
2. *Is the time right?* Do you have enough time to work things out now, or should you wait? Do the participants need to cool off first? Is it too soon to talk things out?
3. *How appropriate is a particular resolution technique?* Is this a simple dispute over resources or a complex conflict of values? Will this technique help solve the problem? Is the technique so sophisticated that the kids need training in it first?
4. *Should the resolution be public or private?* Would the participants be embarrassed by a public resolution? Would the class benefit from seeing this conflict resolved? Could they help with the resolution? Do you have the time to resolve it publicly?

Some solutions to conflict within the classroom include

- introducing games and activities that encourage cooperation
- discussing the advantages and disadvantages of conflict (constructively handled, conflict can make a student feel better about herself, provide new friends, and help everyone get along better)
- role-playing hypothetical conflicts to see how students might resolve certain issues through mediation techniques
- breaking students up into groups of five, and having them tackle an issue by:

1. Defining the problem: have them focus on the problem, not on who is causing the problem
2. Producing solutions: have them come up with as many ways they can to solve the problem
3. Choosing and acting: have them choose a solution, then let them act on it (this step is crucial, obviously, because ideas for wonderful solutions do no good if no action is taken)

Like the peer-controlled classroom behavior suggested earlier, conflict resolution is valuable not only because it gives students another option besides fighting to settle disputes, but because it empowers them to solve problems on their own terms. Most important, when students are given this choice (among others you may present), they take it seriously. An unexpected outcome of this type of classroom management is a boost in student self-esteem, because when they feel that their ideas are taken seriously they view themselves more positively.

Elements of Moral Discipline

Moral discipline, which uses discipline as a tool for moral growth, has the following elements (Lickona, 1991):

1. the teacher as the central moral authority in the classroom
2. cooperative rule setting, or discussing with students how the classroom rules express mutual respect and serve the good of the classroom community
3. an educational approach to consequences, using the occasion of rule enforcement to help students understand and voluntarily follow the rules
4. logical consequences for rule infractions to help students gain self-control, understand why their behavior was inappropriate, and make reparation
5. where appropriate, consequences that are decided on a case-by-case basis
6. individual conferences to promote teacher-student understanding, uncover the cause of a problem, and work out a plan for correcting it
7. situational supports for self-control, including methods that help students gain control through self-awareness
8. positive or negative incentives to improve behavior where they are needed for motivation
9. group and individual incentives that support rather than undermine the moral foundation of classroom rules
10. a holistic approach that sees students as persons and searches for solutions that help them succeed as members of the classroom community.
11. involved parents: send home the classroom-discipline plan, contact them about positive as well as negative behavior, and recruit their cooperation in dealing with problems

Establishing Classroom Goals

All classroom goals boil down to four aspects of teaching and learning. They are:

1. imparting knowledge (this is a given)
2. clarifying values and attitudes that empower students
3. developing a wide range of teaching approaches to present issues and facts
4. developing an ability to integrate all of the above for intelligent decision making and problem solving

In an earlier day, traditional health education in schools stressed only knowledge, in part because the other three goals were achieved to an acceptable degree at home or in some other environment outside of the classroom.

In contrast, when planning activities to carry out the basic goals of health education today, it is helpful to take into account the wide variety of human behaviors that lead to learning.

Establishing Classroom Ground Rules

Using guidelines established by the Boston Area Educators for Social Responsibility (1993), empowering students to establish ground rules requires that educators help them

- define the rationale for establishing ground rules
- share two to three ground rules that are important to the teacher (e.g., "We are essential members of the class community and our voice needs to be heard")

Benefits of Cooperative Rule Setting

Involving students in setting classroom rules and in taking personal and group responsibility for following them benefits students in these ways (Lickona, 1991):

1. It forms a partnership in which student and teacher work together to create rules that serve the good of the classroom community.
2. It fosters students' feeling of ownership of the classroom rules and a moral obligation to follow them.
3. It treats the child as a moral thinker and invests time in helping him develop better moral reasoning.
4. It helps students to see the values (e.g., respect and responsibility) that lie behind rules and to value rule following beyond the classroom.
5. It helps students think critically about rules and develop competence at making good rules themselves.
6. It emphasizes internal rather than external control and so fosters *voluntary* compliance with rules and laws.

- work in cooperative groups and identify two essential ground rules that they want to share with the class community
- come together as a class and share the ground rules while the teacher lists them
- categorize the ground rules and then prioritize them with the teacher
- revisit the list of ground rules the next day and make necessary revisions
- post the ground rules so they are visible in the classroom (older students should receive a typed copy)

Steps to Good Discipline

Based on the concepts of reality therapy, schools (or other learning environments) can be good places to teach and learn the fundamentals of effective discipline (Glasser, 1977). Some basic concepts are as follows:

1. *Be personal.* Use personal pronouns, i.e., "I care enough about you to be involved, to be your friend."
2. *Refer to present behavior.* Awareness of behavior is the first step. Avoid references to the past. Emphasize behavior, not feelings.
3. *Stress value judgments.* Ask students to evaluate their own behavior. The decision to behave better than they have been must be theirs.
4. *Plan.* Work with students to formulate alternatives. Keep the plan simple and within a short span of time. Build success into the plan.
5. *Be committed.* Build in a way to check back and follow up. Give positive reinforcement. (Students need to accept some responsibility for this; a written form may be helpful.)
6. *Don't accept excuses.* Eliminate discussion of excuses to show you know students can succeed. Work with them. Don't give up.
7. *Don't punish.* Punishment lifts responsibility from students. Instead, set rules and sanctions with them. They have to understand they are responsible for themselves. This takes time and consistency.
8. *Never give up.* Each of us must define "never," but hang in there longer than the students think you will.

Additional Techniques for Community Building

At the end of every class, try and bring the group back into a full circle. Give students the opportunity to tell you their feelings about the activities and information you've shared. Some things that should always be part of this discussion are:

- **Practicing compliments and appreciation.** Offer students an opportunity to share their appreciation of other students in the group.
- **Creating an agenda for the next class.** Discuss topics students would like to follow up on based on what was discussed in the day's activities.
- **Developing communication skills.** The circle of sharing encourages all students to share.

An Exercise on Feedback   Once a week, set aside ten minutes of class time to have the students fill out the following form and submit it to you. At the next class meeting, summarize the feedback, noting general trends and pointing out dissenting opinions. Let students know how you are going to use the feedback, what things you can and can't do given that change is a difficult and uncertain thing, and ask for their help, cooperation, and understanding when necessary.

Feedback Form

How satisfied were you with this week's sessions? (Circle one)

1   2   3   4   5   6   7   8   9

very
satisfied

very
dissatisfied

2. What was the high point of your week in class?

3. What factor(s) contributed toward your level of satisfaction?

4. What can I do to make these sessions better for you?

5. What can you do to make these sessions better for you?

6. What are some of the special issues, concerns, or questions that you would like to see raised in class next week?

7. Free comments, suggestions, and questions:

_____   _____
Name (optional)   Date

- **Learning about students' different realities.** Allow students to share ideas from their own gender or cultural perspective with the whole group.
- **Solving problems arising from the issues discussed.**
- **Applying logical consequences.** Discuss the classroom-initiated standards of acceptable behavior, those who may have breached the rules, and the consequences issued.

Exercise: Peaceable-School Assessment

Every school has its own culture. Just as with the culture of a town or a country, a school's culture can increase the likelihood of its citizens engaging in violence, or it can increase the likelihood that they will find peaceful ways to settle their inevitable conflicts. A school, through its staff, students, parents, and support community, can organize itself and teach the skills that increase peacefulness and respect.

The chart below highlights five characteristics of a school's culture that can encourage a more peaceful learning environment. Use it to assess how intentionally and how well your school's culture engenders peacefulness and respect. Illustrations of these aspects of culture can include *rules and policies* (such as discipline codes, schedules), *language* for dealing with conflict and prejudice, *icons* (posters, buttons, mascots), *relationships* (staff to staff, staff to students, ethnic group to ethnic group), *customs and traditions* (holidays discussed, speakers and events), *roles and jobs* (for students in classes and around the school), *the content and skills of the curricula* (what problems are highlighted, what avoided), *physical structures* (location of offices, seating arrangements in classes), *governance* (school councils, mediation programs). There are many other examples as well that you can use to illustrate your school culture's effectiveness in encouraging peacefulness and respect.

Rating
1 = low
5 = high

Communication						Illustrations
Taught	1	2	3	4	5	
Modeled	1	2	3	4	5	
Cooperation						
Taught	1	2	3	4	5	
Modeled	1	2	3	4	5	

From *Creative Conflict Resolution*. Cambridge, MA: Boston Area Educators for Social Responsibility, 1993.

Synthesis

One of the greatest challenges facing us in health education is teaching the very real issues of responsibility to self and others (e.g., cigarette smoking, drinking and driving, and unsafe sex), compassion, and the other values so desperately needed in today's society. Our position as health educators must be toward promoting cooperation and commitment. The way to achieve these two important objectives is through classroom involvement not only in developing these qualities but also in adherence to their goals. Students must be allowed to be involved in making the classroom work if we are to expect them to make their own decisions and regulate their own behavior.

References

Boston Area Educators for Social Responsibility. *Creative Conflict Resolution.* Cambridge, MA: BAESR, 1993.

Drexler, Madeline. "Fatal Habits." *Boston Globe Magazine,* 27 February 1994.

Garbarino, James, et al. *What Children Can Tell Us: Eliciting, Interpreting, and Evaluating Critical Information from Children.* San Francisco: Jossey-Bass, 1992.

Glasser, William. "10 Steps to Good Discipline." *Today's Education,* November-December 1977.

___. *The Quality School: Managing Students without Coercion.* New York: Harper & Row, 1990.

Kilpatrick, William. *Why Johnny Can't Tell Right from Wrong.* New York: Simon & Schuster, 1992.

Kreidler, William J. *Creative Conflict Resolution: More than 200 Activities for Keeping Children in the Classroom K–6.* Glenview, IL: Good Year Books, 1984.

Lee, Harper. *To Kill a Mockingbird.* Philadelphia: J.B. Lippincott, 1960.

Lickona, Thomas. *Educating for Character: How Our Schools Can Teach Respect and Responsibility.* New York: Bantam Books, 1991.

Additional Resources

Abrami, Philip C., et al. *Using Cooperative Learning.* Montreal, Quebec: Concordia University Education Department, 1993.

Judson, Stephanie. *A Manual on Nonviolence and Children.* Garden City, New York: Waldorf Press, 1984.

Kreidler, William J. *Creative Conflict Resolution.* Glenview, IL: Scott, Foresman and Company, 1984.

Nelsen, Jane, Lynn Lott, and H. Stephine Glenn. *Positive Discipline in the Classroom.* Rocklin, CA: Prima Publishing, 1993.

Shor, Ira. *Empowering Education: Critical Teaching for Social Change.* Chicago: University of Chicago Press, 1992.

7　The Exploratory Stage

The major task at the exploratory stage is to look at some ways to bring about behavioral change in those with whom you are working. Before beginning, we need to explore some of the conditions that encourage students to take responsibility for their own leadership, their own decisions, and the refinement of the processes in which they are engaged:

> Instead of looking to a professional elite for the solution to any social problem, look to the greatest resource available—the very population that has the problem. Many of us tend to have a low opinion of people, those wretched masses who don't understand, don't know what they want, who continually make mistakes and foul up their lives, requiring those of us who are professionally trained to come in and correct the situation. But that is not the way it really works. The fact is that some drug addicts are much better able to cure addiction in each other than are psychiatrists; some convicts can run better rehabilitation programs for convicts than do correctional officers; many students tend to learn more from each other than from many professors; some patients in mental hospitals are better for each other than is the staff. Thousands of self-help organizations are doing a good job, perhaps a better job, at problem solving than is the profession that is identified with that problem. People who have the problems often have a better understanding of their situation and what must be done to change it. What professionals have to do is learn to cooperate with that resource, to design the conditions which evoke that intelligence (Farson, 1969).

Establishing the conditions that allow for democratic participation in behavioral change is not simple. The teacher must decide not to lead in traditional

We shall not cease from exploration, and the end of all our exploring will be to arrive where we started and know the place for the first time.

—T. S. Eliot

ways, and the group members must learn to overcome their expectations of what teachers are supposed to do. We have long relied on authorities of one sort or another for the final word in questions of responsibility and decision making; it takes a *new experience* to accept that another kind of responsibility, shared responsibility, is both possible and effective.

Gaining Understanding

Prior to teaching, you must gain some knowledge about where your students are in terms of knowledge, attitudes, and behavior. After teaching, you must also reevaluate to see if you have achieved your established goals. Do this in two separate stages, the first dealing with health knowledge and the second dealing with attitudes and behavior.

The health-knowledge part should be age-specific. The form used can be developed by the health educator and need not be extensive, but it must be accurate and direct:

Health-Knowledge Questions

Answer "True" or "False" to each of the following questions:

1. Physical exercise, such as running, can reduce the risk of coronary heart disease, but only if it is vigorous enough to stimulate the heart.

2. A healthy young adult has a blood pressure of about 110/80 or lower.

3. A person's health is determined partly by genetics and partly by external factors.

Multiple choice: Circle all responses that apply to each of the following questions:

4. What are the most important benefits of regular stretching?

   a. reduces muscle tension and makes the body feel more relaxed
   b. improves coordination by allowing for freer movement
   c. increases range of motion
   d. prevents injuries, such as muscle strains

e. promotes circulation
f. helps loosen the mind's control of the body
g. makes strenuous activities easier
h. feels good

5. The "perfect" exercise is

a. running
b. weight lifting
c. swimming
d. basketball
e. job-walking

6. Why should you quit smoking?

a. your personal risks
b. risks to others
c. if b, to whom?

After the students have completed the test, collect the results. Do *not* go over the answers in class, but tell them they will have a chance to see their results at the end of the semester. Then, look over their responses to gain some understanding of where they are in terms of health knowledge.

The attitude and behavior aspect of evaluating students is more complicated and requires a certain degree of trust. Here, you want to allow students to share their beliefs and actions in all areas of health but also let them know their responses are private and *for their eyes only.* This shows your respect for their honesty and openness.

To guarantee this sense of trust, provide each student with an envelope. Have them place their name on it, date it, and seal it with their answers inside. Either collect their responses, or let them keep them. The attitude and behavior form you come up with might look like the following:

Attitude Questions

1. In general, are you concerned about your health?

a. no, not at all concerned
b. yes, somewhat concerned
c. occasionally concerned
d. yes, very concerned

(continued)

2. How do you feel about casual sex within your age group?

   a. it's morally wrong
   b. it's much too dangerous
   c. it would be acceptable if proper precautions were taken
   d. it's not a problem because (fill in the blank):

Behavior Questions

1. I consider my current weight to be

   a. perfect
   b. a little over the ideal
   c. a little under the ideal
   d. a lot over the ideal
   e. a lot under the ideal

2. Have you changed your eating habits to avoid heightened cholesterol levels?

   a. yes
   b. no
   c. no, but I am considering it

At the end of each teaching unit, have the students do both checklists again. Give them their original checklists so they can compare their responses. Finally, discuss results. When compiling your forms, keep in mind that each area of concentration (e.g., personal health, sexuality, AIDS, and self-esteem) should contain questions that touch on both knowledge and attitudes and behaviors.

Self-Goals

As a final step in gaining knowledge of students (and ultimately, in their gaining knowledge of themselves), you may want to offer them a questionnaire in which they can be open and honest about their personal goals for your class. Ask them to fill out a response to the following questions. Have them seal their responses in an

Contract with Myself

1. In terms of your own health behavior, what areas would you like to change? Be specific.

2. What would it take for you to make these changes?

3. In what ways do you want to change your behavior?

4. What are your time limits in terms of meeting these goals?

envelope, date them, and turn them in to you. At the end of the year, return it to them so they can decide whether they fulfilled their contract with themselves or not.

Let each individual know that you will do everything possible to help them, but it is up to them to achieve their goals. Finally, allow students to assess their own health awareness by filling out the assessment card shown in Figure 7–1.

Exercise: Assessing Health	These statements are designed to help you assess your health and add to your awareness and understanding of your overall health. Circle the number before each statement that you believe to be an accurate description of yourself.

Section 1: Nutrition

1. I limit my consumption of high-fat foods (eggs, dairy products, fatty meats, fried foods).
2. I limit my consumption of salt and salty foods.
3. I eat fish and poultry more often than I eat red meat.
4. I eat five servings of fruits and vegetables a day.
5. I limit my intake of sweets, sodas, and snack foods.
6. I drink several glasses of water a day.

Section 2: Emotional Well-Being

1. I laugh often and easily.
2. I can ask for help when needed.
3. I include relaxation time as part of my daily schedule.
4. I have someone with whom I can discuss personal problems.
5. I can express concern and love to those I care about.
6. I can express my angry feelings rather than hold them in.
7. There is a healthy balance between my work (school and job) and leisure time.

(continued)

Section 3: Fitness

1. I am within the normal weight range for my gender, height, and age.
2. I keep in shape by doing vigorous exercise (biking, swimming, running, sports, aerobics, etc.) for at least thirty minutes three times a week or doing moderate exercise (like walking) an hour a day.
3. I stretch, do yoga, or move my body regularly in a variety of ways to keep it supple and flexible.
4. I regularly engage in activities (weight training, work that involves moving heavy objects, sports that work the whole body) that develop overall strength.
5. I am pleased with the way I look and feel.
6. I have enough energy to do the things I like to do.

Section 4: Family History

I have a family member who:

1. Had a heart attack.
2. Had or has high blood pressure.
3. Developed diabetes as an adult.
4. Had or has breast cancer.
5. Had or has a drug or alcohol problem.

Section 5: Alcohol, Nicotine, and Other Drug Use

1. I do not smoke cigarettes or chew tobacco.
2. I do not use alcohol.
3. I do not use marijuana or other drugs.
4. I ask about the side effects of any prescribed medications.
5. I read and follow the instructions on all prescribed or over-the-counter medications.
6. I ask about the effect of taking more than one medication at a time.
7. I am aware of the dangers of alcohol, nicotine, and other drugs.

Section 6: Accidents

1. I do not accept rides from drivers who have been drinking or taking drugs.
2. I wear a seat belt whenever I am in an automobile.
3. I wear a helmet when I ride a bicycle or motorcycle.
4. I obey all traffic and safety rules.

Section 7: Human Values

1. I take part in activities that stimulate me intellectually.
2. I participate in family, church, or community events.
3. I stand by my own values even when they are different from those of my friends.
4. I use my thoughts and attitudes in life-affirming ways.
5. I accept other people's ideas and values even though they may be different from my own.
6. I believe in a positive force that supports my well-being.

Section 8: Self-Care

1. I have yearly dental and medical check-ups.
2. I get at least eight hours of sleep a day or sufficient sleep for me to awaken feeling rested.
3. I am aware of bodily changes that might indicate a health problem.
4. I know how to do self-examinations.
5. When I am ill, I rest and follow the doctor's treatment.
6. I know what to do in case of illness or injury.
7. I do not participate in behavior that could be dangerous to my health.
8. I know how to prevent the transmission of STDs and HIV-AIDS.

Use your responses for each section to complete the graph in Figure 7–1. The results will give you an overall picture of how you view your health. In each section, shade one box for each statement you circled.

Evaluation Key: *Completely shaded sections*—Healthy behavior and life-style choices. Keep it up! *Partially shaded sections*—A little more effort and attention to these issues can improve the quality and length of your life. Work a little harder! *Barely shaded or nonshaded sections*—There is significant room for improving your health in these areas. First, work on areas where you feel confident of success. Then, attack the areas that are more difficult for you.

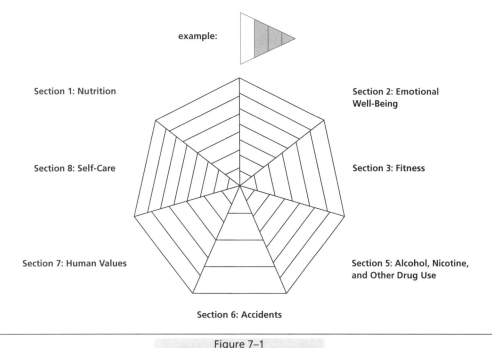

Figure 7–1

A Portrait of Your Health

Note: This graph does not include Section 4, Family History, since you have no control over this area of your life. However, it is helpful to be aware of health issues that may be hereditary and use this awareness to pay particular attention to preventative steps that can help you avoid these conditions.

COURTESY HEALING AND THE MIND WITH BILL MOYERS, TEACHERS GUIDE, © 1993 THIRTEEN/WNET, Prepared by The Educational Publishing Department at Thirteen/WNET, based on a concept developed by the editors of Wellness Letter, University of California at Berkeley.

(continued)

Write the number of statements you circled for each session:

Section	1	2	3	4	5	6	7
				(omit)			

Where Self-Evaluation Leads

Over the years, the classes that were found to be most effective, open, and productive were those that empowered students to perform at their best. Many teachers want a learning community that inspires students to take more responsibility for and control over their lives.

Bruno Bettelheim urged teachers to encourage students to question their experience in school:

> You must arouse children's curiosity and make them think about school. For example, it's very important to begin the school year with a discussion of why we go to school. Why does the government force us to go to school? This would set a questioning tone and show the children that you trust them and that they are intelligent enough, at their own level, to investigate and come up with answers (Meier 1990).

Both a school year and a class lesson that begin by questioning can be a remarkably democratic and critical learning experience for students.

Checking out matters of knowledge, attitudes, and behaviors also gives students a sense of their progress in terms of personal growth. In their book *Passion for Life: Psychology and the Human Spirit* (1991), Muriel and John James stated that

> the challenge to grow is threefold: to get in touch with the urges that come from our inner core, to set goals that are compatible with the human spirit, and to develop the personal qualities that are needed to reach those goals. To meet this challenge, we need to become aware of how our urges get blocked, drained, or restricted and to learn what is needed to release these energies so that we have strength for the spiritual search.

Change through Understanding

To understand how students handle the topic of modifying behavior and the amount of resistance they feel toward change, you may need to discuss how the process works, outline the responsibilities of both yourself and the student, and point out how positive results can be achieved. For example, if you are talking about the negative effects of cigarette smoking to a group of students and you have a student in class whose close relatives smoke, it will take a very different approach to convince this student that smoking is harmful. The same can be said about excessive drinking or eating. All positive and negative health habits start with the family. You, as the teacher, must take this into consideration.

Risk and Personal Change

Dr. David Viscott (1977) sees the concept of risking as central to growth: "If you cannot risk, you cannot grow. . . . If you cannot grow, you cannot become your best. . . . If you cannot become your best, you cannot be happy. What else matters?"

The fact that self-improvement risks are often inhibited by a fear of failure isn't surprising, since these risks usually involve putting yourself on the line in some way. Self-improvement risks can spark a fear of rejection by your peers (e.g., getting off drugs); rejection by your family (e.g., changing your eating habits); disapproval from others (authority figures or teachers); failure (e.g., trying to stop smoking and not succeeding); making a commitment (the fear of being wrong).

Getting people to take risks that can assist them in growing is not simple. The tendency in our educational system is to blame the individual for failing to solve a problem effectively, when in fact the system or environment may be at fault. To help change this, creative approaches to the teaching-learning process must be sought. We will now explore two such possibilities: a rational-emotive therapy (RET) approach, and a reality-therapy approach.

A Rational-Emotive Therapy Approach

People rarely understand that our symptoms *work* (Bandler and Grinder, 1979). Often, we neither appreciate the purpose underlying a troubling pattern nor recognize how the pattern accomplishes that purpose, because the entire process is largely unconscious. For example, an anorexic woman feels that her eating behavior, her life, and her body are perfectly normal. Focus on the positive aspects of personal change, not the negatives. Don't deny the negatives, but give your time and energy to the positives. Some cognitive techniques that focus on positive change rest on three key ideas.

1. The Way You Think Influences the Way You Feel and Behave

Distorted, irrational thinking leads to erroneous conclusions and inappropriate, negative feelings. These feelings then lead to self-defeating, self-limiting, or over cautious behavior.

One of the most dynamic and popular cognitive-behavioral thinkers is Albert Ellis (1967, 1971). His rational-emotive therapy (RET) is usually considered part of existential-humanistic psychology because of its optimistic view of humankind.

Changing your behavior is not as simple as it sounds. A successful plan must be explicit. If vague intentions were all it took to change unhealthy behavior, you wouldn't need the full range of techniques discussed in this book. Of course, sometimes you can change your behavior simply by alerting yourself of the need to do so. But, for serious health issues, a more deliberate plan is called for. To help in this process, use the following plan for change:

1. State your goal. What one change would you like to make in your personal health behavior? If it is a complex goal or one that will take a long time to achieve, state a short-term goal instead. Be specific so you know exactly what must be accomplished.

2. List the specific steps you will take to achieve this goal. What behaviors will need to be altered? List each step separately. Consider alternatives.

3. Will you have a deadline for achieving this goal? If so, when is it?

4. Will you ask for help from others? If so, be sure that you get accurate observations and feedback from them along the way.

5. Now put your plan into action. Then refer back to this list to answer the last question.

6. Did you achieve your goal?

   Yes: _____   No: _____   Somewhat: _____

   How do you feel?

Recently, due to its systematic thinking, it has been embraced by behaviorists. RET focuses more on thoughts than on feelings. It is Ellis's view that people have made themselves victims by their own incorrect and *irrational* thinking patterns. While taking an essentially optimistic view toward people, Ellis criticizes humanism as being too soft at times and failing to cope with the fact that people can virtually self-destruct through irrational and muddled thinking. The whole theory surrounding RET is to correct thought patterns and rid people of irrational ideas.

Perhaps Ellis's most important contribution is his A-B-C theory of what shapes the personality:

A. the objective facts, events, and behaviors an individual encounters

B. the individual's belief about A

C. the emotional consequence; how the individual feels about A

Many believe that A causes C (facts cause consequences), and that B is not a factor. Ellis challenges this equation as naive, since it fails to consider that what people *think* about an event determines how they feel. Using the A-B-C model, for example, we find that

A. the objective fact is the possibility of being overweight

B. the beliefs that the person has about being overweight. In this case, the person believes being overweight is bad, therefore,

C. as an emotional consequence, the person experiences guilt, loss of self-esteem, and self-doubts

In this case, the individual has short-circuited B and thinks, "If I am overweight, I am unacceptable to myself and others."

Time Out for Personal Thoughts

Think about some times in your past when you were rejected or felt less than who you were.

Example:

I *did not make the swimming team* _____

Therefore, *I am a loser* _____

Your turn:

I _____

Therefore, _____

The goal of RET is to attack the belief system. What the person in the example thinks about being overweight is causing him anxiety *not by the objective, cognitive facts of the situation.* There are obviously numerous people, both heavy and thin, who believe that "fat (or thin) is beautiful," and so do not come to the same conclusion that this person does. Ellis's approach is to challenge the person's logic: "If I *were* overweight, I would be a total loser." It clarifies the "A causes C" assumption of the statement by challenging the irrationality of the person's logic. It isn't the specific belief that is challenged, but the *unfoundedness* of that belief that leads to illogical conclusions. The emphasis must be on changing the way a person thinks about his behavior.

In Ellis's view, something happens—a stimulus event of some sort—which he calls an activating event (A). This activating event has consequences (B) for the individual. The individual may think that "A" causes "C." The individual's interpretation (B) of the activating event is what provides the consequences for him or her. These irrational beliefs reflect one of three false ideologies (Ellis and Greiger, 1977):

1. I must win approval for my performance or I will rate as a rotten person.
2. You must act kindly and justly toward me or you are a louse.
3. The conditions under which I live must be such that I get practically everything I want without too much effort and discomfort, or the world turns damnable and life hardly seems worth living.

A: Event stresses	B: Perceptual filters	C: Coping responses
Pressure	Past experience	Guilt
Demands	Expectations	Fear
Changes	Evaluation	Negative self-thoughts
Challenges	Beliefs	Do nothing

Applications in Health Education. Basic to using this therapeutic model in health education is the ability to identify and understand the students' irrational feelings and thoughts, to free them from irrational thinking, and to equip them with beliefs that are satisfactory and functional for everyday life. For example, it is not enough to get young girls to take more responsibility for contraceptive use; we also need to get them to understand that their lack of contraceptive care belies a deep-seated desire to become pregnant to satisfy needs and beliefs not at all connected to their original belief model (Cassell, 1984; Lawson and Rhode, 1993; Sanford and Donovan, 1985). You also must empower them to understand that they have choices. They have the power to

- say no to sex without feeling guilty; they do not have to prove their love for their partner by having sex
- say no to intercourse but allow other sexual activity
- insist on contraceptive use; a condom for their partner, and a diaphragm for themselves

For many young women, confusing sex with love is an irrational idea. Teachers must emphasize replacing irrational ideas with rational ones. Among the irrational beliefs that Ellis identifies as extremely common are (Ellis, 1971):

> you . . . must have sincere love and approval almost all the time from all the people you find significant . . . because something once strongly influenced your life, it has to keep determining your feelings and behavior today . . . people and things should turn out better than they do; you have to view it as awful and horrible if you do not quickly find good solutions to life's hassles . . . you must have a high degree of order or certainty to feel comfortable.

Most of these irrational beliefs involve rigid preconceptions of how we must behave or how events should happen. All lead to negative judgments about ourselves and our existence.

Rational-emotive therapy emphasizes that people are responsible for their at-risk behaviors. Consequently, they are capable of rearranging their lives in ways that will enable them to break away from these unprogressive behaviors. Action-oriented, RET makes use of many scientifically based procedures that work to create significant philosophic, emotional, and behavioral changes. The aim of RET is to help individuals integrate their intellectual and experiential processes, to enhance their growth and creativity and to rid themselves of unproductive and self-defeating habits (Ellis, 1967).

2. You Cannot Change Reality, but You Can Change the Way You Think, Feel, and Act on Reality

For example, you can't make someone like you if he or she doesn't; but you can remind yourself that your happiness and sense of self-worth doesn't depend on your popularity with one particular person. Similarly, you can't remove the element of risk from asking someone out on a date, but you can reassure yourself that the survival of your self-esteem doesn't hinge on whether or not your invitation is accepted.

Beck (1972, 1976) hypothesized that our self-defeating beliefs and attitudes are not completely irrational but overstatements of reality: too extreme, too broad, or too arbitrary. Once a self-defeating idea is identified, we must test the limits of its rationality. He pointed out several ways we're especially likely to distort our ideas about ourselves: discussed *dualistic thinking,* interpreting a mild rebuff as total rejection; *jumping to conclusions* without evidence to back it up; and *overgeneralizing,* concluding from one mistake that we'll never do anything right. Beck also mentions *errors of omission,* emphasizing a detail while ignoring its larger context, and *personalizing*—incorrectly referring an outside event to ourselves: "The teacher is really angry—it must be something I did."

When we are stuck in self-defeating attitudes and behaviors, another person can be helpful. Bandler and Grinder (1979) described how therapist Carl Whittaker reframed his clients' complaints:

The husband complains, "and for the last ten years, nobody has ever taken care of me. I've had to do everything for myself. . . . " Carl Whittaker says, "Thank God you learned to stand on your own two feet. I really appreciate a man who can do that."

Time Out for Personal Thoughts

Have students choose a partner they trust and get them to sit facing each other. Decide who goes first. The first person begins by revealing a negative attitude he holds about himself—some unfavorable evaluation or feeling of who he is or how he handles some aspect of his life.

The other person is his reframer. The reframer will guess at the positive intent underlying his behavior or look for anything else positive she can find, and will articulate that to him.

For instance, the first student says, "I am angry with myself for getting upset with my girlfriend so much. I just don't know what is happening to me." The reframer might reply, "Your girlfriend is very important to you." He responds by saying either "No, that doesn't strike home," or "Yes, that's right." If his response was no, the reframer tries again. If it was yes, he reveals another negative attitude to his reframer.

After five or so minutes, have students reverse roles and repeat the exercise.

3. Equip the Learner with Beliefs that Are Satisfactory and Functional for Everyday Life

For example, it is not enough to help free someone from irrational thoughts and fears about homosexuality. This person must also have the opportunity to explore a new set of beliefs and actions to test their rationality and workability. RET theory does not support or challenge any particular belief system; rather it tends to be unusually open to alternative life-styles and variations among people.

To place this in a health-education context, the health educator must focus on moving the student toward a rational, acceptable belief system. In the case of homosexuality, once having identified the irrational belief, RET theory could support both the active adoption of a homosexual life-style or the equally active rejection of it. The issue is the logic and rationality of the person's belief system rather than the objective behavior.

The power of RET and Ellis's work is increasingly recognized by the helping professions, most notably by the behaviorists who are realizing the importance of cognitive patterns in overt behavior. One example of a new synthesis between behavioral approaches and RET is that of Lange and Jakubowski (1976), who combine the two in an assertion-training model. They suggest (1) identifying the situation where assertion is needed clearly and precisely; (2) adding the methods of RET to bring out irrational beliefs underlying the lack of assertion; and (3) defining the rights and wishes of the individual in the assertion situation. In this way, two major tasks are accomplished simultaneously—situation-specific behaviors are learned, and the underlying belief system relating to behavior is discovered. The combination of thoughts and actions can lead both to more effective assertion and to a higher probability of the learning being applied in other situations.

RET could be summarized as an action therapy. The health educator using this approach is active, confronting (in a positive, challenging way), and involved with the learner. Further, when combined with other approaches such as role playing, open-ended questioning, or small-group interaction, there is some evidence that their effectiveness is increased. As in all such procedures, the ethical competence of the health educator is critical.

A Reality-Therapy Approach

The goal of applying reality therapy (RT) to health education is to free the learner from irrational thinking and equip her with beliefs that not only are need-satisfying but also lead to positive health choices. Whatever health issue you are discussing, the crux of the matter is the logic and rationality of the student's belief system rather than the objective behavior.

Using the RT model in health education requires action, confronting, and, most important, classroom involvement. The lessons should be fast-paced, encourage large-group participation, and have a heavy emphasis on the daily lives of the learners. In a sense, RT is very "American" because of its pragmatism and goal of making things "work" as quickly and efficiently as possible. And, as most of us in health education know, time is of the essence.

In the introduction to William Glasser's text *Reality Therapy*, O. Hobart Mowrer delineates the essence of this powerful tool, which has been popular in schools, rehabilitation settings, youth work, and prisons:

> . . . *human beings get into emotional binds, not because their standards are high, but because their performance has been, and is, too low . . . the objective of this (radically non-Freudian) type of therapy is not to lower the aim, but to increase the accomplishment* (Mowrer, 1965).

Reality therapy presents a clear approach to human growth and change that has won acceptance from those who work with a wide variety of individuals under difficult circumstances.

In describing the basic beliefs of reality therapy, Glasser stated that clients often select ineffective behaviors to meet their needs that virtually assure their failure.

> *[A]ll patients have a common characteristic: they all deny the reality of the world around them. Some break the law, denying the rules of society; some claim their*

neighbors are plotting against them, denying the improbability of such behavior. Some are afraid of crowded places, close quarters, airplanes, or elevators, yet they freely admit the irrationality of their fears. Millions drink to blot out the inadequacy they feel but that need not exist if they could learn to be different; and far too many people choose suicide rather than face the reality that they could solve their problems by more responsible behavior. Whether it is a partial denial or the total blotting out of all reality of the chronic backward patient in the state hospital, the denial of some or all of reality is common to all patients. Therapy will be successful when they are able to give up denying the world and recognize that reality not only exists but that they must fulfill their needs within its framework. . . . A therapy that leads all patients toward reality, toward grappling successfully with the tangible and intangible aspects of the real world, might accurately be called a therapy toward reality, or simply reality therapy (Glasser, 1965).

Reality therapy is a common-sense approach to the facilitation of learning. Find out what the learner wants and needs, examine her failures and her assets, and consider factors in the environment that must change if her needs are to be satisfied. Students cannot meet their needs outside the real world; they must face a world that is imperfect and not built to their specifications, and they must act positively in this world. The basic tenet of reality therapy is that people can do something about their fate if they consider themselves and the environment realistically.

The most basic human need is to find one's identity. The major psychological routes toward fulfilling this need are being loved and feeling that we are worthwhile to ourselves and other people. Reality therapy helps people learn who they are, how they interact with others, and how they can be accepted more fully by others. Secondarily, it helps people find activities in which they can help both themselves and others. If these basic needs are not met, the person will seek substitutes, and his thought patterns will dictate how he meets those needs. Wrong thinking can lead to poor school performance and many other problems. Reality therapy seeks to help individuals find an identity and straighten out these faulty thinking patterns.

As might be anticipated, reality therapy focuses on conscious, planned action and gives little attention to underlying dimensions of transference, unconscious thought processes and the like. *The goal is to consider the past as being done with— the present and the future are what is important.* In contrast to the Rogerian approach (Rogers, 1961), feelings and attitudes are not important, but behavior is. Reality therapy does not emphasize applied behavioral analysis or the detailed plans of assertion training or systematic desensitization. Rather, similar to RET, reality therapy focuses on responsibility and value judgments. Clients examine their lives to see how their behavior (health behavior, specifically) is destructive. The more important step, however, is to take responsibility for this behavior. Glasser defines this as "the ability to fulfill one's needs and to do so in a way that does not deprive others of the ability to fulfill their needs" (1965). Learning responsibility is a lifelong process.

Reality therapy focuses on taking responsibility. A health educator leading a discussion on teen pregnancy would never hesitate to discuss the realities of unprotected sex, to emphasize the total lack of responsibility of this type of behavior, and to open up a discussion on why young people do not practice safe sex (including abstaining). This requires skill on the part of the teacher to examine with the learners the likely consequences of their choices and the benefits of responsible decision making. Such discussion is passionate (without being judgmental) and noncoercive. "Ultimately, no one can make anyone do anything," as Glasser said.

Because reality therapy is often applied in street clinics, to prison inmates, and to schoolchildren, trust is particularly important. The institutions in which young people struggle are not often conducive to building the automatic trust relationship that comes when a student enters the world of the helper. The health educator as a person becomes especially important. The qualities of warmth, respect, and caring, positive regard, and interpersonal openness are crucial. Moreover, the self-in-teaching approach (see Chapter 5) is much more likely to provide pupils with an informal and productive learning situation.

Some Thoughts on Reality Teaching

1. Ask yourself the question, "Do I want to be involved with my students?" Authenticity, genuineness, and willingness to be yourself and be with others is required of the teacher interested in reality in health education. It is difficult to be a reality teacher if you hide behind facts, coming out only to call a student's name or recognize a raised hand. Ask yourself if you are willing and able to take time to be "out front" and with students.

2. Ask yourself, "Am I responsible, and do I understand what responsibility means?" Do you believe that you are the manager of your own life, that you are in charge, and that you take responsibility for your own actions?

3. With a friend or in a journal, explore specific instances where you were or were not responsible for your behavior. Apply the Glasser concept of responsibility to yourself, your past, and your present.

4. Do you believe that it is possible to help others relearn new ways of living and coping with the daily problems of life? If you would rather work on past events and the internal psyche, search for the warmth and caring of humanistic, self-actualizing teachers or some other approach; reality teaching may not be for you. Reality in health education requires a rigorous and direct approach to students coupled with an ability to be equally rigorous and direct with yourself.

5. As a final step, test your ability to use the reality approach by having a role-playing interview with a class that you are teaching. Give the class a situation where you saw irresponsible behavior (e.g., in a news report). Examine that behavior with the class in the framework of reality therapy, and engage the class in planning for more effective, responsible behavior in the future.

Reality in health education involves a deeper teacher-student relationship. It requires that teachers be themselves and model responsible interpersonal behaviors. The following ideas may help you gain some sense of the possibilities of a reality approach in teaching.

Control Theory in the Classroom

Control theory, Glasser's term for the psychology of behavior (1984, 1986), is an attempt to encourage quality work by moving from the inside to the outside. Teaching health is not hard; helping a student want to change her behavior from unhealthy to healthy is the hard part. The good reality teacher is a skilled manager of this change:

> If we want students to be motivated to work hard in school and to follow rules, we must discard the stimulus-response theory of human behavior on which all education is based (the idea that the behavior of all living creatures is their best response to some external event that impinges on them) and turn to new psychology—control theory, which explains that living people are motivated from within themselves and that what happens outside of us is never the cause of anything we do. . . . Basic to control theory is the concept that our genes instruct us to attempt to survive, to love and belong, and to struggle for power, fun, and freedom. If what is offered in school is not seen by students as related to one or more of these built-in needs, they will struggle against, and/or withdraw from, any or all of a curriculum that is not satisfying. . . . Without expanding existing resources, we can use this theory to begin to make some lasting improvements in our schools. We can stop trying to motivate students with externally imposed programs and face the control theory fact that the only thing we can teach them is that working hard and following rules will get them what they want (Glasser, 1985).

The reverse of what Glasser is talking about is a defensive classroom setting, in which student and teacher do not support each other's self-worth. They criticize, backbite, and withhold compliments. Each student feels bad and becomes more defensive—withholding important information, covering up problems and mistakes, and avoiding responsibility. Over time, students feel more powerless, unsupported, lonely, and frustrated. According to Glasser (1985), "Control theory states that the worst behaviors we see are chosen by people who have lost control."

To put this theory into practice is to establish a learning environment in which each student feels like a key person in the group and where teacher-student interactions validate and support self-esteem.

The five basic needs of control theory are

- **Love.** Students feel worth and human caring. Warmth and caring are done *with* students, not to or for them.
- **Power.** Students are made to realize that knowledge is power. Winning is among the most effective ways to satisfy the need for power.
- **Freedom.** Students are able to make choices about what they do.

- **Fun.** Students who are able to make choices have fun. Fun is enjoying what one is doing, and that includes making choices.
- **Survival.** Students feel a sense of personal power because they have control over their lives and their choices.

The learner who supports others gets better responses from people, who in turn feel better and do better work. Trust builds, and students become more supportive and validating of each other. All this takes a new approach to teaching.

Effective Teaching

Glasser defined an effective teacher as "one who is able to convince not one-half or three-quarters but essentially *all* of his or her students to do high-quality work in school. This means to work up to his/her capacity so that there is no need to divide students into tracks and reserve a large number of spaces in a low track for those who 'lean on shovels'" (1990).

He also felt that teachers were being treated more and more as nonintellectual things and less and less as capable professionals. As Linda M. McNeil in *Contradictions of Control: School Structure and School Knowledge* stated,

> [Some] reforms render teaching and the curriculum inauthentic. If we are to engage students in learning, we must reverse this process. When school knowledge is not credible to students, they opt out and decide to wait until "later" to learn "what you really need to know." Mechanical teaching processes knowledge in a way that guarantees it will be something other than credible. Centralized curriculum, centralized tests of outcomes, and standardized teacher behaviors can only frustrate those teachers whose passion for teaching has shown students (and the rest of us) what education should be about.

Control theory can persuade teachers to use cooperative learning to replace lecturing and individual seatwork. Cooperative learning works well because it gives students personal power (Glasser, 1986).

The Learning-Team Model

An important element of control theory is the emphasis on cooperative learning. Having each student work as a member of a team satisfies the students' need for power and for belonging, much as team sports instill the excitement and commitment that students display on the field. Cooperative learning also replaces lecturing and individual seatwork, processes that are often counterproductive to real learning.

Synthesis

Changes in health education must come first. Special programs created to address crisis issues like drugs and teen pregnancy almost always cost a lot of money, and they usually have little or no lasting effect on the problem. What we need are health educators who are willing to adopt different teaching practices, which in turn will require a very different way of viewing the whole teaching/learning environment.

The most important part of a strategy to implement change is to realize that to reach the goal we have to alter certain behaviors. Some old behaviors that contribute to the problem need to be eliminated, and some new ones that help reach the goal need to be developed.

The second step in developing a plan for change is to get students to specify their behavioral goals in particular situations. They can't work toward a goal until they specify the things they have to do to reach the goal.

Finally, and probably most important, to get students to want to change their behavior, the teacher must modify his own behavior. Unfortunately, many teachers are unable to do this and, consequently, have difficulty modifying the behavior of their students.

Time Out for Personal Thoughts

Think about two negative health behaviors you would like to change. Identify them, then briefly describe how you would go about improving them.

Negative health behavior:

Change to:

How?:

Negative health behavior:

Change to:

How?:

References

Bandler, Richard, and John Grinder. *Frogs into Princes.* Moab, UT: Real People Press, 1979.

Beck, Aaron. *Depression: Causes and Treatment.* Philadelphia: University of Pennsylvania Press, 1972.

Cassell, Carol. *Swept Away: Why Women Fear Their Own Sexuality.* New York: Simon & Schuster, 1984.

Eliot, T.S. "Little Gidding," in *The Complete Poems and Plays of T.S. Eliot.* New York: Harcourt and Brace, 1952.

Ellis, Albert. "Rational-Emotive Psychotherapy," in D. Arbuckle (ed.), *Counseling and Psychotherapy.* New York: McGraw-Hill, 1967.

___. *Growth through Reason: Verbatim Cases in Rational-Emotive Therapy.* Palo Alto, CA: Science and Behavior Books, 1971.

___, and R. Grieger. *Handbook of Rational-Emotive Therapy.* New York: Springer, 1977.

Farson, Richard E. "How Can Anything that Feels So Bad Be So Good?" *Saturday Review,* 6, September 1969.

Glasser, William. *Reality Therapy.* New York: Harper and Row, 1965.

___. *Control Theory: A New Exploration of How We Control Our Lives.* New York: Harper & Row, 1984.

___. "Discipline Is Not the Problem: Control Theory in the Classroom." *Theory into Practice,* Autumn 1985.

___. *Control Theory in the Classroom.* New York: Harper & Row, 1986.

___. *The Quality School: Managing Students without Coercion.* New York: Harper & Row, 1990.

James, Muriel, and John James. *Passion for Life: Psychology and the Human Spirit.* New York: Dutton, 1991.

Lange, A., and P. Jakubowski. *Responsible Assertive Behavior: Cognitive/Behavioral Procedures for Trainers.* Champaign, IL: Research Press, 1976.

Lawson, Annette, and Deborah L. Rhode. *The Politics of Pregnancy: Adolescent Sexuality and Public Policy.* New Haven: Yale University Press, 1993.

McNeal, Linda M. *Contradictions of Control: School Structure and School Knowledge.* New York: Routledge, 1986.

Meier, Daniel. "Take Children's Opinions Seriously: A Talk with Bruno Bettelheim." *Teacher,* August 1990.

Mowrer, O. Hobart. "Foreword," in W. Glasser, *Reality Therapy.* New York: Harper & Row, 1965.

Rogers, Carl. *On Becoming a Person: A Therapist's View of Psychotherapy.* Boston: Houghton Mifflin, 1961.

Sanford, Linda T., and Mary Ellen Donovan. *Women and Self-Esteem: Understanding and Improving the Way We Think and Feel about Ourselves.* New York: Penguin Books, 1985.

Viscott, David. *Risking.* New York: Pocket Books, 1977.

___. *Cognitive Therapy and the Emotional Disorders.* New York: International University Press, 1976.

Additional Resources

Baranowski, Tom. "Beliefs as Motivational Influences at Stages in Behavioral Change." *International Quarterly of Community Health Education,* 1992–93.

Currie, Elliot. *Reckoning: Drugs, the Cities, and the American Future.* New York: Hill and Wang, 1993.

Greene, L.W. "Modifying and Developing Health Behavior." *Annual Review of Public Health,* 1984.

Jonas, Gerald. *Visceral Learning: Toward a Science of Self-Control.* New York: Viking Press, 1973.

Payne, Buryl. *Getting There without Drugs: Techniques and Theories for the Expansion of Consciousness.* New York: Ballantine Books, 1973.

Shore, Ira. *Empowering Education: Critical Teaching for Social Change.* Chicago: University of Chicago Press, 1992.

Hundreds of statements have been made about the purpose of health education. But the best statement must come from you, the health educator. So ask yourself these questions:

- Why am I here?
- Where am I going?
- What is the purpose of what I am doing?

These questions have in common a longing for a sense of purpose in health education. As health educators, we have an insatiable need for assurance that what we are doing has meaning. Our dilemma is that we have been thrust into a world in which health's meaning and our educational response to it has been diminished by a system in which our choices may not be motivated so much by what is healthy but by what is quick and easy.

Novelist Walker Percy warns that it is the time of *thanatos*—of the living dead—in which "people who seem to be living lives which are good by all sociological standards . . somehow seem to be more dead than alive. . . . There is something worse than being deprived of life: it is being deprived of life and not knowing it" (Percy, 1991).

We all need to know that what we are doing has some spiritual, intellectual, behavioral, and physiological importance in the lives of those we are working with. Thus, the quest for meaning as a goal gets to the essence of what health education is all about.

Clarity of Purpose

The essential ingredient of an effective educational program is the clarity of a teacher's goals. Many health educators don't know what kind of classroom they want or to what particular goals they should

To be human is to keep rattling the bars of the cage of existence hollering: "What's it for?"

—ROBERT FULGHUM

**Time Out
for Personal
Thoughts**

How would you respond to the question, "What is health education all about?"

direct themselves. Safe sex, drug-free kids, and violence-free environments are all issues that demand a clear educational purpose.

How can you create a specific learning objective when you aren't certain how a learner needs to grow? What sometimes happens is the health-education experience gets watered down to the lowest common denominator. Teachers often feel constrained when addressing a limited number of behavioral skills. Some teachers focus on isolated lessons and activities whose effects frequently undercut each other.

Let me present you, the teacher, with a situation requiring you to set certain goals. Remember, you want to start with the principal goal—the outcome of your lesson.

You must teach a lesson on AIDS/HIV to a high-school class. The principal goal of many teachers would be to teach the facts rather than further the students' awareness of their at-risk behaviors. But all of health education must begin where students are. Students will be interested in learning when they realize that they have a stake in the outcome of the learning process, and when they recognize that what they learn today impacts how they live (and behave) tomorrow. In the film *Stand and Deliver*, Jaime Escalante made no secret of the amount of work that would be involved if his students were to pass the advanced placement exam in calculus, but since the work was need-satisfying, most of his students were willing to go the extra mile to do it. As Glasser states in *The Quality School* (1990),

> *I am not saying that what happens outside of us means nothing; far from it. What happens outside of us has a lot to do with what we choose to do, but the outside event does not cause our behavior. What we get, and all we ever get, from the outside is information; how we choose to act on this information is up to us. Therefore, the information that students get from the teacher, which includes how this information is given, is very important . . . but the students are the ones who make the ultimate judgment about how important it is to them. The more important they think it is, the more they will do what they are asked and the better they will do it.*

Establishing Goals

One way to establish goals that are need-satisfying and, therefore, realistic and acceptable to all is to involve students in the process. You don't believe students want more involvement? A recent survey conducted in the Boston public schools showed that students wanted to evaluate their teachers and help decide controversial issues such as condom distribution in schools. And, despite public perceptions to the contrary, they want more challenging work (Robinson, 1992).

The Youth Mobilization Project in Roxbury, Massachusetts, encouraged young people to get involved in school activities and governance. During the summer, the students were paid a small stipend to conduct a survey of other students and community members that focused on improving teaching and the curriculum and on dealing with racist educators. The survey showed that more than 80 percent of the student respondents wanted classes that dealt with AIDS prevention, drug use, and violence, while 61 percent supported a multicultural curriculum. Fifty-two percent of the respondents said the system for evaluating teachers needed revamping, while 44.5 percent said that teachers who exhibit racist behavior should be fired (Robinson, 1992).

What all this says is that education today needs to become participatory. Students want to have input. We also need to minimize the teaching of rote cultural practices and the mastery of isolated facts. Instead, we should strive to help students attain a rich understanding of the concepts and principles underlying bodies of knowledge. In essence, the student who deeply understands a concept has the capacity to explore its meaning using complementary and personal methods. The test of understanding (as opposed to the test for knowledge of facts) involves neither repetition of information nor performance of mastered practices. Rather, it involves the appropriate application of concepts to behavioral maintenance and change in the student.

We empower students to make judgments and seek answers that fit them. Good teaching is a collaborative relationship. Reality-based teaching does not and cannot do things *for* the student. The student has to be willing to risk seeing the world a new way and trying something different. As a respected teacher of mine explained to me long ago, it's more like a figure-skating coach or a piano teacher: you suggest changes or things to try, but the *doing* belongs to the learner.

Finding Out Where Students Are

Getting to know where students are prior to teaching a unit in health is essential to successful and meaningful learning. Before you devise an educational goal, you must ascertain the following:

- major student concerns in the area to be discussed
- students' knowledge of the subject
- their attitudes toward the subject
- their behavior in situations related to the subject

Identifying these four areas will give the teacher a better grasp of what the major problem areas might be. This knowledge will, in turn, help the teacher set goals that produce a much more rewarding learning experience. It will also help the teacher allocate time and depth of study specific to the topic under discussion.

All these steps will be covered in more detail later as they relate to a specific health-topic area (e.g., AIDS or sex education).

Shared Expectations

A health-education class should help young people become more health-aware and empowered by involving them in the total classroom process. According to Glasser (1990), this should include

- asking students to make a written evaluation of all their work before turning it in
- posting examples of quality work and encouraging students to judge the quality of their own work
- allowing students to retake an examination they have failed until it is passed
- showing students that grades will be used to empower, never as a weapon or as punishment
- defining the classroom as a place where students believe if they do some work they will satisfy their needs enough so that it makes sense to *keep* working
- providing students with a noncoercive, need-satisfying classroom atmosphere

Realistically, the goals listed above are noble, at best. Yet they are the central determinants of positive behavioral maintenance and change. Research tells us a noncompetitive, shared-goal approach to teaching can make a difference in terms of behavior, and that all students in a noncompetitive classroom have improved self-esteem at the end of study (Read, 1968). However, self-determination and autonomy are not synonymous with self-expression and willfulness. Nor does a permissive environment with the absence of expectations or an authoritarian environment with the absence of freedom promote healthy autonomy. Students should be held to very high expectations and goals.

The Goals to Seek

How can the process of health education drive the formulation of educational goals, curriculum development, instructional strategies, assessment mechanisms, and the motivation and engagement of students? How can we educate so that students make what they learn a meaningful part of their lives and see that positive health choices are life-enhancing? How do we guide the development of character as well as intelligence to enhance students' capacity to experience their feelings and empower them to take control of their health behavior?

No single approach can respond to all the subtleties of learning. Our enthusiasm for new ideas can create new orthodoxies and rigidities, so it is good to be skeptical at the same time that we explore new approaches. Keeping this in mind, the question for the health-educator is when and how to intervene to support the student in the educational process.

Whatever the goals you explore and the process you use to achieve them, the focus must not be on the past so much as on the present and future. Remember, *we are not focusing on pathology but rather on health; we are not focusing on problems but more on possibilities, on the potential of our students for creativity, self-generated ethics, and goal attainment motivated by the positive urges of their own desire to change.* Our goals and objectives *must* be in sync with those with whom we are working. Otherwise, we lose them.

About Goals: Questions to Ask Ourselves

Sometimes the process of education seems to illustrate the classic aphorism about not seeing the forest for the trees; we get so busy teaching the required curriculum that we forget the most important question: What is health education about? Thus, we need to ask ourselves,

- Am I teaching students what they need to know?
- Am I teaching students what they want to know?
- Am I teaching process rather than memory gathering?
- Am I giving students information that is useful for decision making?
- Am I teaching students how to solve interpersonal problems?
- Am I teaching students to think about their own personal health issues?
- Am I teaching students how to learn for themselves?
- Am I teaching cultural relativity?

Meeting Goals through a Comprehensive Program

First, let's define a *comprehensive program*. The 1992 Conference on Comprehensive School Health Education provided us with a good working definition:

> *Comprehensive school-health instruction refers to the development, delivery, and evaluation of a planned curriculum, preschool through grade 12, with goals, objectives, content sequence, and specific classroom lessons, which includes, but is not limited to, the following major content areas: community health, consumer health, environmental health, family life, mental and emotional health, injury prevention and safety, nutrition, personal health, prevention and control of disease, and substance use and abuse* (*Journal of School Health*, 1993).

The following list outlines some characteristics of a comprehensive program.

1. The classroom has defined its basic purpose, goals, and objectives as behavioral outcomes or as additions to behavioral potential.
   a. It uses a taxonomy of objectives that is comprehensive and inclusive of human behavior:
      1. knowledge, generalizations, concepts, and structures
      2. values and attitudes
      3. skills
      4. self-esteem and motivation

5. ability to cope with environmental situations
6. modes and patterns of behavior and self-direction
7. self-realization and self-actualization
   b. It strives toward goals. Although goals are independent, they all cross at a single point: the student. Look for teaching strategies that direct students toward self-evaluation and questioning based on these five tenets:
   1. as *organisms*, we strive toward health
   2. as *psychosocial beings*, we strive toward adjustment
   3. as *moral beings*, we strive toward rightness
   4. as *existential beings*, we strive toward meaning
   5. as *spiritual beings*, we strive toward reconciliation
   c. These goals serve as the basis of a comprehensive school-health instruction program.
2. All the staff involved in health promotion are fully and deeply committed to a holistic-humanistic curriculum in health education as evidenced by the following:
   a. Those involved have fully discussed and explored the concepts of wholeness and humanness as they apply to health education.
   b. Those involved have evaluated and appraised their individual and collective efforts by the criteria of wholeness and humanness.
   c. The entire staff has demonstrated the belief that every human being has the potential for greatness.
   d. There is a commitment to support and engage all faculty in a comprehensive health-instruction program.
3. The students are allowed to become proactive members in the construction of the curriculum and learning environment:
   a. They are given as large a measure of self-direction as is feasible on the basis of their individual educational plans and their self-reliance.
   b. The teacher uses a wide variety of appraisal and personality-study methods to ascertain the talents and capabilities of each student.
   c. The teacher is as free to share feelings during individual and group activities as the student.

In sum, students should be provided a changing and expanding range of choices among the goals they (and the teacher) have selected. Students should be vividly aware that they have options, that they are included in and important to the learning process. A narrative of inquiry should be initiated and every effort given to keeping this personal inquiry open. Each student should be kept aware of his progress toward his goals in an atmosphere of *intrinsic reward*. Above all, the student should be afforded dignity; he must know that teachers and peers believe in him so he can believe in himself.

Synthesis

The classroom atmosphere must be perceived by the students as open and autonomous; that is, they must know they have the freedom and responsibility to pursue the goals that they helped choose. The curriculum in such a classroom can

Time Out for Personal Thoughts

Using the information in this and the previous chapter, how would you go about setting goals for drug education? Be specific.

First, I would:

Second, I would:

Finally, I would:

What specific behaviors do you consider most important in a health-education program? (List ten starting with the *most* important.)

1.
2.
3.
4.
5.
6.
7.
8.
9.
10.

How would you go about identifying goals?

How would you go about determining whether you have reached these goals?

How much of a role should the learner play in goal setting?

come from interactions between students and the teacher, from independent reflective time, or from the scope and range of students' personal interests.

Students should be provided with a changing and expanding range of choices when it comes to setting classroom goals. They should know they have personal responsibility for their education, that their performance is valued, and that learning is an active process. A narrative of inquiry should be initiated and every effort given to keeping this personal inquiry open. Every teacher should be concerned enough with her students to keep them personally aware of their progress in an atmosphere of intrinsic reward.

References

Fulghum, Robert. *All I Need to Know I Learned in Kindergarten.* New York: Villard Books, 1988.

Glasser, William. *The Quality School: Managing Students without Coercion.* New York: Harper & Row, 1990.

Percy, Walker. *Signposts in a Strange Land.* New York: Farrar, Straus and Giroux, 1991.

Read, Donald A. "The Influence of Competitive and Noncompetitive Programs of Physical Education on Body-Image and Self-Concept." Doctoral dissertation, Boston University, 1968.

Robinson, Lauren. "Boston Students Want a Bigger Voice." *Boston Globe,* 23, September 1992.

"The Comprehensive School Health Education Workshop: Background and Future Prospects." *Journal of School Health,* January 1993.

Additional Resources

Auter, Jim. "Closing Session Comments: Making It Work." *Journal of School Health,* January 1993.

Dodd, Anne Wescott. *A Parent's Guide to Innovative Education.* Chicago: Noble Press, 1992.

Kolbe, Lloyd J. "Developing a Plan of Action to Institutionalize Comprehensive School Health Education Programs in the United States." *Journal of School Health,* January 1993.

McGinnis, J. Michael. "Closing Session Comments: Making It Work." *Journal of School Health,* January 1993.

Seffrin, John R. "Opening Session Comments: Laying the Groundwork." *Journal of School Health,* January 1993.

Shor, Ira. *Empowering Education: Critical Teaching for Social Change.* Chicago: University of Chicago Press, 1992.

9 The Working Stage: An AIDS Education Model

When Robert Frost wrote "The Road Not Taken," he may not have had self-management in mind. Yet, the message of his poem surely applies to our present quest. In describing the mechanics of behavioral control, we are presenting students with a choice—a choice between a self-managed life-style and whatever their present orientation is. The self-managed life-style is, by all criteria, the less traveled road. Most people do not even get close to their potential for self-management. They engage in behaviors that are hazardous to their own and others' health, fail to attain important personal goals, and generally experience much unnecessary frustration. Effective self-management is simply not the prevailing life-style in our culture. This chapter describes exactly how a class unit in AIDS education can apply the principles of self-management through the thinking, feeling, and acting model. It also incorporates the work of Lawrence Kohlberg (1967), who theorized that different choices, life-styles, and decisions can be viewed as stages of moral development (see Chapter 11).

As in previous chapters, I wish to stress that it's not enough to stuff information about the dangers of negative health behaviors into students' heads. What the health educator must do—and what we as a society must work to achieve—is to make sure students grow as much personally and emotionally as they do intellectually. Teaching methods that engage students in active learning will help them develop self-esteem and a sense of belonging, qualities that students need to avoid destructive habits and behaviors. Teachers have to encourage students to grow as individuals *at the same time* that they help them to gain academic knowledge and skills.

This is really the most critical chapter for bringing it all together in terms of defining the task of the teacher. The teaching-learning model about AIDS described herein will show educators how to:

Creative people use knowledge we all have and make the leap that allows them to see things in new ways.

—Bobbi DePorter and Mike Hernacki

- use active learning methods of instruction
- encourage students to discuss sexual behavior with parent(s)
- include activities that address the social and media-related pressures to have sex
- focus on values and moral decision making when teaching about unprotected sex, postponing sex, sexual alternatives, high-risk partners, etc.
- provide interactive activities that give students the opportunity to practice empowering skills

Probably the most underused prevention-strategy program is that of peer education. This as well as other strategies will be the focus of this chapter. As we move forward, you will see all of the strategies described covered in depth.

A Cognitive-Behavioral Approach to AIDS Education

The evidence supporting the effectiveness of a cognitive-behavioral approach to teaching in such critical areas as AIDS is mounting. Often, in the area of AIDS and sex education in general, the dynamics of what and how to teach are determined not so much by needs as by parental and political pressures. For example, one school district in Massachusetts ruled that health educators could discuss AIDS and other STDs via the facts, but they could not mention their being contracted through sexual intercourse. (Condom distribution would be out of the question in such a school.)

An article by R.J. DiClemente entitled "Preventing HIV/AIDS among Adolescents: Schools as Agents of Behavior Change" that appeared in the Journal of the American Medical Association, strongly made the point that " . . . while cognitive, affective, and skills domains are reflective of successful HIV/AIDS behavior-change programs, only three states currently provide school-based programs that address all three domains. Condom use skills, in particular, are often omitted and seldom practiced" (DiClemente, 1993). Students need to be more involved (via behavioral expression) if any preventive program in AIDS is to be successful.

Educational Note: Contraceptive Education

America is particularly afflicted with an exaggerated need to avoid adequate contraceptive education and practical help. Carole Joffe (1986) produced a devastating examination of the taboos against mentioning a condom in American schools. This—at the time of an AIDS epidemic—is shocking to a European audience, in which there is as much sex among teenagers as there is in the United States. That is because Europeans generally have a more wholesome attitude toward sex. They recognize that teenagers are sexually active and give sex education to young people in schools. They also make contraception easily available.

Additionally, Joffe's article cited these important aims of a successful HIV/AIDS program: School-based HIV/AIDS prevention programs need to be implemented before middle/junior-high school—before high-risk behavior patterns become firmly established and students are less amenable to change (AAPCA, 1990); and HIV-prevention programs must be longer in duration (two to three class sessions) if any lasting, concrete behavioral change is to be hoped for (DiClemente, 1993).

A review of the literature (Kirby and DiClemente, 1994; Solomon and DeJong, 1986) gives the following key elements to enhance program effectiveness:

- use social-learning theories as a foundation for your program (e.g., cognitive-behavioral theory or social influence theory)
- maintain a narrow focus on reducing sexual risk-taking behaviors
- provide modeling and practice of communication and negotiation skills
- strive not to be moralistic
- recognize the enormous anxiety AIDS evokes, and develop strategies that acknowledge this stress and provide the means for coping with it
- conduct adequate preliminary research that takes into account existing knowledge, values, attitudes, beliefs, and practices of the specific target population
- focus on underlying attitudes, behavior change, and communication and interpersonal skills development rather than disease etiology or other rote factual information
- make explicit the often complex and obscure relationship between specific behaviors and subsequent health or disease outcomes
- when a given medium allows for elaboration, emphasize not only what to do, but also the precise circumstances under which to do it, the benefits of doing so, and the consequences of failing to do so
- realistically acknowledge the obstacles to change, and build in supports and reinforcements for adopting new behaviors
- without whitewashing the difficulties, establish a positive tone in which fear-arousing information is balanced by constructive suggestions for purposeful action
- strive to characterize the desired behavior as normative by referring to appropriate role models and associating the target behavior with other qualities considered desirable by the target audience
- develop strategies that engender identification between the target audience and the message
- deliver a clear, coordinated, consistent message through a variety of reinforcing channels of communication
- seek out intermediaries who are accessible to the audience and lend credibility to the project's message

What the Working Stage Attempts to Achieve

The major task at this stage is to help students resolve their concerns and move toward more healthy behavior. This may require the teacher to provide emotional support, encouragement, and reinforcement of newly gained insights. She may want to use one particular teaching strategy or a number of different strategies, but they must cover the three major areas necessary to effective cognitive-behavioral teaching. The program must be:

1. Cognitively focused
   a. establish goals
   b. have students take a pretest of cognitive knowledge
   c. have students take a pretest of affective feelings and behaviors
2. Affectively focused
   a. get students personally involved
3. Cognitively focused
   a. present the facts
   b. posttest
4. Affectively focused
   a. discuss the facts
   b. select a goal; consider
      1. measurability of the goal
      2. internal vs. external goals
      3. positive vs. negative goals
   c. deal with feelings
      1. use activities
   d. deal with behaviors
      1. use activities

The program should also include a pretest to ascertain how students think and feel about the subject.

Establishing Goals

First and foremost, goal setting should be collaborative. In this way, students will feel they are an important part of the process. It will also give them a chance to more closely relate classroom goals for AIDS education to their own reality.

Second, it is important to focus on specific areas about AIDS that you (and the class) want to study. Too often, you may fail to inspire the changes you want because your goals are too abstract and general, and there is no way of adequately evaluating the degree to which your ideas are being taken seriously. Here are some examples of overly general and unmeasurable goals:

- to learn more about HIV/AIDS
- to understand more about how AIDS affects my age group
- to learn how to protect myself from getting AIDS
- to learn how to say no to unprotected sex
- to learn how to say no to sex

While these are legitimate, it would help to break these abstract statements into concrete behaviors that could be focused on in class. For example, "to understand more about AIDS" provides no specific link between understanding and behavior. "To learn how" begs the question. What has learning to do with behavior? We know it has very little to do with behavior, unless (and this is the major qualifier) it is coupled with a corresponding attachment to how one *feels*. Thus, the health educator must focus on ways students react to what is being presented.

Some concrete cognitive and affective goals might include these:

A. Cognitive goals
1. **HIV transmission knowledge.** It has been hypothesized that personal knowledge of the risk factors in HIV transmission is necessary to determine personal risk accurately and to develop perceptions of personal susceptibility (Emmons et al., 1986).
   a. identify and list four ways in which AIDS is contracted
   b. compare effective vs. ineffective methods of AIDS prevention
   c. define at-risk sexual behavior
   d. list factors that identify high-risk individuals
B. Affective goals
1. **Perceived susceptibility.** Although knowledge of behaviors that transmit HIV is of fundamental importance, some individuals, despite high levels of transmission knowledge, feel they are invulnerable to or have successfully fought off HIV infection (Coates et al., 1987).
   a. help students become increasingly sensitive to their own at-risk behavior
   b. let them objectively discuss their at-risk behavior (if any)
   c. have them practice decision-making and peer-resistance skills (Botvin et al., 1980)
   d. increase their self-awareness so they have a chance to make free choices

Giving thought to students' personal goals is a step forward in behavioral teaching, for these goals help students clarify what *they* want from the learning experience and help them frame how *they* will use class time.

Remember, there is value in regularly asking yourself what you and your students want from your course and how well you are using available resources. This can be accomplished easily by having students on occasion write brief comments to you about what is being covered.

Instructional Note: Remain Flexible

While a cognitive-behavioral agenda is useful in focusing on topics and issues to bring up for exploration, it's important to be flexible and remain open to working on new goals and objectives as they come up. Keep an open agenda, one that will allow you to explore whatever issues seem meaningful as you progress in your class. Above all, continue to collect data from students as you move along. For example, suppose you bring up the subject of AIDS having a world impact, and students inform you that they covered this in another class. Instead of rigidly adhering to your agenda, it may be more valuable to you (and the class) to move on to other important issues, which now can be given more time.

Pretesting with a Cognitive Focus

Step one in the cognitive-behavioral process is having students take a pretest of their cognitive knowledge. You should do this before presenting any information. This test of their knowledge need not be long but must relate to their age level. Stress that their responses will not be used in grading and that if they don't know the answer they should guess.

Exercise: Sample test of Cognitive Knowledge

Name: _____ Date: _____

Directions: Respond to each question, even if you need to guess. For the first ten questions, put a check in front of each statement that you think is true.

1. AIDS is caused by a virus.

2. AIDS was not heard of before the 1980s.

3. You cannot get the AIDS virus by kissing a person who has AIDS.

4. You can get the AIDS virus by receiving the blood of a person who has AIDS.

5. You can get the AIDS virus by having sex with a person who has AIDS.

6. The number of children who have AIDS is increasing.

7. When someone has AIDS, his body cannot fight off other diseases.

8. There is no cure for AIDS and no vaccine that prevents the disease.

9. Many people are infected with the AIDS virus but don't know it.

10. People who are infected with the AIDS virus may be able to work or go to school.

Directions: Fill in the blanks or circle the letter of the most appropriate response. NOTE: If you don't know the answer, guess.

11. The acronym AIDS stands for

12. AIDS is a
    a. bacterium
    b. disease
    c. fungus
    d. vaccine
    e. other (list):

13. AIDS is caused by
    a. antibodies
    b. bacteria
    c. a virus

d. a bug bite

e. other (list):

14. HIV is the name of a

    a. blood type
    b. virus
    c. cure for AIDS
    d. vaccine to prevent AIDS
    e. other (list):

15. The only way a doctor can determine if a person has been infected with HIV is by

    a. finding antibodies in a blood sample
    b. determining heart rate
    c. checking urine
    d. taking blood pressure
    e. other (list):

16. HIV attacks cells in the body's ___ system:

    a. digestive
    b. nervous
    c. immune
    d. reproductive
    e. other (list):

17. HIV can be found in which body fluid?

    a. saliva
    b. blood
    c. semen
    d. all of the above
    e. other (list):

Please Respond: For which of these questions did you guess the answer? Circle the number:

1   2   3   4   5   6   7   8   9   10   11   12   13   14   15   16   17

Collect the student responses, again telling them that they are only to help you and them in further classes.

You have now gained information about student knowledge concerning AIDS. Here is an opportunity to focus on cognitive information based on class responses. How much guessing occurred in students' responses? Were their nonguessing responses any more accurate than their guessing responses? Return their pretests to them later in this unit.

Pretesting with an Affective Focus

Here, the object is to gauge students' feelings and behaviors. Step one in this process is having students fill out an attitude-behavioral questionnaire. Unlike the knowledge pretest given earlier, you will want to provide students with an envelope in which to seal their responses. This is important, for you want the most honest responses you can get. Because these questions require personal answers concerning attitudes and behavior, you do not want to inhibit students by suggesting that someone else will see the results. Stress that the questionnaire is for their eyes only. (Note: this test is aimed at the high-school level.)

■
Exercise:
Sample Test
of At-Risk
Behavior

Directions: Circle all answers that apply unless otherwise indicated (you may circle more than one):

1. What do you consider safe sex?

    a. abstinence
    b. monogamous sex with a long-term partner
    c. use of a condom
    d. no anal sex
    e. oral sex only
    f. other (list):

2. Are you afraid that you will contract AIDS?

    a. yes, very concerned
    b. yes, somewhat concerned
    c. no, not at all concerned

3. In general, how much do you worry about becoming HIV positive?

    a. not at all
    b. somewhat
    c. very much
    d. constantly

4. What are your chances of being infected with the AIDS virus?

    a. no chance
    b. low
    c. moderate
    d. high
    e. I am currently infected

5. Have your feelings about AIDS changed during the past few years?

    a. no, I've been consistently worried about AIDS
    b. no, I've never been worried about AIDS
    c. yes, I'm more worried than ever

d. yes, I'm tired of hearing about it

e. yes, I want to hear more about it

6. Have you ever had your blood tested for the AIDS virus?

a. yes, more than once

b. yes, once

c. no, but I'm considering it

d. no, I probably never will

7. How do you feel about casual sex?

a. it's morally wrong

b. it's much too dangerous

c. it's okay if you take precautions

d. it's not a problem because (fill in the blank):

8. How do you feel about casual sex within your age group?

a. it's morally wrong

b. it's much too dangerous

c. it's okay if you take precautions

d. it's not a problem because (fill in blank):

9. If you were considering having sexual intercourse, which of the following would you do concerning your partner?

a. discuss your sexual history

b. ask him or her whether he or she has AIDS

c. request that he or she be tested for AIDS

d. trust your judgment

e. not have sex

f. have yourself tested

g. none of the above; I don't even think about AIDS

h. none of the above (but I would do this):

10. Do you carry condoms with you or use them?

a. yes, I carry them and use them

b. yes, I keep them but do not always use them

c. yes, but not consistently

d. no

11. Have you considered or changed your sexual behavior to avoid exposing yourself to AIDS?

a. yes

b. no

(continued)

c. no, but I'm considering it

d. no, and I'm not considering it

e. does not apply; I am not sexually active

12. If you have changed your sexual behavior or are considering it to avoid AIDS, you would

a. not applicable

b. limit sexual contact to one sex partner

c. take more time and care in my choice of a sex partner

d. avoid sex

e. avoid homosexual or lesbian sex

f. refuse surgery that would require a blood transfusion

g. not use intravenous drugs

h. take other precautions (fill in the blank):

Getting Students Personally Involved

Before presenting cognitive material, you need to get students personally involved in the subject under discussion. The idea behind this is that by getting students personally involved you are often able to isolate particular elements of student concern that you may not have been aware of. And, although you must make the ultimate judgments concerning cognitive information, student input must be considered. The following technique can make this process easier.

Exercises for the Classroom

Exercise 1

Take three 3 × 5 index cards. In the upper lefthand side of one of the cards, place a small dot. On the second card, place two small dots. On the third, three dots. Mix these cards in with other cards so that they equal the number of students in your class. On one side of all cards (on the reverse side of the cards with the dots), draw three lines on which students can sign their names. Number these lines 1, 2, and 3. (Complete this prior to class.)

Now, hand out these cards to your students and ask them to find three other students who they would like to have as partners. Each should then sign the other's card.

Now, have the students who signed on line 1 get together to respond to the following question. Give them time to think about it and discuss it.

1. What are the *most* startling facts you know about AIDS?

Now, have the line-2 students get together and discuss question number 2:

2. Do you see the media (i.e., MTV, rock music, movies) as having any influence on the sexual behavior of your age group?

Finally, have line-3 students get together and discuss question number 3:

3. What suggestions do you have for your age group concerning AIDS?

When all the groups have finished, have a whole-class discussion of these questions. Keep the discussion focused on feelings.

Now, ask students to turn over their 3 × 5 cards and look for the single dot in the upper lefthand corner. Ask the student with the dot to come forward and identify those students he had a discussion with (i.e., the group that addressed question 1, 2, or 3). Then, have the student with the two dots come forward and identify his discussion group. Do the same with the student who has the card with three dots.

Now, share these facts:

The student who has the card with one dot has AIDS and has infected those students he had contact with

except

that student with two dots, for he practiced safe sex using a condom,

and

that student with three dots, for she abstained from sex.

Bring the class back to a full circle and discuss the exercise. Open it up to a full range of ideas and feelings. This exercise should open up some critical issues that must be discussed.

Now, it is your turn: What do *you* see as the critical issues brought up by this exercise?

How would you handle a homophobic response from two same-sex students when one found that the other had given him AIDS?

(continued)

Exercise 2: Imagery

Have students in a class sit quietly, get relaxed, and close their eyes. Then play the Bruce Springsteen song "Streets of Philadelphia." Have them imagine that that person Springsteen is singing about is them. After the song is over, allow them time to write down some feelings. Play the song again, having them imagine that he is singing about a loved one. Again, allow them time to write down some feelings. Have them pair up and discuss their feelings about being the person in the song.

Then have them change partners and discuss feelings about it being a loved one. Finally, get the class into a circle and talk about the exercise.

Cognitive Presentation of HIV/AIDS

Once the students have completed the pretests, move on to the knowledge-based aspect of HIV/AIDS education. Remember, you do not want to go over their test responses in class; save that for a posttest at the end of the unit on AIDS.

Here are some creative ways to present cognitive material. Bobbi DePorter and Mike Hernacki (1992) offer some good suggestions for helping people retain factual data. They suggest that people remember information best when it is characterized by these qualities:

- sensory association, especially visual
- emotional context, such as love, happiness, family, and sorrow
- outstanding or different qualities
- intense associations
- personal importance
- repetition

After presenting the factual material, you want to get students interacting creatively with it. *Creative thinking* is very often employed when a solution to a problem cannot be resolved by deductive-reasoning alone. To free the creative potential that is inherent within each person, various methods have been suggested. These include the use of metaphors (Gordon, 1978), lateral thinking (DeBono and DeSaint-Arnaud, 1983), and imagery (Wolpin, Shorr, and Krueger, 1986). Typically, the creative process involves having students recall previous experiences that relate to the issue being discussed (i.e., AIDS). Have students use both analogous and inductive thinking to brainstorm and obtain new insights into situations, problems, or issues (unprotected sex or multiple partners, for example). Break out of the traditional ways of doing things to reach a new and perhaps unconventional solution to the problem. Creative thinking requires a fairly thorough knowledge of the subject by the teacher. For example, an educator who has studied cognitive and behavioral approaches to teaching and who has experience using a variety of its techniques soon discovers that each student is different, and that although one can employ a particular intervention, the application of that intervention often requires novel approaches.

Teachers who want to foster analogous, inductive, and creative thinking in their students can use a variety of methods. Asking students the following questions may help this process:

1. Which fact that you learned affected you the most?
2. What meaning does this information have for you, your boyfriend or girlfriend, and your friends?
3. What suggestions would you offer to avoid the increase in AIDS among teens?
4. If you were asked to teach a class of students who were three years younger than you, what would you emphasize?

Use question 4 again to encourage problem solving. Have students brainstorm to generate as many ideas as possible. Then ask some open-ended questions to foster imaginative new lines of thought. (The ideas can be a little wild, fragmented, unconnected, or unconventional.) Instruct students to defer judgment on all of the responses. The emphasis is to break out of the typical ways of thinking and open students up to new thought patterns.

Instructional Note

If you plan on using a video to add to your presentation of cognitive information, be sure it is presented interactively. Interactive videos enable students to get actively involved in what is being viewed. To facilitate this, first preview the film (you may have to do this more than once), picking out situations, questions, moral issues, statistics, or subtle facts that can be discussed during or after the film. You may want to write them down and present them to students as a typed list of questions and issues to look for as they view the film. Leave space for them to write down their responses. When the film is finished (or during a pause), have a class or small-group discussion of their observations.

You may also want to develop in students both cognitive and affective knowledge about what is being presented. Cognitive questions would be factual and specific; affective questions might ask students, "What would you do or say? How would you feel? How would you change the script?"

Posttest: Cognitive Knowledge

Have students take a posttest (the same as the pretest), and go over the answers. Be careful not to judge or allow emphasis to be placed on correct or incorrect responses. The idea is that students learn from the responses and the coverage of the material.

Classroom arrangement should, if possible, be done in a group fashion (students and teacher sitting in a circle). Major emphasis should be on students' questions regarding pre- and posttest results. Most of all, you want to deal with questions in which students guessed at answers. You want to find out what their guesses were based on (if anything).

Finally, ask students to identify those areas in which they feel they would like further information. You can do this through class questioning or through student communication via personal letter.

Summary

These strategies are based on the concept that human beings are rational and their cognitive processes exert a strong influence on all their endeavors. Cognitively focused strategies are designed to help students acquire and retain accurate and relevant factual information; learn how to choose among alternative courses of action to make satisfactory decisions and solve personal problems; learn to think more logically about themselves and the world around them; and use their resources in more analogous, inductive, and creative ways. As the teacher, your major function will be to help the student learn new material and different ways of handling various situations.

Affective Presentation of HIV/AIDS

As was presented in previous chapters, active participation by students involves cognitive as well as affective development. Empowering education is not merely rationalistic, as Peter Elbow (1986) argued in a critique of Freire's (1970, 1973, 1978, 1987) work.

Don't think that cognitive and affective teaching are like black and white. To work, they both have thinking, feeling, and behavioral elements, as does traditional, teacher-centered education. This is because all education is a social experience (Dewey, 1963).

In affective teaching, where the focus is on feeling and acting, the general approach to a topic such as AIDS is somewhat different from the customary convergent approach to subject studies. The methodology focuses around learning by doing—relating cognitive information to the student's life-style, teaching her how to learn, and, more importantly, developing her decision-making skills based on how she feels and what she wants to do. In this stage of teaching, the teacher is basically an organizer who selects problems of interest to students, helps them to plan an attack on the problems, and provides suitable materials and guidance to enable them to make satisfying progress.

This process also helps in the development of what William Glasser (1986) called the learning-team model, where students working in groups strive for common goals or objectives. It renders a great service to students if we, as teachers, can provide an environment in which they can not only discover their gifts but also develop them. (The author recommends one text that presents the concept of cooperative learning extremely well: Philip Abrami's book, *Using Cooperative Learning.*)

A Starting Point

Don't let the cognitive information you've passed along dwell out there somewhere. Instead, bring it right into the process of dealing with feelings and behaviors. Start with an exercise that touches on the cognitive information with which you introduced the subject, and bring it into a group-centered process whereby students interact with the material presented. See the exercise that follows for an example.

Exercise: Multisensory Imagery

In this exercise, several sensory images are suggested to both sides of the brain (thinking and feeling). These include images of sight, hearing, taste, smell, and touch. It is designed to make students more aware of their senses.

Have students sit in a comfortable position, close their eyes, and focus on their breathing. (Pause.)

As they breath at a relaxed rate, ask them to release any tension in their body, so they're feeling more and more relaxed. (Pause.)

Now have students focus their attention on their brain, imagining how wonderful it is and how much control they have over it. (Pause.)

Then have them focus on the left side of their brain (the abstract-logic side), and ask them to think about those times in which they allowed themselves to be influenced by another person, even when they knew it was wrong, hurtful, or against their values. Ask them to focus on one specific situation. (Pause.)

Next, have them focus on the right side of their brain (the holistic, feeling side), and ask them to think about how they felt in that situation, and how they felt after. (Pause.)

Now have them assign a negative and a positive feeling to each side of their brain; that is, what side of their brain felt good about the situation, and which side felt bad? Or, did both sides feel good (or bad)? Start with the left (thinking) part of the brain. Now move to the (holistic, feeling) right side. How do they feel about their reactions? (Pause)

Have students go back to their left side. Given all the information they now have, how would they have responded? (Pause.)

Now have them move to the right side. Given the same information, how do they feel? (Pause.)

(continued)

Ask your students to let those images go, and imagine that their bodies and their minds are one. Have them imagine they are in total control of both. Let them feel that sense of power. (Pause.)

When the exercise is over, have students sit in a circle and share their imagery (or parts of it) with the rest of the class.

The critical issue is to keep the students involved in what they have cognitively learned by placing it within their reality, involving them in the process and keeping them involved. Here you are not just a teacher, but a therapist, coach, gatekeeper, and friend all in one. You must accept dual roles if you hope to be effective. This process is about the positive and negative feelings students can develop toward the educational process. In positive educational environments, the classroom encourages students' input, is student driven, is student focused, and is about their reality. As we move on, give the following ideas some consideration. How would you feel about a class in which the majority of students decided *against* your opinion or ideas? For example, suppose your students believed

- AIDS is really a gay/lesbian issue
- AIDS has to do with older, sexually promiscuous people
- AIDS simply can't happen to me
- condoms are an embarrassment

How would you respond to these beliefs?

Your Responses

AIDS is really a gay/lesbian issue:

AIDS has to do with older, sexually promiscuous people:

AIDS simply can't happen to me:

Condoms are an embarrassment:

Using these four questions, ask the class to divide themselves into four groups, each discussing one of these statements. Tell them that their choice of topic should be based on their interest in the outcomes of the discussion. Have them compare and contrast their different opinions and thinking their way through to their own conclusions.

Using this process to develop a classroom discussion may seem limited to some, but you must start from a small bit of information before you move on to more important, personal discussion. You, the teacher, must remain impartial so you do not sway or direct the discussion. With this goal in mind, the teacher helps students

- learn the facts about AIDS (cognitive presentation)
- consider all points of view concerning AIDS, identify the assumptions behind the different viewpoints, and identify the values behind the assumptions
- identify three main points that impact on their well-being with regard to AIDS

For all of these goals, the class interaction should be focused on problem solving in ways that foster high levels of respect and responsibility. This requires a number of teaching techniques such as role-playing, in which students are asked to act out a situation they feel strongly about; a class project on AIDS; creating an AIDS education book; and a discussion of the pros and cons of condom use.

Role-playing: Developing Positive Assertiveness

Role-playing is an effective way of preparing for the real thing. There is merit in getting the feel for a new behavior before attempting that behavior in an actual situation. If role-play is too advanced, you can always engage the class in covert reinforcement exercises. For example, you can have them imagine themselves in a sexual situation in which they must assert themselves; then have them imagine the positive social and personal consequences and their sense of establishing and maintaining personal boundaries.

Discuss the final question in Exercise 1, paying attention to the positive results of the behavior behind each reason as they relate to AIDS prevention. What does it take to live up to the list? Is it realistic?

Interactive Video

The film *Philadelphia* with Tom Hanks and Denzel Washington can be used as a classic example of how the issue of AIDS hits home personally. To use this film, teachers must develop the interactive script discussed earlier—a set of questions to give to the viewer prior to showing the film. The time spent is worth it, for what you have is an interactive-video learning experience that will capture your audience and provide some very critical discussion of AIDS discrimination. (See Appendix E.)

A new way of doing something may feel unusual for some students in the beginning, just as adapting to a new situation or a new way of learning does. With

Exercise 1:	Have students pair up (boy/girl) and sit facing each other. Odd-numbered stu-
Role-Playing	dent(s) can act as observers and discuss their observations. Ask students to take
	the role of first-date partners. Have the girl take the role of sexual aggressor, and
	the boy takes the role of resister.

When they are done, have them reverse the roles. Give each the same amount of time.

Now, ask the class to sit in a circle and discuss which role was most realistic, what was learned, how they felt about their roles. Have students who did not partici-pate share their observations.

Ask the girls what their usual coping style is for dealing with unwanted sexual advances.

Withdrawal: putting off any action that would reduce the pressure for sex (i.e., can we talk about this later?).

Helplessness: the person simply freezes and hides. As a consequence, she never gets what *she* wants, thus never experiences a sense of personal power.

Fear of rejection: the girl gives in because she fears that if she doesn't, the boy will go find some girl who will.

Empowered: the girl can say no, because her action is based on what *she* feels is right for her.

Conclude by having the whole group come up with ten of the best reasons why they should not have sex (a) on a first date, and (b) on subsequent dates.

continued use of role-playing, it comes more naturally to students. But, while the feeling of unusualness lasts, students often get something extra. It's easier to be aware of what's going on inside when first learning something, before it becomes routine. The intense awareness can be a rich event.

Another exercise you might try may seem small, but big learning often comes from small lessons. As Lao-tzu said, "big things of the world can only be achieved by attending to their small beginnings . . . a tower nine stories high begins with a heap of earth" (1961).

Follow-up

Ask students to assess their AIDS risk level using the scale that follows. You do not want to collect the data. Let the students know this evaluation is private, and that it is meant to help them get in touch with themselves.

Exercise 2:
Role-playing

Invite five students from the class to play out roles within their school:

1. principal
2. health-education teacher
3. nurse
4. concerned parent
5. student representative

Second, establish a committee of concerned students (from eight to ten) who want a very realistic, unconstrained approach to AIDS education in their school that includes how to use a condom, condom availability for students, etc. Have this group get together after class and come up with a "Bill of AIDS Rights to Know," which they will present to the above "staff." Have the group select one spokesperson to present their list.

Give them an acceptable amount of time to present their requirements for an AIDS education program. Ask them to be specific and to back up their request with some specific data related to their age group. During all of this, you want nonparticipating students to be observant but not to comment, just listen.

When the student committee is finished, let the role-play staff respond to the student presentation. After they have done so, call for a short period of give and take. At some point, shut down the debate and ask the observing students to make comments (during this time, participants should not make comments). Finally, ask nonparticipants to stand behind that person (principal, health teacher, student committee member, etc.) they feel most represented their own feelings. Ask them to share the reasons for their choices. Now open the issue up to a full class discussion.

Exercise:
Assessing
Your AIDS
Risk Level

Thinking not only about AIDS but about all STDs, how would you rate your overall level of risk taking? Circle the number which best represents your risk level.

Low   High

| 1 | 2 | 3 | 4 | 5 | 6 | 7 | 8 | 9 | 10 |

If you feel you're in a high-risk category, reflect on the things in your life that may cause high-risk behavior. Briefly respond to the following questions concerning your risk-taking tendencies.

1. Are you taking too many risks of the wrong kind? (In other words, are you behaving recklessly and foolishly?)

(continued)

2. Although you may not be risking foolishly, you may be taking psychological risks that prevent you from having more meaningful and satisfying relationships. Is this true of you? How?

3. In what way (if any) would you like to change your risk behavior(s)?

4. Finally, what's stopping you?

My Personal Values and Priorities Checklist

What priorities to counteract your risk-taking behavior do you want to set? In other words, of the various risks you are now taking, which would you like most to address? To help you to focus more specifically on some life goals, fill out the checklist using the scale provided. On the space next to each item listed, write the number that reflects its importance to you.

Scale

0 = not important at all
1 = minimally important
2 = somewhat important
3 = quite important
4 = extremely important

In my life I want

1. ____ gratifying relationships
2. ____ the peace of mind that comes from knowing myself fully
3. ____ to shape and lead my life as I choose
4. ____ to practice healthy/safe sex
5. ____ an opportunity to settle down with one partner
6. ____ to change the way I am sexually
7. ____ the self-assurance that comes with being true to who I am and what I value
8. ____ to not rely on others to choose what I do or feel
9. ____ to be comfortable enough with myself to let others know who I really am
10. ____ to understand that what I have been is not what I am or can become
11. ____ to feel I can say no to sex without fearing guilt or loss
12. ____ what others? list:

Sample Questionnaires

Sample questionnaires can help the teacher formulate a general set of questions about a topic, which, in turn, can provide an agenda for discussion. After the class fills out the questionnaire, ask students to sit in a circle and discuss their answers. This can be in specific terms or in general ones (e.g., What did this questionnaire make you think about in your own life?). Discuss the questionnaire in depth, for if you don't, students will begin to feel they aren't important and will not take them seriously.

Time Out for Personal Thoughts

How do you, the reader, rate your own knowledge of AIDS? In making this inventory, respond quickly with your most honest reaction. Indicate your response by circling the corresponding letter. You may choose more than one response for each item or, if none of the responses fits you, you may write in your own response.

1. How would you identify your first awareness of AIDS?
   a. Reading or hearing about it in the media
   b. Learning about it in classes
   c. Being confronted with it in a personal way
   d. Learning about it from my peers
   e. Other:

2. How would you evaluate your first reaction to AIDS?
   a. No reaction at all
   b. Somewhat concerned
   c. Very concerned
   d. It changed my life-style somewhat
   e. I have been forever affected by it
   f. Other:

3. How have you been motivated to change your life-style?
   a. I have been motivated by what I am doing
   b. I have been motivated by what my friends are doing
   c. I have been motivated by what my peers are doing
   d. I have been motivated by what I have learned (e.g., through school, TV, reading)
   e. Other:

(continued)

4. Given the amount of information on AIDS, have you changed *your* sexual behavior in any way?
   a. Did not need to
   b. Not at all
   c. Somewhat
   d. Totally
   e. Other:

Look over your responses, and then decide which of the following questions are meaningful for you.

1. Suppose you are an elementary-school student who has received current information on AIDS. How do you think it would affect your attitudes and behavior?

Answer the same question, imagining you are a high-school student.

2. What effect, if any, has AIDS education had on you?

3. If you do not like the kind of AIDS education that is currently offered in your school, what would you suggest?

4. What do you see as the really important issues that should be addressed in AIDS education?

5. What do you see as the one major behavior that *must* be addressed in AIDS education?

Your responses reveal a bit about you, your attitude toward certain information, and your own learning style. If you were brought up in an environment in which AIDS was not a problem, you will probably not see it as a personal problem today. But if you were a product of a high-risk environment, you are likely to be more sensitive to the issue and more aggressive about teaching it.

What is critical for teachers is that they go beyond merely repeating what they know or what they have been taught. Anyone is capable of overcoming limits *if they can openly examine them*. Participatory classroom teaching allows that to happen. Productive learning must be a social experience (Dewey, 1963).

In-Class Projects

A Class Project on Aids Education. Tell students that their class has been selected to establish an AIDS education program for students three grades below them. This curriculum should be structured in such a way that it will take up at least three standard class periods. Tell the students that they can choose from one of four teams dealing with different aspects of the AIDS education project.

Team 1: This group will work on the informational aspect of the curriculum. The facts about AIDS must be appropriate to the age, grade level, and culture of the students they are targeting. This is the cognitive aspect of the educational program. It must be short but precise and factual (i.e., five-to-ten minutes).

Team 2: This group will develop a series of questions, experiences, and activities that will actively involve the younger students in the various issues surrounding AIDS.

Team 3: This group will develop an age-appropriate knowledge, attitudes, and behavior checklist for the students.

Team 4: This group will develop age-appropriate goals and objectives for the program. These should be clear and concise, and include concrete methods for achieving them (activities, tests, etc.).

Each group should be given the opportunity to present their material to the younger class. Opportunity for questions and interaction must also be provided.

Creating an AIDS Education Book for Elementary-School Children. Another class project is to have your students develop and produce an AIDS education booklet for elementary-school children. This book will provide your students with experience in creative thinking, interviewing, writing and drawing, as well as researching AIDS facts for younger children. Begin by breaking the class into three groups:

Group 1: These students will compile factual knowledge about AIDS for the elementary level and write it in age-appropriate language. They may want to test their material by presenting it to some elementary-school children and modifying where necessary.

Group 2: These students will develop age-appropriate questions to be used as a pre- and posttest of students' knowledge. Again, they may want to try out their questions on elementary-school students.

Group 3: These students will provide drawings to help elementary-school children better understand how AIDS is contracted, how it affects the body, etc. Here students can elicit elementary-school children to do some of the drawings with their guidance.

This booklet should be put together, edited, and produced by the students and then actually presented for publication, with the hope it will be used in the local elementary school.

Additional Activities

A number of other activities can stimulate students' thinking, feeling and acting. These include:

- **Changing the learning environment.** Break away from the classroom so students realize that learning takes place anywhere and everywhere. Try taking them to a halfway house for AIDS patients, to an AIDS clinic, etc.
- **Having kids talk to kids.** Find (or have students find) some young people who have AIDS to talk to the class. It is important here that students can relate to them. It gives them a sense that AIDS is not only for "old" people, and that they, too, can get AIDS.
- **Having students make their own AIDS-awareness film.** In this age of camcorders, invite students to make a video that can be used by other classes. It is important that you, the teacher, leave this as unstructured as possible. Let the students figure out what and how they want to do this.
- **Using interactive video.** Allow students to either view the film *Philadelphia* in class or request that they rent the film. Provide them with a series of questions concerning the film that requires them to interact with it. (For more on interactive video, see Appendix E.)

Synthesis

Lewis and Lewis (1977) pointed out that it is naive to assume any one program or set of services will be sufficient to improve a situation. While a program of AIDS education can be useful, it does not attack larger, institutional issues such as the media, which extols free, unprotected sex. Similarly, developing a more participatory program in AIDS education does not solve all educational concerns. What is needed is a set of multifaceted services shaped to meet the needs of a particular group of people that is amenable to change as the group matures and develops. A true school or community health-education approach must consider remediation of problems, but its major thrust must be positive health behavior achieved through a psychoeducational, preventive, value-oriented, and self-esteem–building point of view.

References

Abrami, Philip C., et al. *Using Cooperative Learning*. Montreal, Quebec: Centre for the Study of Classroom Process, Concordia University, 1993.

Botvin, Gilbert, A. Eng, and C. Williams. "Preventing the Onset of Cigarette Smoking Through Life Skills Training," *Preventive Medicine,* January, 1980.

Coates, T., et al. "AIDS Antibody Testing: Will it Stop the AIDS Epidemic? Will it Help Those Infected with HIV?" in Joseph A. Catania, Susan M. Kegeles, and Thomas J. Coates, "Towards an Understanding of Risk Behavior: An AIDS Risk Reduction Model (ARRM)." *Health Education Quarterly,* Spring 1990.

Committee on Adolescence. "Contraception and Adolescents," American Academy of Pediatrics. *Pediatrics,* July 1990.

DeBono, E., and M. DeSaint-Arnaud. *The Learning-to-Think Coursebook.* Larchmont, NY: DeBono Resource Center, 1983.

DePorter, Bobbi, and Mike Hernacki. *Quantum Learning.* New York: Dell, 1992.

Dewey, John. *Experience and Education.* New York: Collier, 1963.

DiClemente, R.J. "Preventing HIV/AIDS among Adolescents: Schools as Agents of Behavior Change." *Journal of the American Medical Association,* 11, August 1993.

Elbow, Peter. *Embracing Contraries: Explorations in Learning and Teaching.* New York: Oxford University Press, 1986.

Emmons, Kim, et al. "Psychosocial Predictors of Reported Behavior Change in Homosexuals at Risk for AIDS." *Health Education Quarterly,* Winter 1986.

Freire, Paulo. *Pedagogy of the Oppressed.* New York: Seabury, 1970.

___. *Education for Critical Consciousness.* New York: Seabury, 1973.

___. *Pedagogy in Process.* New York: Continuum, 1978.

___, and Donald Macedo. *Literacy: Reading the Word and the World.* Westport, CT: Greenwood, Bergin-Garvey, 1987.

Glasser, William. *Basic Concepts of Reality Therapy.* Los Angeles: Institute for Reality Therapy, 1986.

Gordon, D. *Therapeutic Metaphors.* Cupertino, CA: Meta Publishers, 1978.

Joffe, Carole. *The Regulation of Sexuality: Experiences of Family Planning Works.* Philadelphia: Temple University Press, 1986.

Kirby, D., and R.J. DiClemente. "School-based Behavioral Intervention to Prevent Unprotected Sex and HIV among Adolescents," in R.J. DiClemente and J.L. Peterson (eds.), *Preventing AIDS: Theories and Methods of Behavioral Interventions.* New York: Plenum, 1994.

Kohlberg, Lawrence. "Stage and Sequence: The Cognitive Developmental Approach to Socialization," in D. Goslin (ed.), *Handbook on Socialization Theory and Research.* Skokie, IL: Rand McNally, 1967.

Lathem, Edward Connery (ed.). *The Poetry of Robert Frost.* New York: Holt, Rinehart and Winston, 1967.

Lewis, Judy, and Michael Lewis. *Community Counseling: A Human Services Approach.* New York: Wiley, 1977.

Paul K.J. Sih, (ed.). Lao-tzu, *Tao the ching* (John C.W. Wu, trans.). New York: St. John's University Press, 1961.

Solomon, Mildred Zeldes, and William DeJong. "Recent Sexually Transmitted Disease Prevention Efforts and Their Implications for AIDS Health Education." *Health Education Quarterly,* Winter 1986.

Wolpin, M., J. Shorr, and L. Krueger (eds.). *Imagery.* New York: Plenum, 1986.

Additional Resources

Brown, Larry K., Lynn Ann Reynolds, and Allan J. Brenman. "Out of Focus: Children's Conceptions of AIDS." *Journal of Health Education,* July/August 1994.

Clark, Noreen M., et al. "Self-Regulation of Health Behavior. The 'Take PRIDE' Program." *Health Education Quarterly,* Fall 1992.

Coates, Thomas J. "Strategies for Modifying Sexual Behavior for Primary and Secondary Prevention of HIV Disease." *Journal of Consulting and Clinical Psychology,* 1990.

Columbia Tristar Home Video. *Philadelphia.* Rated PG-13. Available on videocassette.

Kennedy, Cassondra Jeanne, Claudia K. Probart, and Steve M. Dorman. "The Relationship between Random Knowledge, Concern, and Behavior and Health Values, Health Locus of Control, and Preventive Health Behaviors." *Health Education Quarterly,* Fall 1991.

Kingery, Paul M., et al. "The Health Teaching Self-Efficacy Scale." *Journal of Health Education,* March/April 1994.

Petosa, Rick, and Kirby Jackson. "Using the Health Belief Model to Predict Safer Sex Intentions among Adolescents." *Health Education Quarterly,* Winter 1991.

Wallerstein, Nina, and Edward Bernstein. "Empowerment Education: Freire's Ideas Adapted to Health Education." *Health Education Quarterly,* Winter 1988.

Walter, Heather J., and Roger D. Vaughn. "AIDS Risk Reduction among a Multiethnic Sample of Urban High School Students." *Journal of the American Medical Association,* 11 August 1993.

Wolfe, Geraldine F. "AIDS Education: How Can We Make It More Effective?" *Journal of Health Education,* May/June 1995.

10 The Termination Stage

Termination is the fifth and final stage in the cognitive-behavioral teaching process. This is an extremely important period in which you will need to focus on accomplishing three interrelated tasks: helping students understand what their responses to the unit meant to *them;* testing to establish grades (performance-based education); and fostering student growth after the class unit has been completed.

Ask yourself, Have you ever been harshly judged by a teacher? If so, how did you feel? Have you ever studied for an examination, *really* studied, and then flunked? Again, how did you feel?

Few things steal more vitality or cast a darker shadow on our lives than failing, being critically judged, or being made to feel that we have produced less than others. To see this for yourself, spend a day being attentive to the judgments and put-downs you hear people make. How do they affect the atmosphere and mood of a situation? How does the judging and condemning affect the people around you? How do *you* feel when you receive a low grade on an examination?

This final stage is about evaluation, but, more important, evaluation that leads to positive growth and feelings of self-worth. *A successful health-education program must have a measurable impact on knowledge and behavior.* Any program that does not is of little value.

The idea that someone is evaluated (and possibly flunked) on her academic performance only is simply unacceptable. Like the whole learning process preceding evaluation, evaluation *must* consider the cognitive-behavioral learning process.

As has been stressed throughout this text, new pedagogical methods of evaluation aimed at involving students on a personal level is the goal. This involves evaluating creative and critical-thinking skills by having students write plays and skits, develop their own

> *Grades must be used to empower, never as a weapon or as punishment.*
>
> —William Glasser

evaluation methods, role play, or practice cooperative learning, all of which lead them to make the positive choices so critical in health education today.

Both teacher and student should be involved in the process of inventing methods of evaluation that allow for the democratic process to be present in the classroom. Some guidelines for establishing a democratic environment in which the critical element is positive cognitive-behavioral change are

implementing an evaluation process that focuses on student-centered, cooperative learning

establishing an assessment process that includes

- performance-based evaluation
- narrative grading
- portfolio evaluation
- group projects
- class behavior
- individual exhibitions
- essay expressions that promote critical thinking

Academic expertise is structured *into* student experience, not set ahead of or separate from it. "The first approach to any subject in school," wrote John Dewey (1966), "if thought is to be aroused and not words acquired, should be as unscholastic as possible." Isolating health-education subject matter from the student's reality is the first mistake that most teachers make when establishing evaluation criteria. The premise of reality-based education (that what you teach must relate to the learner's reality and thus must be sensitive to his needs and interests) must also relate to evaluation (Glasser, 1990).

Performance-based Evaluation

In the 1990s, students are measured not by what they recall but by how they show what they have learned (Bloom, 1987; Fiske, 1992; Gardner, 1985; Sinetar, 1991). Allan Bloom, who first studied the preponderance of low-order, recall questions, and Howard Gardner, architect of the theory of multiple intelligences, have furthered the trend toward performance-based education—moving away from memorization, paper-and-pencil tests, and traditional grades and letting students demonstrate their know-how.

Performance-based evaluation takes into account students' values, diversity, and ability to make environmentally sound decisions and healthy personal choices. How students react to various issues within the classroom mirrors what they would do in real life. As such, in evaluating students, teachers must incorporate performance-based evaluation along with traditional paper-and-pencil tests.

To begin the evaluation process, you and the students should determine whether the desired goals were met in the unit. The major responsibility for accomplishing this task should be placed on the students. One way of doing this is to ask the students to prepare a report indicating how (and if) the goals were reached. This may entail having the student state how he has changed, what new learning has occurred, or how he is better able to deal with specific situations or significant others with regard to, for example, sex, unprotected sex, or personal values. To consolidate this report with other materials in the unit, the teacher may want students to keep a portfolio of their work (including attendance, participation in class projects, etc.) to be presented to the teacher at the end of the unit.

Evaluating and Analyzing

The purpose of self-evaluation and analyzing is to help students become more aware of themselves and the information they have presented about themselves, to conceptualize and crystallize the patterns that appear in their concerns, and to gain an understanding of the progress they have made during the learning process.

Getting students to do quality work involves inviting them to become a part of the quality process (Glasser, 1990):

- Examples of quality work should be posted for other students to see
- Students should be encouraged to judge what they do and evaluate it
- Students should be encouraged to work in teams when taking examinations
- Students should be encouraged to retake examinations until they are 100-percent correct
- Students should be given the opportunity to develop their own examinations

The following are some important additional points to consider about grading and evaluation.

Use evaluation to help students focus on their individual strengths and progress in school. Remember, every student is good at something, so find that strength and reward it. Good teachers take the time to make each of their students feel like he excels in something.

When students are failing, teachers should take the opportunity to bring student, parent(s), and teacher together to show the student he has adults who support him. Just saying "I know this grade is hard for you" gives the student the sense the teacher is there to help him.

Recognize the power of grades, but downplay them. Teachers should stress learning for knowledge and the joy of learning. In the best of all worlds, the teacher would deemphasize grades and use anecdotal reports.

Don't use grades to reward or punish students or put them in competition with each other.

Use the evaluation period to set new and realistic learning goals. A student who got good grades and enjoyed the unit on AIDS, for example, might decide to go for a higher level of learning.

Take advantage of the grading period to schedule a parent-teacher conference.

Student evaluation should be a learning process in which all students feel they have achieved, learned, and moved forward. Remember, grading is very much tied into self-esteem.

Narrative Grading

Ira Shor defined narrative grading as encouraging "serious dialogue between student and teacher about the quality of the work" (1992). He felt strongly that, in participatory education, there should be a dialogue that goes on between student and teacher, and the teacher should be able to determine from this dialogue the level of the student's knowledge. The dialogue should not be teacher but rather student generated; that is, the student should carry or direct the dialogue.

Narrative grading would certainly include asking students critical questions about the subject matter, but these questions should not only be seeking specific responses; rather, they should elicit a dialogue that includes creative options, critical thinking about alternatives, and short answers in addition to specific answers to specific directives.

Narrative grading is based on a student's ability to integrate new facts into her current knowledge and to discuss these facts in such a way that they are structured into her own experience rather than separate from it. In essence, facts should not be isolated from personal experience. This is a critical factor in health education, and one that the teacher should be prepared to use in evaluating students.

Throughout this process, the teacher should also encourage students to respond to each other's contributions. Ask interactive questions such as "Can we have a reaction to Marci's idea that saying no is what one should do to respect oneself?" or, "Who has a point of view that's similar to or different from Bob's?" Invite all students to participate, and focus on one or two who have some leading ideas that are structured and focused on the point being discussed.

Portfolios

Each individual has a complex and continuous interior language, a constantly flowing stream of words, images, and ideas that needs to be considered a valuable source of evaluation. A portfolio may be able to capture this constant internal flow of information. It differs from a personal diary, which may be a daily written account of activities, yet a portfolio can include a diary. More important, a portfolio can contain written activities completed in class, articles handed out in class, examinations returned, and student self-evaluations. In short, a portfolio can contain anything and everything that the students deem relevant to them, and as such it can be used as an evaluation tool.

Additionally, the portfolio is one of the most useful instruments we have for long-term self-development. It contains personal experiences and a record of what we see, feel, and think. Something above and beyond ordinary communication takes place when we record our thoughts and feelings.

Portfolios as Self-Exploration

By keeping a portfolio, students have all classroom material in one place and are able to review it from time to time. They can compare via pre- and posttests how they felt at the beginning of a unit with how they felt when it was completed. For example, a pretest activity on self-esteem might ask that students respond to the following questions:

- "I was born . . ."
- "When I was five . . ."
- "My mother . . ."
- "My father . . ."
- "My favorite teacher . . ."
- "Who am I?"
- "What is the most positive thing happening in my life?"
- "What is most important to me right now?"
- "What do I want?"
- "What do I have to do to get it?"
- "What do I need to do to get started?"

Students can keep their written responses to these questions in their portfolios and refer to them from time to time as well as compare them with their posttest responses.

Some additional materials for a student portfolio might include the following:

- A daily log: Students record their daily activities, including those in class.
- A life history: Have students write a life history, including relevant health information.
- Entries about their health and physical activity: This might include diet, exercise, or sports—any information they deem is important to their health.
- Entries about their behavior: Students can relate the response patterns they deem healthy or unhealthy to them.

This list can most certainly be expanded based on class activities or student requests for additional information.

At the end of the class, suggest that students reread all the material they have included in their portfolios and have them respond to the following questions:

- Have I said what I really think and feel or what I've been taught to think and feel?
- Have I told not only what happened but how I feel about what happened and what it meant to me?
- Am I hiding behind impersonal facts or borrowed opinions?
- Am I keeping a distance from myself by focusing on the external world in my writing and thinking?
- Am I too critical of myself or other people?
- Have I been as open as I could be with myself?
- How consistent have I been in my thoughts, feelings, and behavior?

Portfolio Assessment

Allow students to turn in their portfolios, including only those materials they feel they want the evaluator to see and review. You should not assign a letter grade to the students' work but rather give them feedback in terms of what they have included.

The bottom line on using portfolios in evaluation is that you want students to become aware of unmet needs so they can make more positive health choices. Through effective interpersonal communication (e.g., personal conferences), the health educator can use this valuable tool to help students connect learning-by-evaluation with self-growth.

Portfolios provide a healthy way of processing feelings and using the energy that comes from feelings and are a good vehicle for challenging students to evaluate how much they have achieved. It is important that a certain percentage of students' grades are based on their personal assessments. Also, your evaluation of the portfolio should be based on the premise that the person who presented it, rather than the content, is the primary concern.

Group Projects

A truly effective health-education program makes a commitment to developing the concept of working with others and concentrates on *cooperative learning*. Cooperative groups can transform an antiwork peer ethic into positive peer pressure to perform well. Some cooperative group-learning experiences would include

Cooperative learning groups. Students form learning groups to study, learn, work on class assignments, etc. Within each group, students elect a group member to be the team captain. Each group member gives themselves a grade based on their input and help to the group.

Cooperative peer-teaching groups. Students get together in interest groups based on subject matter and plan, teach, and colead a group of younger students. (See Chapter 9.) Each group, with a team leader or captain, develops a set of questions that can be used in evaluating a certain unit that has been taught. Those students who develop the questions will not take the specific exam but instead will be evaluated based on the quality of the exam. At the end of each teaching unit or at the end of a class, students should give themselves a grade along with a brief discussion of what criteria they used in their self-evaluation.

Class Performance

If you accept that there are very different learning modalities, e.g., visual, auditory, or kinesthetic (see Chapter 14), then you must also accept that these learning styles require various evaluation styles.

To judge class performance fairly, you should evaluate each student based on the three modalities just mentioned. This takes into account divergent thinking ability; i.e., the teacher evaluates on the basis of more than one set of standards. Come up with alternative ideas and explore them. Generate student input to explore different approaches to grading.

Rating classroom performance should take into account such things as

- individual participation
- group participation
- critical-thinking skills
- creative thinking
- verbal feedback
- test results (both essay and cognitive knowledge)
- cooperative assignments

Essay Expressions That Promote Critical Thinking

Bobbi DePorter (1992), defines critical thinking as "exercising or involving careful judgment or evaluation, such as judging the feasibility of an idea or product." The bottom line for any successful program in health education would be applying that knowledge to one's own personal life. There is a saying from the Middle East: "He who tastes, knows." We must help students get more of the taste of their own education and make the educative process more alive, and also allow them to express their personal feelings about the learning experience.

Essay papers embrace the philosophy that each individual student should have the opportunity to express his own individual learning experience. In this vein, the teacher may want to direct the student to address the following issues in his essay:

- What were the most critical issues that affected me? Why? How?
- What changes do I see in my own behavior based on this new learning?
- What is one change I see myself making?

Synthesis

Termination is often a hard step, but when the tasks of this stage have been accomplished, the student should be ready to move on. During this final session of a teaching-learning unit, students should be informed that the information covered does not end there but is just beginning; it is now the role of each and every student to carry over what has been learned into their own lives.

Researchers and educators who have addressed the problem of motivation have a pretty good idea of what needs to be done so that students not only learn but, more important, *want* to learn: They must provide a curriculum that is rich and engaging; move away from standardized assessments and extrinsic inducements; promote collaboration among learners; support teacher autonomy; and create caring learning environments where students feel empowered and connected to others. In this way, students will be willing to risk developing the skills to help them choose more healthy behaviors. It will also make a difference in how students feel about themselves, because they will be acting on their own personal values.

In reviewing current conventional health-education literature you will find that much of what has been discussed in this and previous chapters is conspicuously absent, in spite of the fact that the conventional, top-down, standards-driving approach makes it more difficult for health educators to evoke the learner's curiosity and help him explore his health choices. Unfortunately, conventional health education focuses only on results, without an understanding of the dynamics of teaching and learning for behavioral change. It is the author's hope that the ideas provided thus far help readers understand themselves a little better and open up more effective communication, adding a new and more personal dimension to the teaching-learning process.

There is, in sanest hours, a consciousness, a thought that rises, independent, lifted out from all else, calm, like the stars, shining eternal. This the thought of identity—yours for you, whoever you are, as mine for me. Miracle of miracles, beyond statement, most spiritual and vaguest of earth's dreams, yet hardest basic fact, and only entrance to all facts. In such devout hours, in the midst of the significant wonders of heaven and earth (significant only because of the Me in the center), creeds, conventions, fall away and become of no account before this simple idea. Under the luminousness of real vision, it alone takes possession, takes value (Whitman, 1945).

References

Bloom, Allan. *The Closing of the American Mind*. New York: Simon and Schuster, 1987.

DePorter, Bobbi. *Quantum Learning: Unleashing the Genius in You*. New York: Dell, 1992.

Dewey, John. *Democracy and Education*. New York: Free Press, 1966.

Fiske, Edward B. *Smart Schools, Smart Kids*. New York: Touchstone Books, 1992.

Gardner, Howard. *Frames of Mind: The Theory of Multiple Intelligence*. New York: Basic Books, 1985.

Glasser, William. *The Quality School: Managing Students without Coercion*. New York: Harper & Row, 1990.

Sinetar, Marsha. *Developing a 21st-Century Mind*. New York: Villard Books, 1991.

Shor, Ira. *Empowering Education: Critical Teaching for Social Change*. Chicago: The University of Chicago Press, 1992.

Whitman, Walt. *The Portable Walt Whitman*. New York: Viking Press, 1945.

Additional Resources

Cleary, Michael J., and David A. Birch. "Using Portfolios for Assessment in the College Personal Health Course." *Journal of Health Education*, March/April 1996.

Glasser, William. *Control Theory in the Classroom*. New York: Harper & Row, 1985.

Hendricks, Gay, and James Fadiman. *Transpersonal Education: A Curriculum for Feeling and Being*. Englewood Cliffs, NJ: Prentice-Hall, 1976.

Psychosocial Issues

In his book *The Psychology of Consciousness,* Robert Ornstein (1977) provides evidence from current brain research that there are two modes of consciousness at work in human beings: one, a rational, logical, and active mode, is associated with the left side of the brain; the other, a mystical, intuitive, and receptive mode, seems to be the function of the right side of the brain. In a sense, this information is not new, since poets and philosophers have been hinting at it for thousands of years; what is remarkable is that science is finding a physical basis for the existence of these two modes.

In this unit, we are going to look at the functions of the right brain more closely (for this book is really focused on right-side thinking). Comprehensive health education requires a very strong focus on the old Delphic precept, "Know thyself." In turning our attention to the inner world of the student, we are discovering a wealth of unsuspected resources. Many current teaching techniques, such as inner imagery, role-playing, self-evaluation, and self-discovery, which are well suited to classroom teaching of health education, are aimed at right-side feeling and behaving. Researchers in this area have indicated that such teaching techniques can have a beneficial effect on physical, emotional, mental, and spiritual well-being. It is important that we give students access to tools that can be used for continuing growth and awareness throughout their lives. In applying the approaches to value-moral issues and self-esteem described herein, both students and teachers can assume responsibility for making choices and develop a sense of inner direction in their lives.

What is important to know is that the first step in applying the ideas from this unit to health education involves shifting the focus from external to internal awareness. As students become aware of their own inner states, they begin to recognize important conditions that affect their learning ability.

Reference

Ornstein, Robert. *The Psychology of Consciousness.* New York: Harcourt Brace Jovanovich, 1977.

11 Developing Students' Moral-Value Awareness

Dealing with moral-value issues is nothing new, but it is undergoing some very important transformations in the 1990s. These transformations include understanding the important role of the teacher in getting back to the basics of moral-value teaching.

Students should learn about right and wrong, respect, tolerance, honesty, diligence, caring, goodness, generosity, sympathy, and forgiveness. A major question is, should we be teaching moral-value issues? If so, whose positions should they be? Or, should the teaching-learning environment be "value-free?"

As Noreen Clark states in her article "Health Educators and the Future: Lead, Follow, or Get Out of the Way" (1994),

> Many of the problems we are confronting as a society are a matter of values. The pro-choice movement is a matter of values. Economic growth versus protection of the ecology—values. Money for the military versus money for health programs—values. Alas, scientific advances only complicate the question of values.

I would like to add that condom distribution in schools, sex education, and gender issues are all about values and moral positions as well.

Before beginning, I feel it is necessary to define some of the terms that will be explored in this chapter.

Values. Values are synonymous with personal beliefs, especially personal beliefs about what is good, just, and beautiful, what propels us to action, or to a particular kind of behavior and life. Thus, if one values the message of Christ, one will try to "love one's neighbor as oneself" (Lewis, 1990).

Virtue. A virtue is a quality of character by which individuals habitually recognize and do the right thing (Woodward, 1994). The often-thought-of virtues are

Schools today must lead the battle against the worst psychosocial epidemics that have ever plagued the children of our society. . . . Schools need programs to protect children against the ravages of social disorganization and family collapse.

—PERRY LONDON

- *fortitude:* the strength of mind and courage to persevere in the face of adversity
- *temperance:* self-discipline, the control of unruly human passions and appetites
- *prudence:* practical wisdom and the ability to make the right choice in specific situations
- *justice:* fairness, honesty, lawfulness, and the ability to keep one's promises

Morality. Definitions of morality can be broadly divided into models of acquisition and models of growth. The first imply that morality is *learned;* through conditioning, individuals acquire the motives of guilt, shame, and concern for others, and these constrain and regulate their behavior. Habits, skills, and values become internalized in the individuals and provide a repertoire of appropriate responses. The students come to monitor their own behavior. According to this model, effective moral development depends on effective reinforcement and a relationship with adults that provides good role models and good conditions for imitation and identification. Development is a slow process of acquiring habits and motives and strengthening conscience (Aronfreed, 1976).

In contrast, according to growth models, moral development progresses through *transformation* and *restructuring.* Development is change, not accumulation. This model has been applied to the study of moral reasoning. Moral reasoning reflects the way an individual makes sense of the world—how he conceptualizes the rules and norms that govern behavior. The individual does not acquire more rules or learn more rights and duties, but develops greater understanding of the *function* of rules and norms, taking into account more factors and points of view on the issues. Progress results in more differentiation and greater integration of these factors and perspectives. Lawrence Kohlberg (1984) proposed six consistent stages of moral development (Table 11–1).

Ethical behavior. Ethical behavior is conscious behavior. If we are unaware of our motives, it is unlikely that we will behave in a consistently ethical manner. If we are not aware of the particular lens through which we view the world, we do not have any true choice about what we see and how we respond. Behaving ethically is behaving with integrity (Lewis, 1990).

Thus, values are the standards and principles by which we judge people, objects, ideas, actions, and situations to be worthwhile and desirable, worthless and despicable, or somewhere between the two. As Muriel and John James stated in their book *Passion for Life* (1991), "Sometimes our values are traditional, religious ones leading to the search for a personal God. Other times they are directed toward trying to understand the universe and other people. Values can inspire us to create a work of beauty that lifts the soul or commit us to living with integrity in some other specific way."

It is important to distinguish between values and *value judgments.* The latter are assertions we make based on our values. A teacher who says "Young people who abuse drugs will ultimately end up addicts" is making a value judgment. Another teacher urging students to "Just say no to drugs" is also making a value

Table 11.1

Kohlberg's six stages of moral development

Basis of Moral Judgments	Developmental Stages	Typical Responses
Moral value resides in external, quasiphysical happening, in bad acts, or in quasiphysical needs rather than in persons and standards.	*Stage 1:* Obedience and punishment orientation. Egocentric deference to superior power or prestige or to a trouble-avoiding set. Objective responsibility.	"I'll do it 'cause I don't want to do more time." "I do it 'cause I want to keep out of trouble."
	Stage 2: Naively egoistic orientation. Right action is that which instrumentally satisfies the self's needs and occasionally others' needs. Awareness of relativism of value to each actor's needs and perspectives. Naive egalitarianism and orientation to exchange and reciprocity.	"I'm number one. I look after me. If you help me out, maybe I'll help you sometime."
Moral value resides in performing good or right roles, in maintaining the conventional order and the expectations of others.	*Stage 3:* "Good-boy" orientation to approval and to pleasing and helping others. Conformity to stereotypical images of majority or natural role behavior, and judgment by intentions.	"Sure I'd help another guy out. I'd be thinking about how he'd be feeling. Any decent person would help him."
	Stage 4: Authority and social-order maintenance orientation. Orientation to "doing duty" and to showing respect for authority and maintaining the given social order for its own sake. Regard for earned expectations of others.	"Look, you're supposed to help others. It's like a rule. Without people doing their jobs, society couldn't function."
Moral value resides in conformity by the self to shared or shareable standards, rights, or duties.	*Stage 5:* Contractual, legalistic orientation. Recognition of an arbitrary element or starting point in rules or expectations for the sake of agreement. Duty defined in terms of contract, general avoidance of violation of the will or rights of others, and majority will and welfare.	"It's a law that the people consented to. We all have an obligation to work through the agreed structure to get laws that appear wrong changed. When an injustice is committed, it is best to work through the system to end it."
	Stage 6: Conscience or principle orientation. Orientation not only to actually ordained social rules but to principles of choice involving appeal to logical universality and consistency. Orientation to conscience as a directing agent and to mutual respect and trust.	"The law should be subordinate to higher principles of justice. One should act in accordance with these superordinate principles rather than maintain simple conformity to the law."

Adapted from Scharf, Hickey, and Moriarty (1973), p. 661. Used with permission.

judgment. What are the values that led to these judgments? One may be that *people never change*. Another may be that life is a *self-fulfilling prophecy*.

Finally, values are of two kinds: moral and nonmoral. Moral values, such as honesty, respect, caring, and forgiveness, carry obligation. We feel obligated to keep a promise, pay our bills, not steal, love others, and be fair in our dealings with them. Moral values tell us what we *ought* to do. We must abide by them even when we would rather not. The key to a moral value is that it always involves the way we deal with other people.

Nonmoral values carry no such obligation. They express what we want or like to do. I might personally value rock music, for example, or reading a mystery novel, or watching television for an extended period of time. But clearly I am not obliged to, simply because it is about myself rather than my relation to another.

Moral-Value Issues in Health Education

Moral-value issues are at the very center of health education today, not so much because we choose to deal with these issues, but because they have been thrust upon us. Current major health issues have a value or moral focus. Now more than ever, students need to learn about right and wrong, respect, tolerance, honesty, diligence, caring, goodness, generosity, sympathy, and forgiveness. Should health educators be teaching about moral-value issues? If so, whose values? Or, should teaching be "value-free?"

Time Out for Personal Thoughts

Take a moment to list what *you* feel are the ten most important moral-value issues facing health education today:

1.

2.

3.

4.

5.

6.

7.

8.

9.

10.

Moral Illiteracy

According to William Kilpatrick, the socially pathological behavior and conduct we see in some young people today is traceable to the lack of a moral component in teaching and education, a vacuum that has developed since the late 1960s (Kilpatrick, 1992). Morality was taught in different ways prior to the 1960s,

> *partly through exhortation, partly through assumptions about how students behave, through assumptions about their (social) environment, through discipline, dress codes, [and] school spirit. The emphasis was not on taking a stand on an issue but on building good habits of behavior. Morality wasn't just in your mind in an abstract way, but it was wired into you through practice and habit. It wasn't a curriculum or a course. It was a general approach to life.*

Beginning in the 1970s, Kilpatrick found that most schools changed from character education to an untested and instinctive process known as *decision making,* called by some value-free decision making. Events of the 1960s and 1970s, including the assassinations of the Kennedys and Martin Luther King, the drug problem, student unrest, and Watergate, combined to subvert ideas that had withstood the test of time.

As disturbing as the moral tone of much of the youth culture is, the decline is not a hopeless proposition and it is not irreversible. According to Kilpatrick, the best way to develop strength of character is to return to the earlier models in education, with their focus on obedience to lawful authority, responsibility, self-discipline, and perseverance. Teachers can imbue young people with a moral sense about the difference between right and wrong (Kilpatrick, 1992).

Time Out for Personal Thoughts

Values are learned. The question for the 1990s is, "Are young people learning good values (honesty, respect, tolerance, etc.) today?" What is your opinion? Briefly respond:

One example of value-based education is a school system in Oregon with a four-year curriculum emphasizing different virtues each year; integrity and honesty in the first, respect in the second, and so forth. The curriculum includes the study of those who have put a particular virtue into practice.

The "self-discovered values" approach has produced certain consequences (Kilpatrick, 1992):

- It has meant that the development of moral-education curricula has been turned over to theorists who have repeatedly expressed disdain for concepts such as virtue, character, and good example; the same theorists have dismissed past culture and history as being irrelevant to the search for values.

- It has created a generation of moral illiterates, students who know their own feelings but don't know their culture.
- It has helped produce a citizenry unable to distinguish reasonable moral arguments from mere rationalizations.
- Finally, it has helped create an educational system with a de facto policy of withholding from children the greatest incentive to moral behavior—namely, the conviction that life makes sense—by preventing them from learning the larger purposes or stories that give meaning to existence. In failing to impart these stories, schools have deprived children of both moral context and moral energy.

So what's a teacher to do when it comes to moral and value issues? Hunter Lewis, in his book *A Question of Values,* states that

all schools transmit value, which are omnipresent in human subjects, whether or not they choose to "teach" about values per se. Over the past decade, however, most colleges and universities . . . have made a conscious decision to teach about values, or rather, how to think about values, since there is no intention to indoctrinate students, but rather to show them how to arrive at reasonable and moral solutions on their own.

Thus, it is realistic to expect health educators to teach about values, but this education must be directed toward equipping our young students for such issues as care for self and others, drug use, and pregnancy, and the inner struggle young people have with these issues. Most important, this education may lead to behavioral change.

Why We Need Moral Education

Moral education aims to stimulate and support students' natural movement toward more mature thinking rather than to teach particular values or habits. By contrast, programs intending to develop good character usually focus on a core set of traits and behaviors. For example, the *Character Education Curriculum* (CEC) developed by the American Institute for Character in San Antonio, Texas, teaches children to identify with values such as honesty and generosity. While not choosing children's values for them, the CEC points out those values that are generally accepted by our society.

CEC avoids lecturing students, relying instead on discussion, role-playing, and small-group activities. For example, to help second graders explore unfairness, the teacher divides the class into two groups based on students' birth months. Children imagine how they feel if a rule permitted only one group to go to school. Third graders talk together about Anna, a little girl who doesn't understand her teacher's directions but is afraid to ask for help, and eleven-year-olds discuss Helen, who receives several dollars extra in change at the grocery store. Should she return the extra money, or keep it? School administrators testify enthusiastically that since their systems have used CEC, attendance is up, vandalism and misbehavior are down, and students like school more.

The Quest National Center in Ohio has developed materials that focus attention on the way young people feel about themselves and about the people around them. The Center's two curricula, *Skills for Living* and *Skills for Adolescence,* contain units on understanding and communicating feelings, building strong family relationships and friendships, and thinking about the future—marriage, careers, and parenting. Some activities seek to enhance students' self-awareness and self-confidence; others develop more concrete skills like money management. A recent independent evaluation showed that junior-high students enrolled in *Skills for Living* progressed more in attitudes toward family, self-esteem, communication, and problem solving than did comparison groups. A semester in *Skills for Adolescence* improved participants' attitudes toward school and helped them resist peer pressure.

Kevin Ryan (Terry, 1993), founder and director of the Center for the Advancement of Ethics and Character at Boston University, stated that "the character-education movement is a very traditional movement in the sense that it says there are certain ideas from the world culture which we think people ought to know . . . young people deserve to know the very best that we have learned about how to live as a community." This community idea is based on words like respect, integrity, trust, cooperation, and collaboration, starting points in the moral upgrading of what has been called a return to *character education.* Character education includes asking ourselves questions like, What type of people will those we are helping be? What decisions will they make? Can they think, can they feel, and can they empathize?

What Now?

Most students spend half again as much time with teachers as with all other adults (many teenagers spend only five minutes a day alone with their fathers). Until the students take jobs, schools provide their main window on grown-ups at work. As they near graduation, many adolescents feel that teachers have helped to set their direction in life.

Thomas Lickona (1992) made the following strong case for teaching moral values and developing good character in the classroom:

1. *There is a clear and urgent need.* Young people are increasingly hurting themselves and others and decreasingly concerned about contributing to the welfare of their fellow human beings. In this they reflect the ills of societies in need of moral and spiritual renewal.

2. *Transmitting values is, and always has been, the work of civilization.* A society needs values education both to survive and to thrive—to keep itself intact and growing toward conditions that support the full human development of all its members.

3. *The school's role as moral educator becomes even more vital at a time when millions of children get little moral teaching from their parents, and where value-centered influences such as church or temple are also absent from their lives.* These days,

when schools don't do moral education, influences hostile to good character rush in to fill the values vacuum.

4. *There is common ethical ground even in our value-conflicted society.* Americans have intense and often angry differences over moral issues such as abortion, homosexuality, euthanasia, and capital punishment. Despite this diversity, we can identify basic, shared values that allow us to engage in public moral education in a pluralistic society.

5. *Democracies have a special need for moral education, because democracy is government by the people themselves.* The people must care about the rights of others and the common good and be willing to assume the responsibilities of democratic citizenship.

6. *There is no such thing as value-free education.* Everything a school does teaches values—including the way teachers and other adults treat students, the way the principals treat teachers, the way the schools treat parents, and the way students are allowed to treat school staff and each other. If questions of right and wrong are never discussed in classrooms, that, too, teaches a lesson about how much morality matters. In short, the relevant issue is never "Should schools teach values?" but rather, "Which values will they teach?" and "How well will they teach them?"

7. *The great questions facing both the individual person and the human race are moral questions.* For each of us as individuals, a question of the utmost existential importance is: "How should I live my life?" For all of humanity, the two most important questions facing us as we enter the next century are, "How can we live with each other?" and "How can we live with nature?"

8. *There is broad-based, growing support for values education in the schools.* It comes from the federal government, which has identified values education as essential in the fight against drugs and crime. It comes from statehouses, which have passed resolutions necessary for good citizenship and a law-abiding society.

9. *An unabashed commitment to moral education is essential if we are to attract and keep good teachers.* If you want to do one thing to improve the lives of teachers, says Boston University educator Kevin Ryan, make moral education—including the creation of a civil, human community in the school—the center of school life.

10. *Values education is a doable job.* Given the enormous moral problems facing the country, their deep social roots, and the ever-increasing responsibilities that schools already shoulder, the prospect of tackling moral education can seem overwhelming. The good news is that values education can be done within the school day, is happening now in school systems all across the country, and is making a positive difference in the moral attitudes and behavior of students. If you want to make a difference in the lives of students, get involved in moral values.

What Needs to Be Done

The core problem facing us in health education is morals. All the other problems are derived from it. Teen pregnancy, drug addiction, and violence represent behaviors that are lacking in self-discipline. If students don't learn respect, tolerance, honesty, caring, and goodness, we will truly fail to prepare them for their future.

When the student's value system is causing her difficulty, the issue is clearly value-dominated. You, the teacher, must establish overall goals that help the student *want* to change certain unhealthy behaviors. You need to help students truly clarify their personal values.

> Schools wishing to do values education, I believe, need to be confident that (1) there are objectively worthwhile, universally agreed-upon values that schools can and should teach in a pluralistic society; and (2) schools should not only expose students to these values but also help them to understand, internalize and act upon such values. To be confident about those two propositions, schools need first to get clear about the nature of values (Lickona, 1992).

Teachers who care, teachers who understand, teachers who are excited when young people value things, must start by helping them to

- explore the scope and depth of their values
- understand the cultural, family, and nonfamily idiosyncratic background of their values
- identify the values they hold with regard to the health issues they are exposed to, and what may require them to change those values
- understand how those value changes will affect their lives

To avoid the mistake of the 1970s—allowing students to decide for themselves what values they should live by—we must become more involved in shaping their values.

To place this within a cognitive-behavioral perspective, a values approach must focus on the individual's appraisal of a situation (his values) and his perception of responsibility for his actions within that situation (moral-ethical behavior).

Time Out for Personal Thoughts

Cognitive-Behavioral Valuing

Fold a blank sheet of paper down the middle. At the top of the lefthand side, write "Cognitive Values." Under this, list in the order that they come to you the dozen or so things you consider your most important values. Then rank the list, putting a 1 by the value you consider most important, a 2 by the next most important, and so on. Don't rush.

Now, on the top of the right side of the paper, write "Behavioral Values." Jot down, as specifically as possible, how you spend most of your time, money, and energy. For example, "I am into shopping, eating, and watching TV." Then, rank this list according to how much time and energy you put into each (a 1 being the thing you spend the most time and energy on).

Finally, compare your cognitive values with your behavioral values. What do you see? The more your cognitive and behavioral values are in sync, the more at peace with yourself you are likely to be.

For example, if someone says that he values peace, we call this a *cognitive value*. When he acts on this belief, it becomes a *behavioral value*.

Three Approaches to Values Education

The most commonly recognized and often-used approach to values education is *values clarification* (basically, a decision-making approach), which is based on the pioneering work of Louis Raths, Merrill Harmin, and Sidney B. Simon (1966). Raths first coined the term, springboarding off John Dewey's thinking about the need to move away from isolated moral lessons and focus on helping students develop the skills to formulate and test judgments and make choices on their own.

The major problems that educators found with the value-clarification approach are that (1) discussion guidelines for the teacher were sparse, thus teachers were not sure what to do after students had clarified their values; (2) the approach made no distinction between what one might *want* to do (such as shoplift) and what one *ought* to do (respect the property rights of others); and (3) values clarification made the mistake of treating kids like adults who needed only to clarify values that were already sound (Lickona, 1992). Values clarification also lacks a framework for considering the worth and moral value of a decision.

In response to values clarification, Lawrence Kohlberg (1984) pointed out that different choices, life-styles, and decisions can be viewed as stages of *moral development*. The most primitive choices are those made on the naive basis of external pressures or immature personal desires. More advanced moral reasoning is guided by legal frameworks, conscience, or principle (see Table 11–1).

Those who adopted Kohlberg's theory found that an experienced group leader could raise a student's level of moral reasoning through small-group discussions. They also found that moral reasoning too far removed from the current moral stage of the student made learning new forms of reasoning extremely difficult. Kohlberg offered educators a nonrelativistic goal: *stimulate moral development*.

A third approach, known as *rational decision making*, was developed by moral philosophers and is based on the Socratic probe-questions technique in which the teacher requires students to go beyond just giving their opinions and asks for the "why's."

Comprehensive Values Education

A new approach to values called *comprehensive values education* contains four important aspects (Kirschenbaum, 1992):

- It is comprehensive in *content*. It encompasses all value-related issues—from personal values, to ethical questions, to moral issues.
- It is comprehensive in *methodology*. Teachers must model values as well as prepare young people for independence by stressing responsible decision making and other life skills.

- It takes place *throughout the school*—in the classroom, in extracurricular activities, in career education and counseling, in awards ceremonies, and in all aspects of school life.
- It takes place *throughout the community.* Parents, religious groups, civic leaders, police, youth workers, and community agencies participate.

Values education offers health educators a comprehensive cognitive-behavioral approach to teaching that effectively involves students in the process of learning about their values and the important behaviors they influence.

A Reality-Based Approach to Comprehensive Values Education

A reality-centered approach to values is a process in which students learn to deal with certain value issues and are then asked to test them against their behavior:

- Is their behavior helping or hurting them?
- Is it helping them get what they want?
- Is their behavior acceptable?
- Is what they want realistic or attainable?
- How do they view the world?
- How committed are they to the process of learning and changing their lives?
- Is their plan of action helpful and realistic?

Second, this approach helps them develop a plan of action to go about changing the self-defeating values that lead to unhealthy choices.

Building a Moral Foundation in the Classroom

Here are some guidelines to help you lay the groundwork for successful moral-value education:

- Discuss values early (elementary grades), before students make life-limiting decisions
- Model the values you are teaching. What students see and hear carries more weight than what you are sometimes trying to teach
- Share what is important to you as a health educator. When we don't talk about values, we give the message they are not important
- Help students consider the needs of others as well as themselves
- Help students feel good about themselves so they won't be as vulnerable to peer pressure
- Teach respect by demonstrating respect for your students
- Use role-play in demonstrating assertiveness skills in the classroom. Some young people want to stand up for their values but don't know how
- Be receptive to their questions. Don't respond with anger or shock
- Teach them to use mistakes as positive learning experiences
- Help them question the values of others. Are friends who get them into trouble really friends?

A Moral Dilemma

Gail and Sharon were best friends. One day they went shopping together. Sharon tried on a sweater, and then, to Gail's surprise, walked out of the store wearing the sweater under her coat. A moment later, the store's security officer stopped Gail and demanded that she tell her the name of the girl who had walked out. The officer told the store owner that she had seen the two girls together, and that she was sure the one who left had been shoplifting. The store owner told Gail that she could really get in trouble if she did not give her friend's name.

> If you were Gail, what would you do? Why?
> When you saw Sharon, what would you say?
> Would you still consider her your friend?
> Why is this a moral dilemma?

The Basic Values

Certain basic values serve as a starting point in understanding the process of reality as it applies to values education (Elkind, 1992). These values all fuse into a sort of existential-humanistic hope for both young and old, as well as future generations. Values are at the very heart of caring.

Some basic values and their definitions are as follows:

Respect: Thoughtfulness about the needs, beliefs, and feelings of others

Diligence: Being attentive and busy

Tolerance: Lack of opposition to beliefs or practices differing from your own

Integrity: Adherence to a code of values

Honesty: Being truthful, fair, and trustworthy

Trust: Reliance on others

Caring: Compassion for others

Sympathy: Ability to understand or share the feelings or interests of others

Goodness: Being well-behaved and kind

Forgiveness: Pardoning others' transgressions

Generosity: Freely giving and sharing

Cooperation: Acting jointly with others

Teaching the Twelve Core Values

To begin with, you want to get a group consensus of what the twelve core values mean. The point is to arrive at a meaning that is acceptable to a diverse group of students.

Divide the class into pairs (this gives students a sense of worth and demonstrates the value of collaboration). Then have each pair discuss what the values in the preceding list mean to them (how they act, think, and feel toward them). Which ones are particularly significant for them? Which ones are not? Which ones can they articulate more clearly than others? Are there one or two that hold a special meaning for them?

Some points to consider during this exercise are as follows:

- Remember, do not turn the process into a competitive game to see who comes up with the best definition
- Have someone record all the responses; acknowledge all the responses
- Advise students that put-downs (e.g., one student telling another that her suggestion or idea was stupid) are not acceptable

The Valuing Process

Before dealing with the twelve core beliefs, we need to understand the process by which each of us comes to value what we value (Figure 11–1).

Step 1: The value is chosen freely—someone makes this choice based on how he feels, what he wants, and who he is. He is not forced to make this choice. (Stress that students should accept outside values without question.)

Step 2: The value is chosen from among alternatives—a value cannot really be a value unless one has been given the option of realistic, acceptable choices.

Step 3: The value is chosen after critical examination—it is based on one's critical evaluation of alternatives.

Step 4: The value is prized and cherished—the person feels good about his choices.

Step 5: The value is publicly affirmed—the person has publicly stated that he approves of the values.

Step 6: The value is acted upon—the person has taken action based on his values. (Example: he has marched in a protest, worked with the homeless, or otherwise spent time helping another.)

Step 7: The value is part of a pattern of repeated action—the person is consistent in what he values. This is the most challenging step, for it requires a commitment as well as a strong sense of self.

Of these seven steps, those of choosing, prizing, and acting should be focused on, for they are really the most cherished goals of comprehensive values education.

The Values Grid

Using the grid in Figure 11–2, have students list the twelve core values in the first column. When they are done, have them put a P ("pro") or a C ("con") in the sec-

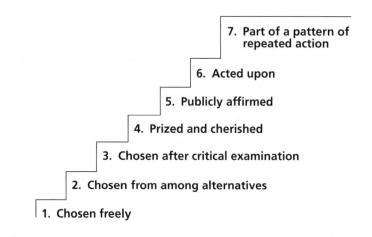

7. Part of a pattern of repeated action

6. Acted upon

5. Publicly affirmed

4. Prized and cherished

3. Chosen after critical examination

2. Chosen from among alternatives

1. Chosen freely

Figure 11–1

The Seven Steps in Acquiring Values

The Seven Steps in Acquiring Values

Value	Pro or Con?	1	2	3	4	5	6	7

Figure 11–2

The Values Grid

ond column to indicate whether they are for or against the corresponding value. Next, have them check the numbered boxes (as they relate to the seven steps in Figure 11–1) that they have completed for each value. (For example, they should check box 6 next to "shows respect for others" to indicate they have "acted upon" that value.) The point of this exercise is to get students to look at the ways they value themselves and others.

Personal Values

Have students list their own values using a similar grid. They should think about things such as friendship, being a member of a gang, money, etc. Let them know they can add to the grid if they find themselves without room.

When they have completed their lists, have them go through the same process as with the core-values grid. When they are done, you may want to have some students share their lists with the class, although this is not required.

A Reality-Based Approach to Evaluating Students' Values

Ask students to look over their core-beliefs grid as well as their personal-values grid. What do they see? How do they feel about their rankings? Ask them to evaluate their own behaviors in response to the value grids based on these seven questions (Wubbolding, 1988):

1. **Are their values helping or hurting them?** Do they serve their best interests? Will what they are doing now hurt or help them in the future? (Don't make this too much in the future, as students do not think in those terms.)
2. **Are their values helping them get what they want?** This is a more specific evaluation. We are not talking about the future but the present. For example, if a value is to lose weight, the behavior is overeating. The value conflict is wanting to lose weight but not wanting to reduce food intake.
3. **Do their values go against the rules?** Do they produce unacceptable behavior? For example, fighting in the lunchroom, calling someone a derogatory name, and so on. Is this realistic, given the rules and goals of the school? Are they protesting by breaking the rules? Do they prevent others from expressing their beliefs?
4. **Do their values allow for realistic or attainable goals?** This question revolves around the attainability of what they want. Can they realistically expect to achieve a given goal? (This should not be a put-down question but rather a reality check.) If not, what is wrong with reevaluating the goal and setting more realistic ones?
5. **Do their values help them look at the world in a positive way?** For example, does the student view the world, the teacher, the school or her parents as the enemy? The idea is to get students to see things more objectively. This is not easily done. But it is important that students know their worst enemy is themselves. When they blame others for their problems, they are not taking responsibility for how they behave.

6. **How committed are they to the process of learning and changing their lives?** Students should think about things they can do to resolve problems in their lives and, more important, take control of their lives. Stress that this is an ongoing process.
7. **Can their values help them change hurtful behaviors?** This question comes after the student has made a plan of action to change certain behaviors. This is "the big C" called commitment. The students are ready to make changes in their lives based on their value choices. Allow them the time and direction to successfully complete their plan.

This type of examination helps the teacher understand the reasons and patterns underlying the overt behaviors of the students. Knowledge of their personal values makes it possible to design behavioral programs that help students understand and want to change their unhealthy behavioral patterns.

Teaching Values to Kids

There are a great number of unique programs now being used around the country. Four of these have been listed in the 1993 *New Age Sourcebook:*

The Mysteries Program is a curriculum designed to help students aged twelve to eighteen develop skills to combat self-destructive behavior. Created by the staff of Crossroads, an innovative private school in Santa Monica, the program involves ninety-minute weekly sessions in which teachers use active listening, group building, movement, art, and play to help teens address the deeper questions of life—the mysteries—such as relationships, sexuality, death, spirituality, and ethics. Teachers can learn to use the curriculum by taking a weekend workshop run annually or by obtaining *The Mysteries Sourcebook*, a 300-page guide to the program. Contact: Peggy O'Brien, Mysteries Program Director, Crossroads School, 1714 21st St., Santa Monica, CA 90404.

Teaching Tolerance, a tool for teaching children to combat racism, is available from attorney Morris Dees and the staff of the Southern Poverty Law Center. It offers a curriculum package, "America's Civil Rights Movement," that includes a video and a biannual magazine focusing on teaching strategies and exercises for increasing racial and religious sensitivity. Southern Poverty Law Center, 400 Washington Ave., Montgomery, AL 36104.

Standing Tall, a program developed by the Giraffe Project, uses stories of real giraffes to inspire kids to stick their necks out for the common good. Standing Tall is available for four different levels, from kindergarten through high school. The program includes a video plus a notebook full of lesson plans, worksheets, and enrichment ideas that will lead students from discussions on courage, caring, and commitment through the planning and implementation of a service project. The Giraffe Project, P.O. Box 759, Langley, WA 98260.

Natural Helpers is a peer-helping program designed for sixth-through-twelfth graders based on the belief that kids in this age group are most likely to turn to a friend first when they have a problem. The program begins with a schoolwide survey to determine which issues are most important to students and which kids are most trusted by their peers. The complete program includes a guide for in-school coordinators and a slew of materials. An introductory video is available free for preview. Comprehensive Health Education Foundation, 22323 Pacific Highway S., Seattle, WA 98198.

Twenty Videos that Teach Good Values

The 1993 *New Age Sourcebook* listed the following twenty videos that focus on moral development. Check out your video store for story lines.

The Long Walk Home	*The Candidate*
Chariots of Fire	*Hoosiers*
Empire of the Sun	*Amazing Grace and Chuck*
Stand and Deliver	*A Tale of Two Cities*
Places in the Heart	*Lilies of the Field*
Breaking Away	*The Right Stuff*
Glory	*The Emerald Forest*
Longtime Companion	*All the President's Men*
Norma Rae	*The Nasty Girl*
Dominick and Eugene	*Au Revoir, Les Enfants*

Developing a Positive, Realistic Plan of Action

Have students again look over their value grids and think about some of the changes they would like to make. There may be just one, or there may be more—the point is getting them to think about these changes. Here are some suggestions to help students in moving forward (Wubbolding, 1988):

1. **Change should be need-fulfilling.** In her plan for change, the student should fulfill certain needs such as enjoyment of the outcome.
2. **Change should be simple.** An easy-to-understand plan of action developed by the *student* is best.
3. **Change should be realistic and attainable.** The student will attain her goals for change more easily if they are reality-based.
4. **Change should be reasonable to maintain.** This is such an important step, I want to quote Wubbolding exactly: "We have all heard someone proclaim, 'My New Year's resolution is to stop smoking . . . to stop yelling . . . to stop oversleeping,' Such statements violate many of the characteristics of a good plan, including that it should be positive. The behavioral system is constantly functioning. Even during sleep, part of the system operates through

dreams. All we can do is behave; we cannot not-behave. Also, the 'picture album' is more receptive to concrete representation than to negative command. For example, probably every parent has experienced a child's spilling the milk after being told [not to] spill the milk. . . . Consequently, the plan must be . . . a positive plan of action."

5. **Change should be dependent on the doer.** The plan the student has for change should be independent of what others do. This is important in terms of establishing an independent base from which to say, "I am doing this for me, not for others!" It is important that the teacher allow for this autonomy.

6. **The plan for change must be specific.** To be feasible, it should also be *exact.* So, words from the teacher like "When?" "How?" and "What change?" are critical to the student's developing a realistic plan for change.

7. **The new behavior must be repeated.** A change in behavior must be repeated over a period of time. It is not enough to do it once. The person has to incorporate it into her daily way of behaving.

8. **The change must be immediate.** The student must not put off making this change. If she actively values something to the degree that she is willing to put energy into doing something about it, she should want to start right away. "What I said yesterday," Gandhi declared, "you can't go by. It's what I say today."

9. **The plan for change must be process-centered.** The reality of life is that we cannot always assure our successes by what we attempt to achieve. The focus must be on what the student wants to accomplish, not on whether she will accomplish it. Remember those lines from Joan Baez: "Yesterday is gone and tomorrow is blind; I live one day at a time." We must get the student to deal with the here and now, because the future is *now.*

10. **The plan for change must be evaluated.** Before a plan for behavioral change is considered, it should (if possible) be reviewed by the teacher. Is it repetitive, realistic, and attainable? Most important, does it fit into the individual student's reality of needs, wants, and achievability? You want to help the student understand that her plan must satisfy her needs by being *specific, attainable,* and *immediate.*

11. **The change should be made firmly.** This is about commitment. The student's resolution to change should be made firmly by whatever method she feels works for her.

Back your students up. Let them know that you care about and support them by creating a learning environment in which each and every student is acknowledged for her efforts toward behavioral change.

Implicit in these suggestions is a concern for the process not only of maintaining positive health behaviors but also of changing attitudes and behaviors. Although the concept of change is perhaps basic to all human life—a fact of our very existence—it is resisted in principle by some. We think change is "good" when we helped design it and "bad" when we feel subjected to it. When asked to change your students' value decisions, the approach of "don't do this because it is unhealthy" is unrealistic. Those who act in unhealthy ways already know that. So, it is important that we focus on the positive—what students can do to improve their lives, move forward, better themselves, and make a mark—and not on how they can stop doing this or that.

The Just-Community Approach to Moral Education

Grounded in the progressive educational tradition of John Dewey, and updated by the use of scientific moral-development principles, is the *just-community* approach to moral education. The key to this approach is the transformation of the classroom into a participatory democracy where students share decision-making rights. Part of this just community is the sharing of some common values among its members. Kohlberg writes, "In traditional schools, it is part of the teacher's role to be a policeman and for friends or students not to be. In a democratic school, it is not desirable for friends to be seen as policemen. It is, however, desirable for friends to have a feeling that at the center of their friendship is a mutual concern about fairness and the sense that their friendship and mutual loyalty exist in some balance within a larger moral community" (Kohlberg, 1985).

To establish a just community, the teacher must start by getting students to agree on a system of classroom rules. These rules require implementing a curriculum based on the discussion of ethical dilemmas. The teacher should pose a dilemma and then encourage an exchange of ideas and opinions while keeping his or her own values in the background (Kohlberg, 1985).

Here is an example:

The class is taking a final exam. The teacher has informed the class that their final grade on this exam will be determined by the class average; that is, the student with the highest grade will establish the grade of A. You are sitting in your chair taking the exam when you notice your best friend using cheat notes. The following day, the teacher informs the class that this student has received the highest grade in the class.

What would you do?

The teacher asks students if cheating was going on in class. Would you tell her? Why?

(continued)

Would you confront your friend? If yes, what would you say to him?

When you present this dilemma to your class, you must decide which discussion model you plan to use:

- informal discussion, in which students are asked to respond to arguments they hear
- getting the class to split on the issue. The split may be either two-way (with a for and an against) or three-way, allowing for an undecided
- assigning different groups to develop different arguments
- assigning different individuals or groups to play different roles
- a moral evaluation of responses to the situation with a final analysis

As the teacher, challenge the class to think about the question, "What are the moral issues raised by this dilemma, and what kinds of questions will elicit discussions of these issues?" Have them ask themselves what kinds of responses are most likely to be represented and what each might sound like. Finally, allow one or two students to come to an agreement on each of these points and have them "teach" their dilemma, sharing their thoughts and responses with the rest of the group. In essence, they will tell the group how they arrived at their own moral assessment of the situation.

Do I Value Myself?

Standing up for what we value sends a strong message: that we value ourselves. Here is a perfect example of this and one you should share with your class:

> This is a story about someone who just wasn't going to take it any more. In 1991, Teresa Fischette, a ticket agent for Continental Airlines, was fired for refusing to wear makeup. It was a simple request but one that Fischette felt had nothing to do with how she performed her job. The story made the front pages, she was on Oprah Winfrey and a Jay Leno sketch. It didn't take Continental long to realize it was outmatched. Fischette was reinstated. She won her fight.

There are a number of wonderful questions you could put to your students based on this example:

1. Like Ms. Fischette, have any of you ever stood up for a belief that was close to you?
2. Would you, in Ms. Fischette's situation, quit your job over such an issue?

3. How many of you support Ms. Fischette's decision? How many of you oppose it?

The most effective way to teach this issue is to point out that internal strength is a sign you feel good about yourself, and that these positive internal feelings translate into positive external actions. Ms. Fischette's decision was based on an inner conviction that she was correct in her feelings. She chose to stand by those feelings as her behavior illustrates.

Another approach is to deal with the issue of respect for authority—examples such as Thomas Jefferson, Rosa Parks, and Martin Luther King, Jr., could make for a discussion on such things as legitimate resistance to authority.

Internal strength is very much related to the efforts all people make toward feeling good about themselves. The contemporary catchword for feeling good about oneself is self-esteem. The following chapters will explore the development of self-esteem through teaching.

One Approach to Moral Choices: Drug Use

Making a moral judgment is really a statement about how we feel about ourselves. Thus, a cognitive-behavioral approach to drug education can help students make the moral judgment that doing drugs is wrong for at least four reasons (Lickona, 1992):

1. drug abuse is self-destructive—a violation of our obligation to respect and care for ourselves, develop our potential, and not throw away our future
2. drug abuse almost always leads to some other wrongful behavior, such as lying, stealing, pushing drugs to pay for the habit, or recklessness and violence
3. drug abuse causes much suffering to those people, especially families, who care about the drug abuser
4. drug abuse by minors or adults contributes to an enormously destructive societal problem. If you're dealing in drugs—buying or selling—you're part of that national problem

Effective programs of drug awareness target those who are most at risk: the very young. These programs are being implemented at the fifth, sixth, and seventh grade level, when students typically begin experimenting with alcohol, tobacco, and other drugs. At this level, we can teach resistance skills that will help students to find their own center of strength. This idea is eloquently expressed in Eldridge Cleaver's *Soul on Ice* (1968).

Effective drug-prevention programs teach people how to make healthy life choices that do not include drugs. Students must first be aware that they have choices even in difficult situations where substance abuse is pervasive. The most successful programs provide practical skills that translate the desire to live without drugs into reality (Falco, 1992).

Moving Students from Value Issues to Moral Thinking

Values present us with a moral foundation on which we can move the learner from how she feels about something toward acting with responsibility. When dealing with value issues, we should allow students to express freely their personal beliefs, even when they may not be willing to act on those beliefs. As Hunter Lewis stated, "Personal values are beliefs, not personality traits, and no matter how interconnected beliefs and personality traits may be, an effort to analyze the former solely in terms of the latter is certain to fail" (1990). The key here is that we start with value issues but move on to moral and ethical issues and how they interact with each student's personal life.

To accomplish this, teachers can use any number of strategies for clarifying specific value issues, including the following:

Exercise: Honesty

Have students briefly respond to the following:

1. You have handed a cashier a ten-dollar bill for a $7.95 item. He gives you change for a twenty-dollar bill. What would you do?

2. You back out of a parking lot and ever so slightly hit a car behind you. You look and see that the other car has a major dent in the door. No one else has noticed the accident. What would you do?

3. You are driving along the highway when you notice two people attempting to break into a car that is parked. One is stripping the car, the other is breaking the window. What would you do?

4. You come to a stop sign, but no one is around. Would you still stop?

5. You arrive at your destination to find a friend of yours being severely beaten by her boyfriend. Would you intervene?

6. Your friend asks you to testify about this incident in court. Would you?

Ask students for nothing more than what *their* responses would be. In the values-clarifying process, you should ask only noncommittal questions that encourage the student to discuss her values more fully. The student could be asked about what the value means, whether she has thought through her response, how she came to adopt this value, or how she feels about the value. You should

- avoid moralizing, criticizing, giving your own values, or evaluating
- exclude all judgments of "good" or "right" or "acceptable"
- not pressure or suggest the moral implications of her choices

The most critical and cautionary process now is to move the student from values clarification to promoting moral growth, which is based on the effect of her choices on others (moral responsibility).

In the previous exercise, for example, honesty and dishonesty should not be seen as two alternatives with equivalent moral status. Honesty is the better value because it shows respect for the rights of others. Acquiring more sophisticated modes of moral judgment means learning how fundamental values like honesty can be implemented and coordinated with other essential values in the total process of moral development.

Time Out for Personal Thoughts

How would you turn each of the value questions in the previous exercise into moral-ethical questions? Rephrase each one individually as a moral-ethical question.

1.

2.

3.

4.

5.

6.

Ideally, this technique creates both an incentive for students to reexamine their own values and a strong awareness that there is a better mode of moral judgment available to them. For example, the student evaluating scenario 1 in which she was given extra change might now feel a need to discuss her reaction more fully. The teacher could present some moral-ethical issues such as:

- Who ultimately pays for the loss: the store or the consumer?
- If the mistake was not yours, whose responsibility is it to report it?
- What if the person who overpaid you had to repay the loss to the store from his own salary? How would you feel?
- What benefits do you personally gain by *not* accepting the overpayment?
- How would you want your children to react to this situation?
- If someone said to you, "I think you have overpaid me on this," how would you react?

The essence of moral awareness is the ability to detect moral issues in complex social situations. Young people naturally develop a degree of moral awareness through their social experience, but few realize their full potential on their own. Thus, there is much that teachers can do, directly and indirectly, to expand a student's moral awareness beyond its incipient state.

The moral education process discussed in this chapter can provide useful tools for enhancing students' moral awareness. In particular, the programs that have taken clear, unequivocal stands on moral choice while encouraging students' active participation have proven most valuable. Moral-discussion groups led by a trained teacher are perhaps the surest means of achieving heightened moral behavior. In such groups, the teacher poses the problem and guides the discussion, but the students express their own views and listen to each others' feedback. Students thus become engaged in the issue because they are presented with—but not forcefed—peer feedback with an adult's moral guidance. This is the principle of respectful engagement in a collective educational setting.

Synthesis

The overall goal of the teacher is to help students become more effectively functioning persons. In this process, the teacher's role is to assist the student in maintaining or modifying his health behavior or in choosing between alternative courses of action, or perhaps to support the student while he is experiencing some trauma in the course of decision making.

As Lickona stated, "How can schools foster an 'I can make a difference' sense of citizen responsibility? It starts in the classroom, where children can see the results of their actions as they work to create a caring moral community. But what can be done to extend students' caring attitudes into larger and larger spheres so that they come to identify compassionately with the mainstream of humanity and do what they can to build a better world" (1992). Those of us who miss this message, with its powerful emphasis on caring about ourselves, our wellness, and the wellness of all humanity, should rethink our own values. In short, our outward expression of caring is an expression of how well we care for ourselves.

Finally, we must be aware of what James Carbarino and Frances Scott say in *What Children Can Tell Us* (1992):

> *Children have concerns about their competence and their acceptance by, or relatedness to, the important people in their lives. These concerns are translated into conscious and unconscious efforts to cope with the stresses and challenges of life, including those situations in which adults seek information from and about children.*

References

American Institute for Character Education. *Character Education Curriculum.* P.O. Box 12617, San Antonio, Texas 78212.

Aronfreed, J. "Moral Development from the Standpoint of a General Psychological Theory," in T. Lickona, *Moral Development and Behavior.* New York: Holt, Rinehart and Winston, 1976.

Clark, Noreen M. "Health Educators and the Future: Lead, Follow, or Get Out of the Way." *Journal of Health Education,* May/June 1994.

Cleaver, Eldridge. *Soul on Ice.* New York: McGraw-Hill, 1968.

Elkind, David. "Spirituality in Education." *Holistic Education Review,* Spring 1992.

Falco, Mathea. *The Making of a Drug-Free America: Programs that Work.* New York: Random House, 1992.

Garbarino, James, and Frances M. Scott. *What Children Can Tell Us: Eliciting, Interpreting, and Evaluating Critical Information from Children.* San Francisco: Jossey-Bass, 1992.

James, Muriel, and John James. *Passion for Life: Psychology and the Human Spirit.* New York: Dutton, 1991.

Kilpatrick, William. *Why Johnny Can't Tell Right from Wrong: Moral Illiteracy and the Case for Character Education.* New York: Simon & Schuster, 1992.

Kirschenbaum, Howard. "A Comprehensive Model for Values Education and Moral Education." *Phi Delta Kappan,* June 1992.

Kohlberg, L. "Essays on Moral Development," in *The Psychology of Moral Development* (vol. 2). New York: Wiley, 1984.

Kohlberg, Lawrence. "The Just Community in Theory and Practice," in M. Berkowitz and F. Oser (eds.), *Moral Education.* Hillsdale, NJ: L. Erlbaum Associates, 1985.

Lewis, Hunter. *A Question of Values.* San Francisco, CA: Harper & Row, 1990.

Lickona, Thomas. *Educating for Character: How Our Schools Can Teach Respect and Responsibility.* New York: Bantam Books, 1992.

London, Perry. "Character Education and Clinical Intervention: A Paradigm Shift for U.S. Schools." *Phi Delta Kappan,* May 1987.

Quest National Center. *Skills for Living.* 6655 Sharonwoods Blvd., Columbus, Ohio 43229.

Raths, Louis, Merrill Harmin, and Sidney Simon. *Values in Teaching.* Columbus, OH: Charles E. Merrill, 1966.

Scharf, P., J. Hickey, and T. Moriarty. "Moral Conflict and Change in Correctional Settings." *Personnel and Guidance Journal* 51, 1973.

Terry, Sara. "Moral Upgrade." *Boston Globe Magazine,* 16 May 1993.

Woodward, Kenneth L. "What Is Virtue?" *Newsweek,* 13 June 1994.

Wubbolding, Robert E. *Using Reality Therapy.* New York: Harper & Row, 1988.

Additional Resources

Bennett, William J. *The Book of Virtues: A Treasury of Great Moral Stories.* New York: Simon & Schuster, 1993.

Damon, William. *The Moral Child: Nurturing Children's Natural Moral Growth.* New York: Free Press, 1988.

Doyle, Robert. *Essential Skills and Strategies in the Helping Process.* Pacific Grove, CA: Brooks/Cole, 1992.

Dubler, Nancy, and David Nimmons. *Ethics on Call: Taking Charge of Life-and-Death Choices in Today's Health Care System.* New York: Vintage, 1993.

Gilligan, Carol. "In a Different Voice: Women's Conceptions of Self and of Morality." *Harvard Educational Review,* November 1977.

Greenberg, Jerrold, and Robert Gold. *The Health Education Ethics Book.* Madison, WI: Brown, 1992.

Parsley, Bonnie M. *The Choice Is Yours: A Teenager's Guide to Self-Discovery, Relationships, Values, and Spiritual Growth.* New York: Fireside, 1992.

Patterson, Sheila M., and Elaine M. Vitello. "Ethics in Health Education: The Need to Include a Model Course in Professional Preparation Programs." *Journal of Health Education,* July/August 1993.

Pietig, Jeanne. "Values and Morality in the Early 20th Century Elementary Schools: A Perspective." *Social Education,* November 1983.

Whitehead, Barbara Defoe. "Dan Quayle Was Right." *The Atlantic Monthly,* April 1993.

Wilson, James. *The Moral Sense.* New York: Free Press, 1993.

12 Teaching for Self-Esteem: Theory

Self-esteem, a popular expression in the 1990s, is defined as an impression one has of oneself that can be either negative or positive. A commonly held theory is that schools (and, more important, teachers and community-health educators) can influence self-esteem in the learner. As such, schools are instituting multicultural programs that feature the historic achievements of ethnic and racial minorities, in part, to boost self-esteem. Leading corporations are hiring consultants to elevate worker morale and productivity via self-esteem enhancement techniques. Companies are forming to teach people how to feel better about themselves.

Foster self-respect, insist some experts (Branden, 1992), and society as a whole will benefit—with decreases in teenage pregnancy, crime, welfare dependency, eating disorders, substance abuse, academic failure, and drop-out rates.

The self-esteem movement in education kicked off in the late 1980s with the formation of the *California Task Force to Promote Self-Esteem and Personal and Social Responsibility* (1989). It instituted classroom discussions about the importance of self-esteem and had students keep notebooks on what made them feel empowered. The effect was measurable, according to Gloria Steinem's bestseller, *Revolution from Within: A Book of Self-Esteem* (1992). In a high school that examined the connection between unwanted pregnancy and self-esteem, the number of pregnancies after the program was employed dropped from 147 to 20 over three years.

The effects of poor self-image can be more subtle. People who judge and reject themselves take fewer social, academic, or career risks (McKay and Flanning, 1987). They avoid meeting new people, opening up to others, expressing their sexuality, hearing criticism, seeking help, and solving problems. And these are the children we teach. They need our self-

We do not see things as they are.

We see them as we are.

—THE TALMUD

esteem support. This support includes our ability to feel good about *ourselves,* because this quality is essential to building self-esteem in the classroom.

The Impact of Self on Self-Esteem

In conducting interviews for their book *Women and Self-Esteem,* Linda Sanford and Mary Ellen Donovan found that "a single positive experience could have an enormous impact on the outlook of a small child from a troubled family. Sometimes, one affectionate, encouraging, and supportive teacher made the difference between self-hate and the start of self-acceptance for a child" (1984).

If a health educator is trying to help a student feel better about himself so they can get him into a personal, cognitive discussion about potential change, it would be naive to merely manipulate the situation according to one or another theory of motivation. Inadvertent "teaching" is already taking place, through the student's perception of the teacher's "silent language"—her feelings, tone, posture, timing, and choice of words. In short, the way the teacher comes across is obvious and just as influential as what she says. We could say that a teacher's principal *effect* is his or her *affect* (Hilgard, 1966; Luft, 1970).

As teachers, feeling good about ourselves is necessary to helping others feel good about themselves. Therefore, unless we have positive self-esteem and communicate this feeling in both verbal and nonverbal ways, we will not be of much use in helping anyone else.

William W. Purkey, in his book *Self-Concept and School Achievement* (1970) states,

> *a basic assumption of the theory of the self-concept is that we behave according to our beliefs. If this assumption is true, then it follows that the teacher's beliefs about himself and his students are crucial factors in determining his effectiveness in the classroom. Available evidence (Combs et al., 1969) indicates that the teacher's attitudes toward himself and others are as important, if not more so, than his techniques, practices, or materials.*

To help students gain more positive perceptions of themselves, we must begin by noticing how we present ourselves to them. The key may be in presenting ourselves as we truly *are.*

What Learners See Is What They Get

In a series of studies, Rhona Weinstein and her associates (1984) concluded that children are highly sensitive to a helpers' behavior and can describe it in a consistent manner as early as first grade.

Elisha Babad (1990) of the Hebrew University used Weinstein's methods for assessing students' and teachers' perceptions to compare what they see. Like Weinstein, he found that students respond quite differently depending on how questions about their teacher are framed. When asked how often they experienced particular teacher behaviors, students had a tendency to report being treated "like the others." But when given descriptions of two hypothetical students—a low and a high achiever—students predicted important differences in how the teacher would act toward each. For example, students believed that the low achiever would receive more learning support from the teacher, because he would approach the student more often to observe and help her with her work. They also thought the teacher would put more pressure on the high achiever, addressing more difficult questions to her and demanding a higher level of work.

Teachers agreed with both these observations, but their answers directly contradicted the students when it came to assessing which child would get more emotional support. The students expected the teacher to be more positive toward high-achieving students, praising them more and being more warm and supportive. In contrast, the teachers believed that low-achieving students would get more emotional support.

How this translates is that students believe teachers often reward pupils with high self-esteem and ignore those with low self-esteem. It is a reverse of what we should really be doing. So, how should we deal with it?

What Is Self-Esteem?

Psychologist Nathaniel Branden (1992), considered to be the father of the concept of self-esteem, defined this quality as "the disposition to experience oneself as competent to cope with the challenges of life and as deserving of happiness." In his view, the self is the mind and its characteristic manner of operation. Unlike that of other species, the mind of the human being can judge what is best for itself and yet *proceed to do the opposite.*

Self-esteem includes feeling lovable and capable, and caring about oneself and others. People with positive self-esteem do not have to build themselves up by tearing other people down or by patronizing less competent people. This quality has two interrelated aspects (Branden, 1994):

1. **A sense of personal efficacy.** *Self-efficacy* means confidence in the functioning of your mind and in the processes by which you judge, choose, and decide. You trust your ability to understand the realities in your sphere of interests and needs; cognitively, you trust yourself and are self-reliant.
2. **A sense of personal worth (self-respect).** *Self-respect* means assurance of your value. You believe you have the right to live and be happy and are comfortable in appropriately asserting your thoughts, wants, and needs.

As health educators, our connections with our students can evoke these positive qualities or at least help us identify those areas where we can evolve creatively and constructively. Feeling like a unique and special person while working in close affiliation with others, however, is sometimes hard. Yet effective relationships include a measure of frustration: they provoke us to confront our contradictions and develop beyond our previous limitations. Even though they may be painful, such confrontations can reinforce our commitment to foster individual growth as collaborators rather than antagonists.

Unrewarded choices lead to low self-esteem and an expectation that life will be difficult—and so it may be. The tragedy—or triumph—is that our sense of self is often a self-fulfilling prophecy. We *become* what we believe we *are*. Thus, self-esteem is central to healthy human functioning. If we believe in free will, we must take responsibility for our choices. "We cannot exempt ourselves from the realm of values and value judgments" (Branden, 1992).

The Sabotage of Self-Esteem

The sabotage of self-esteem starts at a very young age. Because they don't want to acknowledge their own confusion and fears, adults often try to disguise their feelings and actions around children, as well as other adults. But, given her innate drive for understanding, the child tries to make sense of the situation on her own. The solution is often "there's something wrong with me" (Branden, 1984). This self-condemnation is a survival strategy. "If I suffer, I must have committed some offense, even though I don't understand what it is. It is too terrifying to imagine that my parents do not know what they are doing. I will disown what I see, express what I feel—and take the guilt upon myself" (Branden, 1984). The problem is compounded by the fact that when she thinks she's bad, the child acts to prove herself right. She hits younger siblings, smashes a friend's toy, or tells lies.

The Negative Effects of Low Self-Esteem

If we look at teenage pregnancy, an area that is very much related to health education, we see that lack of self-esteem is an important component behind the problem. A number of studies support the finding that teenage females who become pregnant have low self-esteem or engage in self-devaluation, regardless of methods used for measuring self-concept (Patten, 1981). Pregnancy was associated with feelings of estrangement and shame, inability to defer gratification, distrust of others, and lack of confidence in the work-employment domain (Protinsky, 1982). Pregnancy at this age is also associated with social isolation (Roberts, 1966) and a sense of anomie (Goode, 1961). Teenage mothers often have an external locus of control—they feel they have no control over their lives or what happens to them; rather, they see themselves as propelled by fate or circumstance and not by their own effort or ability. This perceived lack of control is tied to an increased willingness to take risks, because personal responsibility for actions is never really accepted (Connolly, 1975; Osofsky, 1988). (One study of 93 teenaged mothers, seventy of whom had at least one child, was conducted on the basis of normlessness—being unaware of dominant societal rules—and powerlessness. This is one of the few studies to report no differences in self-esteem between teenage mothers and nonmothers) (Streetman, 1987).

How can we approach this problem? No answers come easy, but some realities can be offered:

- *teenage girls who become pregnant are betraying themselves*
- they are love "junkies" with a false, romanticized perception of their sexual encounters and those they are getting involved with
- they are desperately seeking love through sex and pregnancy
- they need to view their behavior realistically

A child with seriously low self-esteem is more vulnerable to negative social pressures (Sattler, 1994):

> When a teen feels unsuccessful in school, extracurricular activities, or fitting in with peers, he (or she) may use drugs or alcohol to feel "older," or to "treat" uncomfortable feelings of anxiety, disappointment, or depression. . . . Since a child with low self-esteem tends to believe he (or she) has no appreciated talents, that individuals are more easily tempted by drugs and alcohol than he or she is by the more challenging path of sports or music in his or her attempt to establish an identity.

Thus, we as health educators must conclude that building self-esteem is critical to positive health education. The process should not be complicated, energy consuming, or require a great deal of extra work, but it does require some understanding (Branden, 1994).

> In working with self-esteem, we need to be aware of two dangers. One is that of oversimplifying what healthy self-esteem requires, and thereby of catering to people's hunger for quick fixes and effortless solutions. The other is that of surrendering to a kind of fatalism or determinism that assumes, in effect, that individuals "either have good self-esteem or they haven't," that everyone's destiny is set (forever?) by the first few years of life, and there's not much to be done about it (except perhaps years or decades of psychotherapy). Both views encourage passivity; both obstruct our vision of what is possible.

Factors in Self-Esteem

Self-esteem is more than merely recognizing your positive qualities. It is an attitude of acceptance and nonjudgment toward yourself and others. If self-esteem is a judgment you make or a feeling you have about yourself, then it most surely follows that having positive self-esteem supports positive caring and regard for others. Self-esteem is the result of a long process and an accumulation of events. It is dynamic and ever-changing. Building and maintaining it is an all-day, all-year, all-the-time endeavor. It flourishes in a safe, caring environment and grows when people with high self-esteem work to promote the same in others.

Much has been written on the attributes and sources of this inner quality, whether it is called self-concept, self-confidence, self-image, or self-esteem. Maslow (1942) researched what he called the dominant personality, then later called it self-esteem. He found that high dominance feeling (high self-esteem) involved

- self-confidence
- self-assurance
- high evaluation of the self
- feelings of general capability and superiority
- lack of shyness, timidity, self-consciousness, or embarrassment

Conversely, he found that people with low dominance feeling (low self-esteem) had extensive feelings of general or specific inferiority, shyness, timidity, fearfulness, and self-consciousness.

Maslow saw the self-actualized person as having achieved a high level of mental health (1968). He and others in the humanistic branches of psychology brought to our attention that every human being carries within his life the only real and possible standards by which to measure adjustment—*the realization of the self.* For some, personal adjustment may take place at the expense of social adjustments. But people who attain self-actualization are neither sociopaths nor anarchists. They are aware that we live in a social environment and benefit greatly from social experiences. Therefore, they "actualize" their selfhood as fully as possible while at the same time maintaining a realistic understanding of the social demands placed on them. Although this often calls for a compromise in behavior, it does not necessitate compromises in thought or attitude. Self-actualization includes the full appreciation of the social relations and needs of each person remaining true to the self without infringing on the selfhood of others. As Albert Schweitzer understood, "I am life affirming itself in the midst of other lives affirming themselves" (1959).

How can we move toward a more positive sense of self? Nathaniel Branden lists several central components of self-esteem (1994):

- **The will to understand.** This is an active rather than a passive response to life, a commitment to thinking as a way of life.
- **The will to be efficacious.** This is an extension of the will to understand. It emphasizes perseverance in the face of difficulties and defeat. We all know times of bewilderment and despair. The question is whether we allow such moments to define us. The will to be efficacious separates those who feel fundamentally defeated by life from those who do not.
- **Intellectual independence.** Often, what people call thinking is merely recycling the opinions of others. Self-esteem is not a given. Rather, it is acquired by thinking independently when it isn't easy to do so and even when it is frightening to do so.

"That which we call 'genius' has a great deal to do with courage and daring, a great deal to do with sheer nerve." (Branden, 1984).

The Core Ingredients in Self-Esteem

To a large extent, self-esteem is formed by what others tell us about ourselves, especially during the formative years of childhood. Whether we develop a basically positive or negative outlook has a good deal to do with what people close to us have said and expected (Mellody, 1989):

Children learn self-esteem first from their major caregivers. But dysfunctional caregivers give their children, verbally or nonverbally, the message that children are "less-than" people. These "less-than" messages from the caregivers become part of the children's own opinion of themselves. Upon reaching adulthood, it is almost impossible for those with "less-than" messages to be able to generate the feeling from within that they have value.

Our sense of self-worth is sometimes so repressed we have to struggle to accept that we are truly lovable and capable.

Low self-esteem also plays a major role in distorting our perception of reality. We repress our feelings and understanding of why we do what we do. Such people, when asked why they smoke, are involved in drugs, or are engaged in unprotected sex, simply say "I don't know." And they truly don't.

Shame and Self-Esteem

Psychologist Nathaniel Branden calls self-esteem the reputation we have with ourselves (1984). When we live our lives out of shame and believe that we are unworthy, that reputation is low—and low self-esteem is the result. Our relationship with ourself is strained and burdensome.

We stand in the midst of an almost infinite network of relationships: to things, to the universe. And yet, at three o'clock in the morning, when we are alone with ourselves, we are aware that the most intimate and powerful of all relationships and the one we can never escape is the relationship to ourselves. No significant aspect of our thinking, motivation, feelings, or behavior is unaffected by our self-evaluation. We are organisms who are not only conscious but self-conscious. That is our glory and, at times, our burden (Branden, 1984).

While the capacity to feel shame is normal, adaptive, and a requirement for the health development of guilt, conscience, compassion, and empathy, it can take on a life of its own that is unrelated to its primary function as an alarm for overstepping boundaries. We must distinguish between shame as a passing emotion, a normal reaction to a sudden, unexpected exposure where we lose face, and shame as an identity, a state in which we feel alienated, deficient, despairing, and helpless in general (Kaufman, 1985):

Contained in the experience of shame is the piercing awareness of ourselves as fundamentally deficient in some vital way as a human being. To live with shame is to experience the very essence or heart of the self as wanting. Shame is an impotence-making experience because it feels as though there is no way to relieve the matter, no way to restore the balance of things. One has simply failed as a human being. No single action is seen as wrong and, hence, reparable.

Shame as an identity—what John Bradshaw calls *toxic shame*—means feeling flawed and diminished, as though we never measure up. With toxic shame, "there's something wrong with *you* and there's nothing you can do about it; you *are* inadequate and defective" (1991). Bradshaw traced how this distorted thinking leads to a whole range of addictive behaviors. Whether we choose to alter our mood and recover a temporary sense of power and connectedness through alcohol, drugs, sex, work, perfectionism, dependent or controlling relationships, or some forms of religious or other beliefs and practices, we are really seeking the same thing: self-respect and a connectedness to a larger frame of meaning. We are searching both for our temporal self (a human being of unique worth) and our eternal self as part of a greater whole. The opposite of this is *healthy shame,* which Bradshaw defines as the permission to be human (1991).

The Two Extremes of Self-Esteem

Pia Mellody (1989) stated that codependents experience difficulty with self-esteem at one or both of two extremes: at one extreme, self-esteem is low or nonexistent; they think they are worth less than others. At the opposite extreme is arrogance and grandiosity; they think they are superior to others. This "other-esteem" is based on external things, including some of the following:

- how they look
- how much money they make
- who they are
- what kind of car they drive
- what kind of job they have
- how well their children perform
- how powerful and important or attractive their spouse is
- the degrees they have earned
- how well they perform activities in which others value excellence

Getting satisfaction or enjoyment for these reasons is fine, but it is not self-esteem (Mellody, 1989). Other-esteem is based either on human "doing" or on the opinions of other people. The source of other-esteem is outside the self; thus, it is vulnerable to change and beyond our control. We can lose it at any time, so it is fragile and undependable.

As those with low self-esteem use external sources to satisfy internal needs, so do codependents seek constant approval to feel good about themselves. They experience a basic sense of shame: "When I make a mistake, it's just another example of what a worthless person I really am. I come from a screwed up family, so there must be something wrong with *me*" (Subby, 1987). This is what Albert Ellis talks about in his concept of rational-emotive therapy (see Chapter 7).

Self-Esteem and Achievement

Have you ever had a heated argument with someone you care for, an argument that left you with feelings of self-doubt, and then had to attend a class the next hour? Consider the following questions:

- How focused were you on the subject being taught?
- How did you respond to the professor's questions?
- Did you feel like you just wanted to be somewhere else?
- Were you happy?

When you enter a classroom every day, ask yourself these same questions about the students facing you. Did they have a fight with one of their parents that morning? Did their friends play a mean joke on them? Did they just have a fight with their boyfriend or girlfriend? All of these situations can be especially debilitating to students with low self-esteem.

Students function in school the same way they do outside. If they feel bad, they act bad in the classroom. If they are angry, they act out this anger in the classroom. If they feel less than zero outside the class, they feel less than zero inside the class. If they have suffered a loss of love and have low self-esteem, little else matters.

Research evidence clearly shows a significant relationship between self-esteem and academic achievement (Purkey, 1970; Wiley, 1961). One study by Peggy Orenstein, author of *School Girls: Young Women, Self-Esteem, and the Confidence Gap* (1994), illustrates this relationship clearly. She documented how, as young girls reach adolescence, their self-esteem plummets. "Girls begin first grade with the same levels of skill and ambition as boys, but, all too often, by the time they reach high school their doubts have crowded out their dreams. They emerge from adolescence with reduced expectations of life, and much less confidence in themselves and in their abilities than boys have."

Self-Esteem, Peer Acceptance, and Social Bonding

Most individuals who are products of dysfunctional families are vulnerable to low self-esteem. This group is often lost to drug abuse, crime, and teen pregnancy (Hamburg, 1992). They are also vulnerable to seeking peer acceptance as a way of building and supporting their self-esteem.

Peer acceptance and social bonding has a lot to do with how young people react to their environment (more specifically, to health issues such as safe sex, drug abuse, cigarette smoking, drinking to excess, etc.). If we look just at cigarette smoking, teens will tell you that it promotes social bonding to smoke, to ask someone for a cigarette (or be asked for one), or to sit around smoking in a group. This is also true of sharing role models such as professional athletes (i.e., Magic Johnson or Larry Bird). One recent study discovered that black teenagers in urban areas perceived most black celebrities as simply being white-owned performers, and that more of those teenagers were listening to Ice-T than to Magic Johnson. The same study found that young urban blacks lived in a world in which many would risk death rather than be ostracized for raising issues of safe sex or not using drugs (MEE Productions, 1992).

Who do young minorities look up to? A recent study conducted by the Educational Testing Service (Senior and Anderson, 1993) found that black students harbor personal respect for the academically inclined:

- Those most respected by others were the "smart but popular" students and male athletes
- Those they *personally* most respected were the "smart but popular," rule-obeying students and nerds

These facts present us with cognitive and behavioral resources that need to be worked into student-centered pedagogy: students respect peer role models who are academically inclined, forward moving, and on a positive course. Health educators need to explore peer role models as an avenue through which to pursue positive health behaviors. Rather than using unrealistic role models such as Magic Johnson, we need to highlight the more realistic achievements of the students around them. This concept makes sense, since students are seeking acceptance and respect from other students and the teacher, not from outside sources.

Self-Esteem, Health, and Positive Performance

Robert Ader, who pioneered the field of psychoneuroimmunology (the study of the link between thoughts and emotions), has been joined by a growing cadre of researchers in documenting the role of the mind in disease and healing. In short, they are studying how the mind affects the body, both positively and negatively. This was covered extensively in Chapter 2, but we need to look at it again in the context of *self-efficacy* (the belief that one can perform a specific task) (Bandura, 1993). Self-efficacy is like self-esteem, but the sense of confidence relates to something specific rather than general. For example, your feeling of self-efficacy may be high in regard to driving—you know you have the skills to get where you are going despite road conditions, etc.—but poor when faced with organizing a given task.

Building self-esteem is a form of cognitive therapy. Cognition, which has been covered in previous chapters, is simply a fancy name for thought. Cognitive therapy is based on the idea that our thoughts and attitudes have a profound impact on our moods. Thus, when we change negative feelings into positive feelings, we are creating some very powerful and profound effects. One of these is a greater sense of self-confidence. Instilling this confidence can translate into the most important progress a teacher makes toward helping people change their lives for the better (e.g., via nutrition, exercise, giving up drugs, and smoking cessation).

A number of studies have raised the following additional questions:

- Does academic success foster self-esteem, or does self-esteem foster academic success?
- Does social status cause high self-esteem, or does high self-esteem help gain social status?
- Do young people abuse drugs because they hate themselves, or do they hate themselves because they abuse drugs?
- Do highly successful athletes like themselves because they are doing so well, or do they do well because they like themselves?

These are classic chicken-and-egg debates, but they all deal with human performance and motivation. Thus, the sole question becomes "Do internal or external forces determine the self? The bottom line is, internal feelings play the most important role in positive self-esteem. External factors may bolster or damage self-esteem momentarily, but the lasting qualities come from within. Supporting this theory are the cognitive-behavioral methods that raise self-esteem by changing the way people interpret their lives. External support for self-esteem is short-lived, based on acceptance and conformity, and ultimately self-destructive (Anderson, 1994).

Providing students with superficial, externally directed programs to bolster self-esteem simply supports the idea that you can gain self-esteem from outside things (e.g., peers, money, or the right clothes, shoes). Reliance on things takes away a person's sense of value, and ultimately her sense of self.

Golden opportunities for self-esteem building come when teachers realize the need to confront learners with their cognitive distortions of self and teach them more accurate and compassionate methods of self-evaluation.

Health Education and Self-Esteem

As we learn to treat ourselves with increasing respect and regard as health educators, we increase our ability to accept the love and respect that others might give us. At the same time, we strengthen our foundation for genuinely loving and respecting others. "Love of one's self is not antagonistic to having satisfying relationships. On the contrary, we are free to love others only as we become free to love ourselves" (Hodge, 1967). Milton Mayeroff agreed with this assessment (1971): "If I am unable to care for myself, I am unable to care for another person." To care for ourselves, we need to be responsive to our own needs for growth; we also need to feel at one with rather than estranged from ourselves. Furthermore, caring for ourselves and caring for others are mutually dependent; we can only fulfill ourselves by serving someone or something apart from ourselves. If we are unable to care for anyone or anything else, we are unable to care for ourselves.

A basic assumption of self-concept theory is that we behave according to our beliefs. If this assumption is correct, it follows that the teacher's beliefs about himself and his students are crucial to determining his effectiveness in the classroom (Purkey, 1970). Additional evidence indicates that the teacher's attitudes toward himself and others are as important, if not more so, than his techniques, practices, or materials (Combs, 1969).

When asked about the purpose of psychoanalysis, Freud replied, "to love and to work." In a broad sense, most helping theories support the idea that effective daily living and positive relationships are the goals of helping and teaching.

Negativism to Positivism

Fact: No one wants to come to school every day and feel like a failure.
Reality: A positive approach to teaching emphasizes the strengths in every student, helping them feel like a winner. Teachers must accept and understand that

many students have the capacity to achieve positive goals in at least some areas of their lives. To develop this capacity, the focus must move away from irrelevant subject matter to students' real-life concerns and experiences. The approach must also be positive; pay attention to how you talk to and behave toward students.

Positivism, as I use it here, is based on the work of Eric Berne and his best-selling book *Games People Play* (1974), in which he developed his theory of transactional analysis (TA). One of the special strengths of transactional analysis is the development of a language system that is about communicating with people rather than hiding behind vague theoretical constructs, thereby demystifying the process of teaching.

> *The worldview of TA can be summarized by the following: Transactional analysis is a rational approach to understanding behavior and is based on the assumption that all individuals can learn to trust themselves, think for themselves, make their own decisions, and express their feelings. Its principles can be applied on the job, in the home, in the classroom, in the neighborhood—wherever people deal with people* (James and Jongeward, 1971).

The belief that people can learn to trust themselves, think for themselves, and express their feelings is based on Berne's "I'm okay/you're okay" philosophy. For educators, it is the belief that students should feel validated and acknowledged as individuals, and that they can form a positive self-identity along with a positive image of the world around them.

To help students feel this sense of okayness, a teacher must offer positive strokes. In *Readings in Radical Psychiatry* (1975) C. Steiner stated, "Children are born princes and princesses, and their parents turn them into frogs." In effect, Steiner is saying that people are born with natural abilities and intentionality, but society (school and community in our context) takes it out of them.

Strokes are delivered to us physically when we are touched with warmth and caring or given to us emotionally through kind words and deeds. However, through carefully controlling strokes, teachers often and without conscious knowledge deny students the most important learning experience of their lives—that they are valued for their contribution to the learning experience. The most validating way to encourage students to feel positive about themselves is in positive interactions with the teacher.

Positive stroking can be described as virtually anything a person does to enhance another (Harris, 1967). Strokes can be active positive regard, respect and warmth, or a shared response that conveys the message that you care. The bottom line is, *when you treat people responsibly, they act responsibly.*

Synthesis

Teachers who habitually judge make the classroom a living hell. Few things steal more vitality or cast a chillier mood than the habit of criticizing and condemning students for mistakes or moments of "creative" thinking. Being habitually critical also affects the quality of the classroom environment. When you put someone down, all are on guard against being the next victim. In this way, you cut yourself off from the other students. A teacher who is a chronic critic becomes harder, more hostile, and more egotistical. Remember, champion one-uppers leave their victims one down. They may evoke admiration and fear but seldom affection.

Roman Emperor Marcus Aurelius once commented, "Men exist for the sake of one another. Teach them or bear with them." When we, as health educators, feel an impulse to criticize learners, we might first ask ourselves if we are willing to take the time to show them a better way and do so nonjudgmentally, so they'll be willing to hear. Do you, the prospective health educator, know a better way? In some instances, I truly believe the answer is yes.

References

Anderson, Elijah. "The Code of the Streets: How the Inner-City Environment Fosters a Need for Respect and a Self-Image Based on Violence." *Atlantic Monthly,* May 1994.

Babad, Elisha. "Measuring and Changing Teachers' Differential Behavior as Perceived by Students and Teachers." *Journal of Educational Psychology,* 1990.

Bandura, Albert. "Arthritis and Rheumatic Disease: What Doctors Can Learn from Their Patients," in Goleman, Daniel, and Joel Gurin (eds.), *Mind/Body Medicine: How to Use Your Mind for Better Health.* Yonkers, New York: Consumer Reports Books, 1993.

Berne, Eric. *Games People Play.* New York: Ballantine, 1974.

Bradshaw, John. "Healing the Child Within" (interview with Joan Borysenko). *New Age Journal,* July/August 1991.

Branden, Nathaniel. *Honoring the Self.* Los Angeles: Jeremy Tarcher, 1984.

___. *The Power of Self-Esteem.* Deerfield Beach, FL: Health Communications, 1992.

___. *The Six Pillars of Self-Esteem.* New York: Bantam, 1994.

California Task Force to Promote Self-Esteem and Personal and Social Responsibility. Sacramento, CA: 1130 K Street, Suite 300.

Combs, A.W., et al. *Florida Studies in the Helping Professions.* University of Florida Social Science Monograph No. 37, 1969.

Connolly, L. "Little Mothers." *Human Behavior* 11, 1975.

Goode, W.J. "Illegitimacy, Anomie, and Cultural Penetration." *American Sociological Review* 26, 1961.

Hamburg, David. *Today's Children: Creating a Future for a Generation in Crisis.* New York: Times Books, 1992.

Harris, Thomas A. *I'm OK—You're OK.* New York: Avon, 1967.

Hilgard, Ernest. "The Human Dimension in Teaching." *Stanford University Delta News-Journal,* Winter 1966.

Hodge, M. *Your Fear of Love.* Garden City, NY: Doubleday, 1967.

James, Muriel, and Dorothy Jongeward. *Born to Win*. Reading, MA: Addison-Wesley, 1971.

Kaufman, Gershen. *Shame: The Power of Caring*. Rochester, VT: Schenkman Books, 1985.

Luft, Joseph. *Group Process*. Palo Alto, CA: National Press Books, 1970.

Maslow, A.H. "Self-Esteem (Dominance Feeling) and Sexuality in Women." *The Journal of Social Psychology* 64, 1942.

___. *Toward a Psychology of Being* (2nd ed.). Princeton, NJ: Van Nostrand, 1968.

Mayeroff, Milton. *On Caring*. New York: Harper & Row, 1971.

McKay, Matthew, and Patrick Flanning. *Self-Esteem: A Proven Program of Cognitive Techniques for Assessing, Improving, and Maintaining Your Self-Esteem*. Oakland, CA: New Harbinger Publications, 1987.

MEE Productions, Inc. "Reaching the Hip-Hop Generation." Princeton, NJ: The Robert Wood Johnson Foundation, 1992.

Mellody, Pia. *Facing Codependence*. San Francisco: Harper Collins, 1989.

Osofsky, J.D., H.J. Osofsky, and M.O. Diamond. "The Transition to Parenthood: Special Tasks and Risk Factors for Adolescent Parents," in G.Y. Michaels and W.A. Goldberg (eds.), *The Transition to Parenthood*. Cambridge: Cambridge University Press, 1988.

Patten, M. "Self-Concept and Self-Esteem: Factors in Adolescent Pregnancy." *Adolescence* 64, 1981.

Purkey, William. *Self-Concept and School Achievement*. Englewood Cliffs, NJ: Prentice-Hall, 1970.

Protinsky, H., H. Sporakowski, and S. Atkins. "Identity Formation: Pregnant and Nonpregnant Adolescents." *Adolescence* 65, 1982.

Roberts, R.W. *The Unwed Mother*. New York: Harper and Row, 1966.

Sanford, Linda T., and Mary Ellen Donovan. *Women and Self-Esteem*. 1984.

Sattler, Ann. "Teens and Self-Esteem." *Wayland Weston [MA] Town Crier,* 27 October 1994.

Schweitzer, Albert. *Light within Us*. Secaucus, NJ: Citadel Press, 1959.

Senior, Ann Marie, and Bernice Taylor Anderson. "A Study on Respect." *USA Today,* 22 March 1993.

Steinem, Gloria. *Revolution from Within: A Book of Self-Esteem*. New York: Little, Brown, 1992.

Steiner, C. (ed.). *Readings in Radical Psychiatry*. New York: Grove, 1975.

Streetman, L. "Contrasts in the Self-Esteem of Unwed Teenage Mothers." *Adolescence* 86, 1987.

Subby, Robert. *Lost in the Shuffle: The Codependent Reality*. Deerfield Beach, FL: Health Communications, 1987.

Weinstein, Rhona. "Perceptions of Classroom Process and Student Motivation: Children's Views of Self-Fulfilling Prophecies," in R. Ames and C. Ames (eds.), *Research on Motivation in Education,* vol. 3. New York: Academic Press, 1984.

Wylie, Ruth C. *The Self-Concept: A Critical Survey of Pertinent Research Literature*. Lincoln: University of Nebraska Press, 1961.

Additional Resources

Orenstein, Peggy. *School Girls: Young Women, Self-Esteem, and the Confidence Gap.* New York: Doubleday, 1994.

Taylor, Jill McLean, Carol Gilligan, and Amy M. Sullivan. *Women and Girls: Race and Relationship.* Cambridge, MA: Harvard University Press, 1996.

13 Building Self-Esteem: Application

In Richard Bach's book *Jonathan Livingston Seagull* (1970), a wondrous story about a seagull who chooses to fly beyond the limits he was taught to believe and accept, the gull is advised, "to fly as fast as thought, to anywhere . . . you must begin by knowing that you have already arrived." This advice is so simple that we can lose sight of its meaning. The major realization for Jonathan was that he was not trapped inside the limitations of his body; rather, his limitations were those he had placed on himself.

A basic premise of this book is that the individual and the environment are mutually influential, acting on one another dynamically to produce development. In other words, development results from encounters between children and their physical, social, and cultural contexts. As the child changes and matures, her caretakers respond and adapt to these changes. In turn, the child's development is influenced by the caretakers' responses. Thus, both adaptive and maladaptive parent-child relationships influence the characteristics and changes in the child, as does the wider environment.

To turn maladaptive behavior around is to first understand that such behavior is often caused by early childhood experiences that result in internalized shame. While guilt is a painful feeling of regret and responsibility for one's actions, shame is a painful feeling about oneself as a person (Fossum and Mason, 1991). A great deal of this shame comes from the people in students' lives.

Health and Self-Esteem

A study conducted in California suggests that health is intimately related to feelings of self-esteem and regard for others. A survey of roughly one-thousand Californians was commissioned by the Office of

To evolve into selfhood is the primary human task. It is also the primary human challenge, because success is not guaranteed.

—Nathaniel Branden

Prevention, California Department of Mental Health, to report on health attitudes, coping strategies, and methods of change. Self-esteem was measured by the subjects' agreement or disagreement with two statements: "On the whole, I feel good about myself" and "I wish I could have more respect for myself." In the final tally, those who felt best about themselves also said they were in better mental and physical shape than those who were low in self-esteem. In addition, low self-esteem went with more reported physical illness, with disturbances such as insomnia, anxiousness, and depression, and with greater frequency of marital conflict, financial problems, and emotional distress (Field Research Corporation, 1979).

The survey, designed to illuminate how beliefs strongly affect well-being, found that respondents considered outlook on life and style of life the factors that most influenced health. Other factors, in order of their importance to respondents, were relations with others, physical environment, heredity, and availability of medical and psychological services. (Persons with low self-esteem were less likely than those with high self-esteem to seek professional help for psychological problems.)

Body Image

We often times think of the body as separate from the mind, but nothing could be further from the truth. They coexist, and as such they are part and parcel of what we call self-esteem. Some researchers believe that how we experience our bodies may have more profound influences on our behavior than how we experience the world around us.

Our body encompasses a sector of space that is uniquely our own. It represents our base of operations in the world, the outward manifestation of our being and identity. No other object is so persistently with us.

Body image certainly affects those of us who, for example, feel overweight, underweight, unattractive, bland, or short. All of these feelings well up into behaviors that include eating disorders and relationship problems, and contribute to feelings of low self-worth.

Body-image problems seem to be more pronounced in girls and women (Rodin, 1992). Unnatural and unrealistic societal expectations give rise to beliefs and feelings that keep women imprisoned by anguish over how they look, whether they are doing enough to be attractive, and feelings of shame for worrying about it. These distortions arise in part from the staggering amount of misinformation the public receives about the physiological determinants of weight.

Body-image conflicts are shared by almost every woman, even those who appear to others to have bodies that are close to "ideal." These conflicts are as complicated and intertwined as our feelings about our bodies.

Self-Esteem and the Learning Process

Self-esteem. It used to be assumed that children came to school with it and that it was the responsibility of parents, not teachers, to build it. Now educators are talking about the relationship between a student's self-esteem and school perfor-

Self-Esteem and Young Women

In *School Girls* (1994), Peggy Orenstein looks at the education system and how it often breaks the precarious confidence of young women and girls. Some schools have recognized this disturbing trend and taken steps to amend it. For example, the Foundation for Seacoast Health in Portsmouth, New Hampshire, a local health organization, has issued a grant to begin self-esteem and assertiveness training for middle- and high-school girls. According to Deb Schnappauf, one of the grant writers, "Girls' perspective of themselves influences all aspects of their lives. And while that includes academics, we are looking at the whole girl and issues like relationships and the future. We're trying to work with girls to make good choices for themselves" (*Boston Globe,* 1994). The training will involve a three-day conference for female students between the ages of fourteen and eighteen and will encourage the young women to become community leaders by featuring local role models. The Portsmouth school board has also agreed to review a proposed all-girl math class at the high school.

Source: The Boston Globe, 25 November 1994. Used with permission.

mance. Children today, in addition to classes, spend ten hours a week or more in after-school programs. It is a documented fact that a child with high intelligence but poor self-esteem will not achieve as well as a child with average ability and high self-esteem and will have a higher incidence of crime and violence, alcohol and drug abuse, teenage pregnancy, child and spousal abuse, chronic welfare dependency, and failure to learn in school (Purkey, 1970; CA Department of Education, 1990).

Some techniques for boosting a student's self-esteem are based on common sense, such as encouraging her efforts, giving her a sense of belonging in the classroom, talking with her about her outside interests, or showing patience with her learning style. According to Robert Brooks, director of child and adolescent psychology at McLean Hospital in Belmont, Massachusetts and author of *The Self-Esteem Teacher* (1994), "the most influential force in determining the effectiveness of self-esteem strategies is the relationship students have with their teachers." We must accept and understand this principle if we are to make the learning environment more positive for those who feel "less than zero."

In the mid 1980s, California assemblyman John Vasconcellos set up a task force to determine if improving young peoples' self-esteem might mitigate social problems like welfare dependency, high drop-out rates, teen pregnancy, and gang violence (CA Department of Education, 1986). The concept has since been called a *social vaccine;* a new organizing principle for solving problems. Today, three-fourths of California schools have some self-esteem component, most social legislation includes it as a curriculum goal, and many other states have self-esteem task forces of their own (*New Age Journal,* 1993).

Self-esteem, however, cannot be directly taught; it must be developed. Special programs and activities, stickers, and gold stars are all nice, but they will not be enough for children who feel worthless because they come from dysfunctional families or have been labeled as failures by their schools.

Developing self-esteem doesn't mean praising students for shoddy work; children are quick to spot and discount false praise. To foster real self-esteem, we must create learning environments where all children feel valued and are provided with enough support and encouragement to be successful. Some children need more "scaffolding" than others. Because schools don't always help children feel good about themselves and achieve results valued by others, many teenagers just drop out. School has actually taught them *not* to have pride in themselves.

All of our behavior is a constant attempt to satisfy one or more of the five basic needs written into our genetic structure: (1) to *survive and reproduce,* (2) to *belong and love,* (3) to *gain power,* (4) to *be free,* and (5) to *have fun* (Glasser, 1990). If teachers can make students feel they belong and are capable, then students will learn because they want to learn. We have only to talk with young people to see that the reasons they drop out or do poorly in class can often be traced to teachers' lack of concern with satisfying these basic needs.

When students believe that teachers and other students care about them, they begin to believe in themselves. Each small success makes them hungry for the good feeling that comes when something goes well, so they are motivated to risk more and try again. When classroom activities require only that they listen or read to get information and spit it back on a test, there are too few opportunities for students to develop their creative and critical-thinking skills, both of which help them discover and demonstrate their unique individual talents and abilities.

The American Association of School Administrators makes these recommendations for establishing a classroom climate in which self-esteem can flourish (1991):

- Make sure that developing self-esteem is a priority in your school or district. Emphasize that all students are capable of academic achievement and are expected to be successful.
- Model the behavior that staff members should adopt with students. Teachers and others who lack a sense of self-esteem are unlikely to instill it in others. When teachers like themselves, they are much more likely to develop healthy self-concepts in their students.
- Provide in-service programs for all school staff members on ways to bolster students' self-esteem.
- Provide a variety of curricular offerings and extracurricular activities. A feeling of competence—whether it is in the art studio or on the football field—can develop self-esteem that leads to improved classroom performance. Find ways to showcase extracurricular activities, perhaps by having a fair or other special event near the beginning of the school year. Make activities available to all children.

- Institute and maintain a school- or district-wide system of rewards and incentives for academic and extracurricular achievements by all students. Such programs should recognize as broad a range of accomplishments as possible: the student who operates the sound system at school assemblies should be honored as much as the student who scored the winning basket.
- Ensure that staff—and, when appropriate, students—participate in school decision making. For example, ask a student committee to review the student handbook, or ask a group of teachers to help develop a new policy regarding substitute teachers.
- Provide training programs for parents. These sessions should include information on child development and appropriate discipline, as well as techniques for enhancing self-esteem.

What Health Educators Can Do to Improve Students' Self-Esteem

What can health educators do to get young people to feel better about themselves, thus gaining a more positive attitude toward learning? Begin by considering some of the ideas discussed in the earlier chapters, particularly those ideas concerned with getting students to know one another and the teacher.

Students aren't the only ones who need a supportive and encouraging environment. When principals act like dictators and use their power to control, teachers expend less time and energy on their teaching. The more administrators concern themselves with rules, regulations, and procedures, the more teachers will hold back their knowledge from students (McNeil, 1986).

You, the teacher, hold the key to helping students feel better about themselves. In conducting interviews for their book *Women and Self-Esteem* (1984), Linda Sanford and Mary Ellen Donovan found that "a single positive experience could have an enormous impact on the outlook of a small child from a troubled family. Sometimes one affectionate, encouraging, and supportive teacher made the difference between self-hate and the start of self-acceptance for a child."

The American Association of School Administrators offers these additional ways for teachers to enhance their students' self-esteem (1991):

- Adopt teaching techniques that help students develop a sense of achievement. For example, teachers might begin each class by asking one or two questions covered in a previous day's lesson. This helps students see that they are making progress.
- Encourage students to work together cooperatively on some activities.
- Offer opportunities for students to make choices, take the initiative, and practice autonomy. A feeling of control over one's environment is an important component of self-esteem at any age. For example, teachers might offer students a range of project options, some designed to appeal to students with varying learning styles. Students could then select the project that would allow them to do their best.
- Help students develop a "success mind-set." Most successful people don't use the word "failure." They talk instead about a "glitch," a "problem," or a "snag."

Successful people look on every experience as an opportunity for learning and growth. When students are unsuccessful, help them focus on learning from their mistakes.

- Use positive reinforcement in the classroom. Say "I like the way Maria is working," or "John has his book open." Praise students for their efforts as well as their achievements. Make an effort to give even more praise to students with lower self-esteem.
- Praise specific behaviors. Saying "I appreciate the fact that you turn your work in on time" is more likely to boost a student's self-esteem than saying, "You're a great kid."
- Don't set children up for criticism by their peers. For example, walk quietly around the room and ask privately who needs extra help rather than forcing a child to raise her hand. A child who often has difficulty understanding material will feel much more comfortable seeking help if she is not put in the spotlight. Make it known that it is okay to ask questions.
- Create a rotating display of students' best work. Let students choose the work they want to share with others.
- Teach students how to set—and achieve—goals. Help them break down large goals into smaller, achievable steps. Success at each level will provide incentive to continue their efforts.
- Telephone or write parents asking them to give students praise. Set goals for the number of positive parent contacts you will make each week.
- Teach students strategies to accomplish new tasks. "I can't" sometimes means "I don't know how." Learning new things renews a sense of success in young people.
- Highlight the value of different ethnic groups. Teach your students to value diversity.
- Encourage interactions with students of different ages, whether by establishing a multi-age classroom or by partnering students with younger or older students in other classrooms. Being able to help a younger student or to emulate an older student can raise self-confidence.

Some Suggestions for Teaching

Remember the five basic needs: survival, belonging, power, freedom, and fun? If your students feel cared for, capable, confident, and powerful, they'll also have a sense of control over what happens to them. They'll be able to confront the routine challenges of life rather than be overwhelmed or paralyzed by them.

Let your students know you care: listen to them, and spend time with them. All of us who feel loved by others find it easier to love ourselves. Whenever possible, give options rather than orders. The opportunity to make choices also fosters a sense of control. Students will care more about outcomes when they have some ownership of a task or project.

Make sure you direct negative statements at students' actions or words, *not* at them. They are not "bad people" even when they make bad choices. Maintain high expectations for students, but make sure goals are within their reach. Try showing the film *Stand and Deliver*, in which the teacher, Jaime Escalante, makes no secret of the amount of work involved in his calculus class, but because the work is need-satisfying the students are willing to do it.

Have students evaluate all work they turn in by placing a grade on it, but let them know you, as the teacher, must be the final judge (Glasser, 1991). Give students responsibility for chores that contribute to the classroom's well-being, and acknowledge their contributions. Suggest that students keep records of their accomplishments: charts, journals, and scrapbooks.

Recognizing Low Self-Esteem

The American Association of School Administrators has a booklet called *Building Self-Esteem: A Guide for Parents, Schools, and Communities* (1991). In it are some of the early warning signals that self-esteem is so low professional help might be needed:

- *withdrawal from family life*
- *spending most free time alone*
- *socializing only with younger students*
- *any signs of drug abuse*
- *dramatic drop in grades*
- *any discussion of suicide*
- *any dramatic change in behavior*

Establishing a Learning Environment Conducive to Positive Self-Esteem

A number of earlier chapters are about establishing an environment for positive learning as well as building self-esteem. The key to positive learning is to help students focus on their accomplishments rather than on their failures. Some classroom techniques include the following:

Give students the message that mistakes are part of learning. Ask students, "Who might make a mistake this year?" Before any student raises his hand, raise yours. This simple exercise is a launching pad for students to take risks (Brooks, 1994).

Create a classroom environment where students feel safe from teasing and put-downs by their classmates. Teasing and put-downs are one of the most destructive aspects of a classroom environment. It can make or break a student no matter what the teacher tries to do. Ask students to recall a time when they were teased and have them write about how they felt. Help students understand how they might hurt others' feelings. Ask them to write down one way in which they might help others feel better about themselves.

Provide opportunities for all students to feel special and to share with classmates their individual talents and interests. It's simple and it works. Allow students to take turns hearing positive comments about each other. Make a poster board filled with positive comments that students make about their peers. Send the board home so parents can add to the list.

Develop positive relationships with parents. Too often, teachers communicate with parents only when there is a problem. Call or write to parents when a student is doing well or showing improvement as a way to reinforce positive behavior (Brooks, 1994).

While reading the material in this chapter, you will have noticed striking similarities between the recommendations of the American Association of School Administrators and those of Robert Brooks. This duality supports the concept that these ideas have widespread acceptance. Taken alone, each of the techniques outlined herein, regardless of the source, might not make a difference. But, if several methods are mixed, the reward may be better feelings for everyone.

Some Exercises to Develop Self-Esteem

Most self-esteem problems arise from the relationship (or lack thereof) we have with our parents, then from a broad base as we move away emotionally from our parents. Most important are those significant other people in our lives. The following exercises may help bring about a discussion of self-esteem and the influence that people have on our feelings about ourselves.

Exercise: People in My Life

This exercise is intended to get students to think about how the special people in their lives (past or present) have influenced them.

Ask them to respond to the following list of situations by giving the first names of those people who most properly fit into the various categories. They can use a name more than once. They can also use people from their past who they may not have seen in some time, or those who may be dead but whom they still remember.

1. List the names of the three people you feel are most important to you in your life right now:

2. List the names of the two people who have had the most important influence on your life up to this point:

3. What person in your life do you feel most secure with?

4. Who are you most able to tell your innermost feelings to without hesitation?

5. Who is the one person that you would like to *shadow* (follow with his knowing) for a day?

6. Is there someone in your life right now who loves you unconditionally for who you are? If so, who?

7. Who do you feel most admires *you*?

8. Who do *you* most admire?

9. If you could retract one negative statement or harsh word that you said to someone, who would that person be?

10. If you could go back in time and spend a day talking with one person, who would that person be?

(continued)

11. When you think about all the special people in your life, who do you consider the most special? Why?

Have students pair up and share the reasons why they named the people they did. Finish by having the class sit in a circle and share some of their responses with you and the rest of the class.

Exercise: People Who Have Had the Greatest Influence on Your Life

Have students think about those people, living or dead, who had the most influence on their lives. Who were they, and how were they influential? Do they still have this influence? (Remind students that the influence can be negative or positive.) Give them time to think about it, then have them list names in chronological order, starting with the first person they can remember on down to the most current person. Let students know it is not a contest to see who has the longest list, but they will get additional questions, so they should be creative in answering.

Next, provide them with a response grid (a sample of which is provided here). You need to set up the grid as shown for there is a coding process that goes along with it. Hand out the grid; it should be a full page long. (You can also have students draw it on their own.)

Example:

Names of significant people in my life	1	2	3	4	5	6
1.						
2.						
3.						
4.						
5.						
6.						

Column 1. Have the students list the approximate length of time each of the people named has had an influence on them (five years, one year, one month, etc.). Even if one of the people is dead (a grandmother, for example) or they have not seen this person in a long while, they should list the time from beginning until the present.

Column 2. On a scale of 1 to 5 (+ or –), how do students value each person in terms of their influence on them?

–								+
5	4	3	2	1	2	3	4	5

A 5 on the negative side would equal a very negative influence; a 5 on the positive side would equal a very positive influence. If students say the influence started out positive but ended up negative, tell them to think of the entire relationship and give it one value (either positive or negative).

Column 3. Have students expressed their appreciation to the people who had a positive influence on them? Have students rate on a scale of 0 to 5 whether they expressed these feelings verbally or otherwise. (A 0 would mean that they *never* expressed their feelings; a 5 would indicate that they expressed them on a regular basis, verbally or through cards, gifts, etc.)

Column 4. Have students place a check in each box corresponding to a person who would put *their* name down as influential if they were participating in the exercise.

Column 5. Using the scale in the instructions for Column 2, have students rate the quality of *their* influence on the people they checked in Column 4.

Column 6. Have students go over their lists and put a check next to the names of those people with whom they have unfinished business (e.g., they have some-thing they would like to say to them or express their feelings about). Then, have students circle the name of the one person they checked that they would *most* like to conclude business with. Next, have them turn their papers over and write a letter to this person expressing their feelings. It is important that this be an expression of *how they feel,* not how they view the other person. It also should not be a negative, blaming letter or a positive, promising one, rather, it should be an expression of how the student feels.

Finally, invite three or more students to read their letters to the class. Allow for an entire class discussion in a full circle.

Let students know that negative experiences often can lead to positive ways of living and being. We often learn more from our negative experiences in that we learn not to repeat mistakes as well as more positive ways of dealing with such experiences.

In all of this, the emphasis should be on positive, forward-moving behavior. Young people need their parents and other peoples' attention, time, affirmation of their feelings, direction, and positive role modeling. When they don't get this, they often feel they are to blame.

Young people need to be valued for who they are, not what they may become (Naylor et al., 1994). Schools are for this purpose. Health education is the most realistic vehicle for making this concept a reality.

**Exercise:
Redefining**

Redefining is a process that allows one idea to be exchanged for a better one. In its broadest expression, redefining invites students to create a new vision of themselves and their relationships.

Throughout life, we continually redefine ourselves, giving new meaning to our experiences (being the best on the team, having a new car, being in love, being accepted, and so on). Redefining, as a creative pathway, is often helpful in broadening personal, educational, and spiritual growth.

Present the following questions to your students. Note that the ages suggested are only an example; you should choose these based on the age group of your class.

How You See Yourself

Picture yourself at each of the following ages; 6, 8, 12, 15, and the age you are now. Recall how you looked, what you felt, where you were, and who the most important person in your life was at that time. Imagine, at each age, answering an interviewer who asks you, What makes you happiest? What do you think happiness is? Write down briefly what you feel and think.

Age 6:

Age 8:

Age 12:

Age 15:

Age you are now:

Briefly express how you feel about the person you are now:

This exercise requires some class discussion, but most of all it requires the teacher's understanding of how positive and negative changes in behavior affect students' personal happiness.

Exercise: "What I Will Miss Most?"	Self-esteem is strongly linked to certain significant people in our lives. "When you are sorrowful, you are weeping for that which has been your delight" (Gibran, 1966). When someone we love dies, our grief is often heightened because we feel we never really told the person how important they were to us. Here is an exercise that helps in that process.

There is an old cultural habit of thinking of people as primarily material, as flesh and blood. In truth, each person who is truly important to us is not an object, but a pattern—something attached to us, something to hang on to. This is probably why grieving people feel such attachment to cemetery headstones and any other material representation of the deceased. And so, the question to ask is, "What is it *about* this person that I miss?"

Ask students to think of five significant people in their lives (living or dead) and write down one thing they will (or do) miss when they are gone. Have them stress the importance of these people in their lives and what it is that made them so significant. |

Significant Person: **What I Will Miss Most:**

To conclude this exercise, invite students to share some of their responses in class. Specifically, you want students to understand that their feelings about themselves are very much linked to their feelings about the significant people in their lives.

Exercise: Relationships	No one needs to tell elementary- or secondary-school teachers how important being "in" is to kids today. It's not what you do but who you do it with that really counts.

Each of the following situations calls for a response from students. The first response is what the person would say to them in the given situation. The second response is their reaction in the same situation. |

(continued)

Situation 1:

Yesterday, my girlfriend/boyfriend called me on the phone and said she/he did not want to see me again. She/he said

I guess she/he does not want to see me anymore because

Situation 2:

My boyfriend/girlfriend of two years told me the other day that he/she needs to date other people because

I guess he/she feels that way because

Situation 3:

When I meet someone I am really attracted to, I wonder if he/she thinks I am

My feeling about this is

Get some of the students to share their responses without focusing on any one student's response. You will find that some students have responded negatively to both sides of a situation; some will have mixed responses, and a few will be all positive.

One of the most important points to be made here is that students who have all negative or partially negative responses are often reacting to situations they have experienced in their past, or they are basing their expectations on what they learned as a child, i.e., that they were no good, not acceptable, or not attractive. The point should be stressed that their past is *not* their present nor their future.

**Exercise:
Our Bodies**

It is amazing how we sometimes totally disconnect from our physical selves. It is as though our bodies are separate entities. To quote from Chungliang Al Huang (1983),

Many people treat their bodies as if they were rented from Hertz—something they are using to get around in but nothing they genuinely care about understanding.

Yet facts indicate otherwise. More and more, the mind-body connection is becoming a reality in health education (see Chapter 3). As such, we need to include the body in self-esteem issues. This exercise attempts to connect the body with feelings about the self.

Unfinished statements: Have students read and respond to each of the following unfinished statements about their bodies. Have them be as specific as they can. Example: "My nose *is too big!*"

1. My hair
2. My eyes
3. My teeth
4. My complexion
5. My nose
6. When I look in the mirror,
7. My chest
8. My body weight
9. My height
10. The part of my body I dislike most is
11. The part of my body I like the most is
12. Looking over all that I have said, I feel my body is

Building Healthy Relationships

Choosing to develop rich and meaningful relationships is a vital survival skill. A supportive network of friends who offer understanding, closeness, and friendship enhances our potential for well-being and self-esteem. Ask students to list the people they know who truly understand who they are. Have them look at their list of supporters and reflect on the different ways they have of letting these people know them (e.g., being open, honest, sharing, or friendly).

Healthy relationships are characterized by reciprocal responsibility and mutual satisfaction. When two people are committed to give and take, to sharing and listening, the needs of both are satisfied in the exchange.

Have students reflect for a moment on the current health of their relationships. Then have them respond to the following questions:

- How fulfilling were your interactions with others this past week?
- Did you feel alone even when you were with others?
- Did you feel rejected? Ignored? Let down?
- Did you feel that people misunderstood or didn't appreciate you?
- Did you feel isolated? Without support?
- Did you feel forgotten? Left out? Uninvolved?
- Did you feel pressured? Overburdened with responsibility to others?
- Did you feel drained, as if you'd given your last ounce of caring?
- Can you summarize how you feel about friendship(s)?

Everyone feels unsupported once in a while. However, if these feelings are frequent, it may be a sign that the student needs to work on improving her support network.

Life Scripts

Eric Berne (1975), founder of transactional analysis, talked about life scripts. In essence, a life script is made up of both parental teachings and the early decisions we make as children. Often, we continue to follow our scripts as adults.

Scripting begins in infancy, with subtle, nonverbal messages from our parents and significant others. During our earliest years, we learn much about our worth as a person and our place in life. Some of the messages we might hear include "Boys don't cry," "Don't be so sensitive," "You are never going to amount to anything," "Don't expect to ever find the right person," or "You are too fat."

According to Berne, our life script forms the core of our personal identity. Our experiences may lead us to such conclusions as "I really don't have any reason to feel anyone wants me" or "Why would anyone want to go out with me?" These basic themes running through our life determine our behavior, and very often they are difficult to unlearn. In many subtle ways, these early decisions about ourselves come back to haunt us in later life.

What teachers need to do is get students to challenge these inner voices; to move from "we are not" to "we are" capable, acceptable, attractive, etc.

In his book, *Making Peace with Your Parents,* psychiatrist Harold Bloomfield (1983) makes the point that many of us suffer from psychological wounds as a result of unfinished business with our parents. According to Bloomfield, before we can resolve any conflicts with our *actual* parents, we first must make peace with our *inner* parent—the voice that reiterates the messages we have accepted from our parents, the feelings and conflicts we still carry with us, and the memories and hidden resentments we still cling to from childhood. The following exercise may help students tap into some of these feelings and conflicts.

Exercise: "What I Have Learned about Myself"

What are some messages you have learned about yourself concerning

your self-esteem:

your potential to succeed:

your intelligence:

your role in the family:

your sex (being male/female):

your choice of a dating partner:

your contribution to the family:

(continued)

your academic ability:

your future:

Because your view of yourself has a great influence on the quality of your inter-personal relationships, it is important that you look at some of the views and consider how you arrived at them. To do this, reflect on these questions:

1. How do you see yourself? To what degree do you see yourself as confident, secure, worthwhile, accomplished, caring, open, and accepting?

2. How would you describe the way you see yourself to a close friend?

3. What is the difference between the way you see yourself now and the way you would like to be? Do you feel hopeful about closing this gap?

4. Do others generally see you as you see yourself? What are some ways others view you differently than you view yourself?

5. Who in your life has been most influential in shaping your self-esteem, and how has he or she affected your view of yourself?

This exercise is designed to stress how much of what we feel about ourselves is learned. If we hope to change negative self-esteem, we must help young people to challenge irrational premises that they have accepted uncritically. Further, we must work toward building self-esteem by allowing the individual to take responsibility for his own self-esteem, focusing health education on replacing self-sabotaging beliefs with positive, constructive ones. If you wish to know more ways of changing this self-indoctrination process, I refer you to Ellis and Harper's *A New Guide to Rational Living* (1975).

Synthesis

Self-esteem-building programs are alive and growing in our public schools today. The major difference from early self-esteem programs is that they were short on success if long on a sincere desire to help. The early efforts were based on the shallow belief that self-esteem could be improved by a word, a star on a student's paper or forehead, or having students tell themselves they were lovable and capable. The new self-esteem programs are more reality-focused, based on the real world in which the students live. The new, successful programs are more hands-on. Young people get in touch with themselves by getting in touch with others; everyone is a part of the process. They give students the ability to get outside themselves and find love, support, and coping skills that help them feel good about themselves.

References

Al Huang, Chungliang. *Quantum Soup.* New York: E.P. Dutton, 1983.

American Association of School Administrators. *Building Self-Esteem: A Guide for Parents, Schools, and Communities.* Arlington, VA: AASA Leadership for Learning, 1991.

Associated Press. "NH Self-Esteem Program Aims at Girls." *Boston Globe,* 25 November 1994.

Bach, Richard. *Jonathan Livingston Seagull.* New York: Macmillan, 1970.

Berne, Eric. *What Do You Say after You Say Hello?* New York: Bantam, 1975.

Bloomfield, Harold, and L. Felder. *Making Peace with Your Parents.* New York: Ballantine, 1983.

Branden, Nathaniel. *The Six Pillars of Self-Esteem.* New York: Bantam, 1994.

Brooks, Robert. *The Self-Esteem Teacher.* Circle Pines, MN: American Guidance Service, 1994.

California Department of Education. *California Task Force to Promote Self-Esteem and Personal and Social Responsibility* (Assembly Bill No. 3659). Sacramento, CA: California Bureau of Publications, 1986.

California Department of Education. *Toward a State of Esteem: The Final Report of the California Task Force to Promote Self-Esteem and Personal and Social Responsibility.* Sacramento, CA: California State Bureau of Publications, 1990.

Ellis, Albert. "The Essence of RET." *Journal of Rational-Emotive Therapy,* 1984.

___, and R.A. Harper. *A New Guide to Rational Living.* Englewood Cliffs, NJ: Prentice-Hall, 1975.

Field Research Corporation. "Survey Finds Correlation between Self-Esteem, Health." *Brain/Mind Bulletin,* 3 December 1979.

Fossum, J., and T. Mason. *Facing Shame.* New York: W.W. Norton, 1991.

Gibran, Kahlil. *The Prophet.* New York: Knopf, 1969.

Glasser, William. *The Quality School.* New York: Harper Perennial, 1990.

McNeil, Linda. *Contradictions of Control.* New York: Routledge & Kegan Paul, 1986.

Naylor, Thomas H., William H. Willmon, and Magdelena R. Naylor. *The Search for Meaning.* Nashville: Abingdon Press, 1994.

Orenstein, Peggy. *School Girls.* New York: Anchor, 1994.

Purkey, William W. *Self-Concept and School Achievement.* Englewood Cliffs, NJ: Prentice-Hall, 1970.

Rodin, Judith. *Body Traps: Breaking the Binds that Keep You from Feeling Good about Your Body.* New York: Morrow, 1992.

Sanford, Linda T., and Mary Ellen Donovan. *Women and Self-Esteem.* New York: Penguin, 1984.

"Taking It to the Streets." *New Age Journal,* January/February 1993.

Additional Resources

Barenblatt, Maida, and Alena Joy Barenblatt. *Make an Appointment with Yourself: Simple Steps to Positive Self-Esteem.* Deerfield Beach, FL: Health Communications, 1994.

Bingham, Mindy, et al. *Choices: A Teen Woman's Journal for Self-Awareness and Personal Planning.* El Toro, CA: Mission Publications, 1984.

Borba, Michele, and Craig Borba. *Self-Esteem: A Classroom Affair.* San Francisco: HarperSanFrancisco, 1982.

Brooks, B. David, and Rex K. Dalby. *The Self-Esteem Repair and Maintenance Manual.* Newport Beach, CA: Kincaid House, 1990.

Burkin, Peggy Dylan. *Guiding Your Self: A Unique Manual for Personal Growth and Success.* Twain Harte, CA: Reunion Press, 1986.

Burns, David D. *Ten Days to Self-Esteem.* New York: William Morrow, 1993.

Fisher, Seymour. "Experiencing Your Body: You Are What You Feel." *Saturday Review,* 8 July 1972.

Hartline, Jo Ellen. *Me!? A Curriculum for Teaching Self-Esteem through an Interest Center.* Tucson, AZ: Zephyr Press, 1990.

Hazelton, Deborah M. *Solving the Self-Esteem Puzzle: A Guide for Moving From Piece to Peace.* Deerfield Beach, FL: Health Communications, 1991.

Jensen, Eric. *Super-Teaching: Master Strategies for Building Student Success.* Tucson, AZ: Zephyr Press, 1988.

Wells, Valerie. *The Joy of Visualization: 75 Creative Ways to Enhance Your Life.* Tucson, AZ: Zephyr Press, 1990.

A Matter of Style

Psychological findings (see Chapters 1 and 2) indicate that our brains function in two ways. The function of the left hemisphere is predominantly linear, rational, and verbal. The function of the right hemisphere is predominantly holistic, intuitive, and metaphoric. Most educational processes have focused on the development of left-hemisphere functions; now we know that the greatest achievements of the human mind require the integrated functioning of both hemispheres. The ability of the right cerebral hemisphere to perceive patterns, possibilities, meaning, and relationships and to create symbolic images is essential both to the creative process and the development of the healthy personality. Yet we are only beginning to recognize the importance of validating these functions within our educational system.

What Jerome Bruner called left-handed knowing (1962) is what we now refer to as right-hemisphere knowing (since the right hemisphere of the brain controls the left side of the body, while the left hemisphere of the brain controls the right side of the body). Although the importance of both modes of knowing has been affirmed in learning theory, the primary focus of theorists such as Piaget and Bruner has been on the cognitive functions of the left cerebral hemisphere.

In *The Crack in the Cosmic Egg* (1988) and *Evolution's End* (1992), Joseph Pearce points out how we create our reality by the way we structure our perceptions of the world: "formal education prevents development of the imagination—children without such development tend toward violence and are often uneducable." We are now beginning to understand how a limited imagination affects reality in terms of the way we teach. New methods of teaching must take into account all the ways that we learn. This part explores those possibilities as well as other issues.

References

Bruner, Jerome. *On Knowing: Essays for the Left Hand.* New York: Atheneum, 1962.
Pearce, Joseph. *The Crack in the Cosmic Egg.* New York: HarperCollins, 1988.
___. *Evolution's End.* New York: HarperCollins, 1992.

14 Styles of Teaching and Learning

According to researchers, each person has a distinct and often idiosyncratic style and preference for learning and remembering. Unfortunately, most teachers teach as if there were only one learning environment—lecturing and note taking. Learning-style research suggests such an environment is optimal for less than half the students. Yet many of us carry that model with us, often because it is the way we were taught.

Not only does this outdated thinking make us feel inadequate, it also dramatically limits our potential. Conversely, once we know how a person learns, we can teach him to teach *himself* anything.

The most influential element of one's learning style is cognitive ability—the way the brain perceives and processes information. The cognitive style depends on which brain hemisphere is dominant. Those with dominant right hemispheres (55 percent of the population) tend to be global thinkers—they process information holistically, preferring to understand the concept before getting down to detail. Those who rely more strongly on the left side of the brain (28 percent) tend to be analytical thinkers—their brains process information step by step, following a logical progression. (The rest of the population are "integrated" learners who favor neither hemisphere.)

In recent years, the idea of being left or right brained has been popularized in a host of self-help books and in holistic medicine. But it has also spawned a substantial body of research with far-reaching implications. For instance, cognitive style often correlates to a number of distinct environmental, social, and biological preferences. If these important needs aren't met, learning may be a struggle (Dunn et al., 1992). What follows are some of the elements of learning styles that other researchers

Creativity requires the courage to let go of certainties.

—ERICH FROMM

have identified. If you would like to learn about your own learning style, try taking the "How do you learn best?" test that follows.

Exercise: How Do You Learn Best?

Studies show that most of us have one preferred mode of learning: visual (by reading), auditory (by listening), tactile (by handling), or kinesthetic (by experience or movement). To determine how you learn best, circle true or false next to each question, then refer to the answer key that follows.

When I learn something new, I like to learn about it by:

T F **1.** reading about it

T F **2.** hearing a record

T F **3.** hearing a tape

T F **4.** seeing a filmstrip (no soundtrack)

T F **5.** seeing and hearing a movie

T F **6.** looking at pictures and having someone explain them

T F **7.** hearing my supervisor or trainer tell me

T F **8.** playing games

T F **9.** going someplace and seeing for myself

T F **10.** having someone show me

Things I remember best are things:

T F **11.** my supervisor tells me

T F **12.** someone other than my supervisor tells me

T F **13.** someone shows me

T F **14.** I learned about on trips

T F **15.** I read

T F **16.** I heard on records or tapes

T F **17.** I heard on the radio

T F **18.** I saw on the television

T F **19.** I read stories about

T F **20.** I saw in a movie

T F **21.** I tried or worked on

T F **22.** my friends and I talked about

I really like to:

T F **23.** read books, magazines, or newspapers

T F **24.** see movies

T F **25.** listen to records

T F **26.** make tapes on a tape recorder

T F **27.** draw or paint

T F **28.** look at pictures

T F **29.** play games

T F **30.** talk to people

T F **31.** listen to other people talk

T F **32.** listen to the radio

T F **33.** watch television

T F **34.** go on trips

T F **35.** learn new things with my hands

T F **36.** study with friends

T F **37.** build things

T F **38.** do experiments

T F **39.** take pictures or make movies/videos

T F **40.** use typewriters, computers, calculators, or other machines

T F **41.** go to the library

T F **42.** mold things with my hands

Once you determine the type of learner you are, you can make adjustments in how you learn new material. Learning-styles consultant Joanne Ingham offers the following advice for how each type should approach a training lecture or discussion:

Visual: Find out what readings the session will be based on, then read the material in advance.

Tactile: Skim through the readings and underline the major headings and important points. Draw charts and diagrams to summarize the material or take notes on your computer.

Kinesthetic: Review the readings before the lecture while sitting in a rocking chair or on a stationary bike. Tape the lectures and listen to them later while you walk.

Auditory: Lectures and discussions are your preferred modes, so tape written material.

Answer Key

Scoring: Mark whether each true answer was an indication of an auditory (A), visual (V), tactile (T), or kinesthetic (K) perceptual style using this key. (Some answers correlate to more than one mode.) The letter that occurs most often indicates your dominant perceptual style. If you have a nearly equal number of each letter, you probably have equally distributed perceptual style preferences.

1. V	10. V	19. V	28. V	37. T, K
2. A	11. A	20. V	29. T, K	38. K
3. A	12. A	21. T, K	30. A	39. T, K
4. V	13. V	22. A	31. A	40. T
5. A, V	14. K	23. V	32. A	41. V
6. A, V	15. V	24. V	33. V	42. T
7. A, V	16. A	25. A	34. K	
8. V, T, K	17. A	26. K	35. T	
9. V, K	18. A, V	27. T	36. A	

Adapted from Bringing Out the Giftedness in Your Child, *by Rita Dunn, Kenneth Dunn, and Donald Treffinger* (John Wiley, 1992). Used with permission.

Learning Styles: Cognitive, Affective, and Psychomotor

Not only do individuals perceive and modify experience in their own unique manner, but attention to these differences in learning styles can be the key to independent learning (Atwood, 1975). The differing learning styles of children must be taken into account; the important thing is for teachers to build on the child's special style (Reissman, 1962).

Anyone surveying professional journals in education would likely conclude that it is vogue to talk about learning styles and their effects on the learning process. Essentially, *learning style* can be defined as a consistent pattern of behavior influenced by individual variability. When persons learn, they use learning styles that are uniquely their own but make moment-by-moment adjustments depending on the nature of the task and the teaching style. These overall patterns give general direction to learning behavior. But, rather than simply looking at learning styles in isolation, health educators need to understand how they are affected by the classroom, where they interact and influence one another in an infinite number of ways.

When discussing learning styles, it is helpful to take into account the wide variety of human behaviors that lead to learning. Systematic surveys of educational objectives have spelled out human behavioral characteristics in what has come to be known as Bloom's taxonomy (Bloom, et al., 1988). It defines three general educational arenas: the cognitive domain (thinking and knowing), the affective domain (feelings, attitudes, and values), and the psychomotor domain (motion controlled by the mind). The cognitive domain is subdivided into the following increasingly complex levels:

1. **Knowledge.** Basic information, facts, and concepts that apply to the learning process and to the learning unit.
2. **Comprehension.** Awareness of the significance of information and its relationship to other information, and the ability to recall the information in a relevant manner when required.
3. **Application.** Using and applying knowledge and comprehension under different conditions. In a reality-centered curriculum, motivation for learning often begins with application and then backtracking to fill in the required knowledge and comprehension.
4. **Analysis.** Dissecting a problem into logical elements; seeing relationships and distinguishing between facts, hypotheses, and principles.
5. **Synthesis.** Putting knowledge into a new form, thereby creating new knowledge or creative behavior.
6. **Evaluation.** Making judgments based on knowledge and evidence. This process involves the use of external criteria and value systems that affect the making of choices and decisions. The evaluation area impinges on the affective domain.

The affective domain is related to feelings, values, beliefs, and attitudes and affects learning in fundamental ways. For example, a child brought up in a home in which excessive drinking is the norm may react to a classroom discussion on alcohol abuse not only with pain but with resistance to the message being conveyed. A student whose family behaves in conflict with the lesson is not likely to enter a class favorably disposed to the message or the teacher.

The following aspects of the affective domain are identified in approximate order of complexity and priority:

1. **Receiving.** The student must first be aware that information is being offered (she may be daydreaming). Then she must be willing to receive it (she may be angry and unwilling to listen). Finally, she must offer controlled or selected attention (she may be unable to pay attention because of other factors such as personal, physical, or emotional problems).
2. **Responding.** The student is sufficiently motivated to respond to information. At the lowest level of intensity is simple acquiescence; at a higher level, she is willing to respond; and at the highest level she obtains satisfaction in doing so.
3. **Valuing.** The student feels a sense of a commitment to certain behaviors that she considers worthy.

Table 14–1

Common verbal cues by modality

Visual	Auditory	Kinesthetic
appears to me	all ears	all washed up
bird's-eye view	call on	boils down to
catch a glimpse of	clear as a bell	come to grips with
clear-cut	clearly expressed	floating on thin air
dim view	describe in detail	get a handle on
eye to eye	earful	get a load of this
get a scope on	give me your ear	get in touch with
hazy idea	hear voices	get the drift of
in light of	hidden message	hang in there!
in person	idle talk	hold it!
in view of	loud and clear	hothead
looks like	outspoken	lay cards on table
mental image	rap session	pull some strings
mind's eye	rings a bell	sharp as a tack
pretty as a picture	to tell the truth	slipped my mind
see to it	tuned-in/tuned-out	start from scratch
short-sighted	unheard of	stiff upper lip
showing off	voiced an opinion	too much hassle
tunnel vision	within hearing range	underhanded

Source: DePorter, Bobbi, and Mike Hernacki. *Quantum Learning.* New York: Del, 1992. Used with permission.

4. **Organizing a system of values.** Certain values are internalized and made an integral part of her system of beliefs and attitudes.
5. **Organizing a complex of values (a philosophy).** The various values are interrelated under a broad philosophy of life that determines what she chooses to learn or even to do.

The third area of learning, the psychomotor domain, includes sensory perception (visual, auditory, kinesthetic, taste, and smell); environmental characteristics (noise level, light, temperature, room arrangement); the need for food; and the times of day conducive to optimal learning (Table 14–1).

Importance of Knowing Learning Style

Every teacher has a learning style. It is likely to have a greater variation than that of students, because the teacher has had many more experiences. But, whatever the teacher's learning style, *it will have an effect on his teaching style.* In a nutshell, we tend to teach the way we learn, unless there is a conscious reason to do otherwise.

The more teachers know about their teaching and learning styles, the easier it will be for them to find specific ways to amplify or modify them. If teachers know that they are visual-kinesthetic *learners* (tending to process information in a global way, often oversimplifying and ignoring details), that they are intrinsically motivated, that they work best in the morning, and that they favor right-brain activities like art, drama, and literature, then they should take these factors into consideration when evaluating their *teaching* styles. Varying teaching style could be a critical factor in relation to their students' success in the classroom. By making explicit their own teaching and learning styles, teachers have taken the first step toward realizing that not all their students learn as they do. Perhaps the problems some students have result from mismatches between teaching styles and students' learning styles.

Once teachers gain an appreciation of the variety of learning styles, they can respect learning-style differences and adapt their teaching for different situations. They may also be more alert to situations in which a students' learning style limits his success in an academic area. (For example, with strongly right-brain learners who have difficulty memorizing, the teacher might suggest alternatives to the rehearsal method for memorizing.) Success in teaching is highly dependent on exposing students to a variety of teaching styles selected for their effectiveness in particular situations.

In the following activity, you are asked to examine your teaching style as a basis for self-analysis. While this skill is important, checking your perceptions against those of a learning partner who is familiar with various teaching styles is also helpful. The comparison between the two sets of perceptions can be fruitful if you are accepting, open, and nondefensive. A careful consideration of the similarities and differences in your two views can give you a more accurate picture of your teaching self.

Exercise: Determining Your Teaching Style

Objectives:

1. to compare your perceptions of your teaching self with those of an observer

2. to consider the implications of any similarities and differences in the two sets of perceptions

Directions: Ask a learning partner to watch a class in which you are teaching a typical lesson. (At a later time, you may wish to use this activity with an atypical lesson.) After the class, both you and your partner should fill in a separate worksheet about how you conducted the lesson. You might wish to add more questions to the worksheet to cover any aspects of your teaching that have not been included. Do not share your worksheets until you are both finished. Then, compare the two worksheets and discuss the results.

Questions:

1. About what aspects of your teaching do you agree? What does this tell you about your teaching? What agreements make you feel good? What agreements make you uncomfortable?

2. On what do you disagree? How do you account for these differences?

3. What factual data did each of you use for your decisions?

4. Which differences make you feel comfortable? Uncomfortable?

5. What did you learn about your teaching from the discussion with your observer? What did you learn about your perceptions of your teaching?

Worksheet

Directions: Using the key below, circle the number that best represents your evaluation of the presentation.

> **KEY**
>
> 5 = Exceptional
> 4 = Good
> 3 = Neither good nor bad
> 2 = Poor
> 1 = Very poor
> 0 = Does not apply

Organization:

1. 5 4 3 2 1 0   Clear purpose

2. 5 4 3 2 1 0   Good introduction

3. 5 4 3 2 1 0   Good conclusion

(continued)

Visual aids:

1. 5   4   3   2   1   0   Has one idea, easy to see

2. 5   4   3   2   1   0   The idea is presented effectively

Delivery (circle the appropriate teaching style):

Flexible	Student-centered	Fair
Creative	Left-brain focused	Humorous
Impatient	Right-brain focused	Visually oriented
Closed	Whole-brain focused	Other:
Didactic	Sarcastic	

Learning to "Flex-Style"

The first step in increasing the range of styles in your teaching repertoire is to *want* to change and to believe that it is possible to do so. Flex-styling—which might include augmenting your map, increasing your options, becoming cognitive-affective, holistic teaching, using both sides of the brain, and cooperative learning—is one way to increase your style repertoire. Be eclectic, not just for variety's sake (although that is not a bad reason in itself), but because different students and tasks demand different styles. By varying your approach, you provide a model of flexibility for students. Each teaching strategy has a parallel learning strategy; by "learning to learn," each student will acquire the lifelong habit of teaching themselves.

Flex-Style Strategies

Following are strategies to use in teaching. Remember, nothing works all the time. The success of a strategy is highly dependent on how, when, where, why, and by whom it is used.

1. Present concepts and skills in a logical sequence, e.g., concrete to abstract, easy to difficult
2. Let students know that you expect them to succeed
3. Use specific examples and concrete models to make abstractions and generalizations clear
4. Plan tasks within a student's range of ability, e.g., so that some success is guaranteed for everyone (this implies that the teacher knows what skills and concepts a task assumes and what skills and concepts her students possess)
5. Match learning tasks to students' developmental levels
6. Reinforce desired behaviors, e.g., eating healthfully or choosing healthy pastimes

7. Give honest, descriptive feedback to students about their performance
8. Relate students' past experiences to new learning, e.g., alcohol abuse to alcohol nonabuse alternatives
9. Give students various kinds of practice experiences, e.g., visual, auditory, or kinesthetic
10. Use varied modes (visual, auditory, tactile, kinesthetic) when teaching concepts and skills
11. Clearly communicate the objectives of a task so students understand its relevancy
12. Give students opportunities to make choices and provide input about their own learning
13. Use a variety of teaching strategies, and change pace as appropriate
14. Involve students actively in a lesson (see Chapter 11 for techniques)
15. Capitalize on student interests; structure learning around interests rather than just teaching isolated skills
16. Act as a model (listening, reading, speaking, writing, and especially *thinking*); demonstrate and practice what you preach
17. Ask open-ended questions using all levels of Bloom's taxonomy
18. Preteach key vocabulary presented in reading assignments
19. Prepare students for learning by
    a. allowing them to introduce each new unit
    b. opening each unit with a brief video that focuses on the need for knowledge
    c. giving students a brief knowledge and behavior test on the subject
20. Structure and organize lessons with clear, concise directions, explanations, and focus questions
21. Provide students with opportunities to pursue interest areas and receive credit for independent study
22. Teach students to self-evaluate and reflect on their learning (routinely ask, "What's one new thing you learned today?")
23. Capitalize on teachable moments when interest and readiness to learn is at a peak
24. Integrate the teaching of skills and content in a given unit
25. Ask students to retell main points of a reading or listening experience
26. Follow direct teaching with practice or reinforcement activities
27. Balance right-brain activities with left-brain activities
28. Teach to students' strengths while remedying weaknesses (we all like to do what we do well)
29. Set an appropriate pace for learning

Can teachers who already have well-established teaching styles learn to be flexible? It depends on the creativity of the individual teacher. Bruce Joyce (1981), a leading researcher in the field of teaching and learning styles, suggests the following procedures to help teachers incorporate new strategies into their repertoire: provide them with

an overview and description of the new model or style, including the theory and rationale supporting it a demonstration of the model or style (in person or on videotape)

practice using the model in simulated or classroom settings

open-ended feedback about performance, emphasizing self-evaluation and goal setting

in-class assistance in the form of direct coaching

Using Storytelling and Metaphor to Convey Facts and Concepts

Great teachers have always been great storytellers. People love to be told stories; their enthusiasm comes from deep in their psyches (Bettelheim, 1975). Storytelling provides an opportunity for the imagination to supply its own images to match the tale. This feeds the powers of visualization, which has become a powerful tool for health and healing within the medical field.

Storytelling in health education ought to be a regular part of a student's learning experience. You can make up your own stories about health issues, or you can get them from books. (For more information on storytelling, see *Creative Storytelling* (1985) by Jack McGuire).

Storytelling is a great way to teach academic material. The following is an example of how storytelling can teach the concept of cause and effect.

> *For want of a nail the shoe was lost,*
> *For want of a shoe the horse was lost,*
> *For want of a horse the rider was lost,*
> *For want of a rider the message was lost,*
> *For want of the message the battle was lost,*
> *For want of the battle the kingdom was lost,*
> *And all for want of a nail.*

One thing is certain: the impossible happens. Look at the moon trips, which moved from fantasy into reality, or how young people take risks that lead to accidents and death. Cause and effect has a whole range of possibilities for health education because how we behave can often have unhealthy consequences.

Stories often employ images that have multiple meanings (metaphors). The mind of the child is innately metaphoric; it requires an approach to learning that is interdisciplinary, multilevel, and nonlinear (Samples, 1976). Metaphors, thus, make wonderful seeds to sow in a child's mind. Instead of passing on dull health-science concepts, create images for these lessons. It's less effective, for example, to explain the laws involved in the formation of rain to a child in purely scientific terms (Harwood, 1958). This is also true of health education. For instance, the important aspect of teaching anatomy should not be in having children memorize the parts of the human body. Help them instead to understand the complex inter-relationship between the human body and the person.

Stephen Sagarin talked about a project he has his eighth grade pupils do: they "model caricatures of human faces in clay or papier-mâché. At this time, when the changes of puberty are rapidly occurring and each student is likely to be painfully aware of her own individuality, it is healthful for students to concentrate on character and caricature. By imaginatively creating or recreating the character of others, students begin the process of sorting out their own personalities." In this exercise, the clay or papier-mâché becomes a metaphor for the learner's inner feelings about herself.

The Use of Visualization

Children with vivid imaginations can generate more problem-solving options than children who have difficulty in fantasizing. In studies of students up through senior levels of high school, visual-imagery exercises have been shown to enhance behavior and academic performance.

Basketball star Bill Russell of the Boston Celtics explained how he used visualization by sitting with his eyes closed, watching plays in his head. "I was in my own private basketball laboratory, making mental blueprints for myself" (Garfield, 1986). Tennis champion Chris Evert also used this technique, as did golfer Jack Nicklaus, who called it "going to the movies" (Garfield, 1984). Positive visualization is an important aid to improving physical and mental health as well as performance.

There are three major qualities of imagery that make its use particularly valuable in mind-body healing and health (Rossman, 1993):

Physiological changes. The mind is capable of controlling a large number of physiological functions such as heart rate, blood pressure, breathing patterns, brain-wave rhythms, and blood flow. To demonstrate this physiological function, talk your students through the following simple exercise (Rossman, 1993).

You are standing in your kitchen in front of a cutting board. Next to it is a good, sharp knife. Take a few moments to imagine the kitchen: the color of the countertops, the appliances, the cupboards, windows, and so on. Also notice any kitchen smells or sounds—the running of a dishwasher or the hum of a refrigerator.

Now imagine that on the board sits a plump, fresh, juicy lemon. In your mind, hold the lemon in one hand, feeling its weight and texture. Then place it back on the board and carefully cut it in half with the knife. Feel the resistance to the knife and how it gives way as the lemon splits. Notice the pale yellow of the pulp, the whiteness of the inner peel, and see whether you have cut through a seed or two. Carefully cut one of the halves in two. See where a drop or two of juice has pearled on the surface of one of the quarters. Imagine lifting this lemon wedge to your mouth, smelling the sharp fresh scent. Now bite into the sour, juicy pulp.

Psychological insight. Imagery can help illuminate the connections between stressful circumstances and physical symptoms when such connections exist. It does this by helping students see the big picture (Rossman,

1993). By using imagery, you can give students a sense of the whole situation: unlike watching cars go by on a street one at a time, with imagery you can place the student high above the street looking down, so that he can see the whole picture. Try this with your class. Have them imagine that they are floating like a balloon above the classroom they are in. Have them describe what is going on.

Emotional awareness. The third significant attribute of imagery is its close relationship to the emotions. These emotions can create changes within the body: "Fear makes our hearts pound, grief make us shed tears, and joy leads to laughter. But the natural ways of demonstrating emotions—especially negative ones, such as anger and sadness—are often socially unacceptable and are suppressed. People may then find unhealthy outlets for such emotions, such as physical symptoms or behaviors (smoking, drinking, etc.) that lead to health problems. Imagery is one of the quickest and most direct ways to become aware of one's emotional state and its potential effects on health" (Rossman, 1993).

Time Out for Personal Thoughts

Here is another brief exercise to illustrate for students the emotional power of imagery.

Get comfortable. Close your eyes. Take a few deep breaths, letting yourself relax as you exhale. Begin to focus inside and recall a room from your childhood. Notice what you see there and any sounds you might hear in the room. Is there an aroma? What does the room look like? Do any feelings come up as you imagine this? Just notice them and let them be there. Then imagine that your mother walks into your room. At that moment, how do you feel? Quickly jot down some first feelings:

Now, your mother leaves the room and you go back to doing what you were doing. Feel yourself again in that same room. Now, your father walks in. Again, how do you feel?

Take a moment to look over your responses. Do you see a different response to each image? Can you respond to these differences? If yes, briefly do so:

In a similar classroom exercise, have students get relaxed, and then read them the following situations and have them visualize the outcome of each. Ask them to let their minds construct detailed, lifelike scenes before answering.

- You and your friends are standing on a street corner when someone approaches you. They offer to sell you some drugs. Visualize what you see and feel and write it down.
- One of your friends asks if others want to purchase some drugs. Visualize what you see or say and write it down.
- The person selling the drugs leaves. Visualize what happens next and write it down.

Invite students to share what they have written with the class. "Visualization" states John P. Miller, "can be used not only in problem solving, but also to help students relax, to help in creative writing, and to make connections between the subject and the inner life of the student" (Miller, 1992). (For another good book on imagery, get Maureen Nurdock's (1987) *Spinning Inward: Using Guided Imagery with Children for Learning, Creativity and Relaxation.)*

Video: Another Way Children Learn

Surveys show that, although more than 60 percent of American parents say they limit their children's television watching, 62 percent of nine-year-olds and 70 percent of thirteen-year-olds watch at least three hours of television each day (Educational Testing Service, 1990). When parents and educators worry about the amount of time children spend in front of video screens, they usually focus on the content of particular programs or games.

The video screen has become omnipresent in our society. Action games are now a mass medium. In one survey, 94 percent of children said they had played video games either at home or in an arcade (Rushbrook, 1986). While national statistics are not available, we do know that as of December 1988, the sale of Nintendo® game sets numbered 14 million.

How can health educators transmit a broad range of specific information via the video screen? What difference does the video screen make in the way children process information? Traditionally, the term *literacy* has been defined as the ability to read or write. Formal education grew up around the technology of print. As a consequence, instead of thinking of print as just one of many forms of communication, we have equated it with education. The screen has developed a new kind of literacy—visual literacy—and children will need it to thrive in a technological world.

Interactive Video

Interactive television does just what it says: it gets students to interact with the programs on the screen. Using interactive television requires work on the part of the teacher, who has to preview the video, evaluate it, and figure out how it might apply to the class. Consider the following options:

- Establish a series of questions for students to answer as they view the video
- Have students search out the moral-value issues in the video
- Have students think about and plan how they would rewrite the plot or reevaluate the issue in the video
- Have students take specific parts in the video and tell you how *they* would have responded

A wonderful film if you are dealing with the issue of self-esteem (it must be previewed because of the language) is *Less than Zero,* based on the best-selling novel by Bret Easton Ellis. It is a tale of Beverly Hills kids that seem to have it all—money, looks, prospects—yet stand to lose it. To make this film work for class use, have students pair up into twos and view the film from the perspective of

1. the kids: why do they seem to have everything going for them externally yet have nothing sustaining them internally?
2. the parents: how did they contribute to the "less than zero" feelings of their kids?

Questions to ask after the film include:

1. How could the parents have acted differently toward their kids?
2. How could the kids have helped each other? (Be specific.)
3. How did each of the kids end up with such low self-esteem?

Socratic Dialogue

An important learning tool for students is dialogue between themselves and the teacher. Socrates spurned writing because he felt it was static, unresponsive, and lent itself to one-way communication. The opposite is true of dialogues. They can give you a lot of wrong answers, but if you help students shape their ideas and experiences—in other words, help them think for themselves—they usually do amazingly well. Children have no hesitation about telling you what they think if you free them from having to be "right." Good teachers empower students to be creative and to express their own opinions in class. Right or wrong can be sorted out later.

Creativity isn't simply about additional ways to learn material. It is about finding new ways to get students to think and act. The problem is the false impression that truth comes only from the *front* of the classroom rather than from all individuals therein.

We know that every teacher has a curriculum and a syllabus to follow, that time is limited, and that we sometimes have as many as thirty students in a classroom. I don't oppose texts, tests, or achievement standards. But creativity is not measured by grades alone. The problem is that the educational system overall is set up to package information and to enforce conformity, so that people become cogs in the economic and social engine.

We need a system that encourages kids to decide whether they want to be bystanders or active participants. Somehow, we have to get young people participating creatively. I would like to see 10 percent of classroom time devoted to creative discussion. I can't think of anything that holds more promise for the future than a teacher who is willing to say to a student, "I don't know the answer to your question, but how do you think you and I together can find it?"

I'd also like to propose that competition in the classroom or on the playing fields be mixed with some compassion. We need to teach young people that winning also has an obligation to recognize how the loser feels, and to remember that winners are sometimes going to be losers.

The following are some important points to remember about dialogue:

- Teachers should ask questions for which they genuinely seek a variety of answers; students will come to care more about the questions (and the teacher).
- Creative questioning raises problems of time, training, and wrong responses. But how much does the alternative cost?
- If the questions at the heart of the lessons have meaning in students' lives, no issue is too daunting.

Additional Learning Styles

Vicarious Learning. This format allows students to observe other group members. For example, students who have quit smoking might talk to the class about why and how they quit. Learning through the experience of others is a valuable adjunct to learning through one's own experience.

Fostering Independence. The group format encourages students to rely on each other for support and direction. Rather than fostering dependence on the teacher, as in the traditional classroom, the group provides an atmosphere of interdependence that is less intense and can more easily be transferred to self-reliance.

Peer Learning. An individual who is similar to another member of the class makes a more effective teaching model. Consequently, group members dealing with certain health issues who are perceived to be coping with and overcoming these obstacles provide excellent models to those who are wrestling with similar issues.

Learning through Helping Others. Helping others in the group (offering support, reassurance, suggestions, and insight and sharing similar problems) creates a mutually shared goal for the class with an emphasis on change.

Public Commitment. Allowing students the opportunity to publicly state their intention to change to the class increases the probability that such a change will occur.

Encouragement through Others' Successes. The perception that other group members are meeting with success can be inspirational to the student, especially where certain health problems are concerned (e.g., when a student with a long history of smoking stops). When a student is able to view the actual changes in another group member and be part of that change system, hope and positive expectations can follow.

Teachable Moments. One of the most effective reality-based approaches to teaching is seizing the "teachable moment." Here, the health educator uses very current events that are related to the topic under discussion.

Synthesis

All teachers and students possess the ultimate learning center: the brain. Each of its approximately twelve-billion neurons has up to five-thousand synapses, making the possible number of interconnections so enormous that it is beyond our comprehension. As Shakespeare said, "We know what we are, but not what we may become." Our potential for "becoming" is unlimited. Research in learning and teaching styles helps us to understand the complexity of learning and to appreciate the role teachers play in the process. Somewhere, right now, a teacher is helping students learn by doing something as simple as making them aware of how their bodies function or how their feelings affect their well-being. Such simple strategies are just two among dozens (Whittrock, 1978):

> . . . *Unlike teaching machines, [these strategies] are easy to construct, transport, and change. They need little maintenance, never rust, and usually last as long as you need them. Their supply is infinite, the more of them you have. But there's one catch: You have to generate them yourself.*

The teacher, however, is only a "bridge": she can take students halfway there—but the last few steps they will have to take alone (Silverstein, 1974).

References

Atwood, Beth. "Helping Students Recognize Their Own Learning Styles." *Learning,* April 1975.

Bettelheim, Bruno. *The Uses of Enchantment.* New York: Knopf, 1975.

Bloom, F.E., A. Lazerson, and L. Hofstadter. *Brain, Mind, and Behavior* (2nd ed.). New York: Freeman, 1988.

Dunn, Rita, Kenneth Dunn, and Donald Treffinger. *Bringing Out the Giftedness in Your Child.* New York: John Wiley and Sons, 1992.

Educational Testing Service. Survey of television viewing by children. Princeton, NJ: Policy Information Center of the Educational Testing Service, 1990.

Fromm, Erich. *The Fear of Freedom.* London: Routledge and Kegan Paul, 1942.

Garfield, Charles. *Peak Performance: Mental Training Techniques of the World's Greatest Athletes.* Los Angeles: Jeremy P. Tarcher, 1984.

___. *Peak Performers: The New Heroes of American Business.* New York: William Morrow, 1986.

Harwood, A.C. *The Recovery of Man in Childhood.* London: Hodder & Stoughton, 1958.

Joyce, Bruce R. (ed.). *Flexibility in Teaching.* New York: Longman Green, 1981.

McGuire, Jack. *Creative Storytelling: Choosing, Inventing, and Sharing Tales for Children*. New York: McGraw-Hill, 1985.

Miller, John. "Toward a Spiritual Curriculum." *Holistic Education Review*, Spring 1992.

Murdock, Maureen. *Spinning Inward: Using Guided Imagery with Children for Learning, Creativity, and Relaxation*. Boston: Shambala, 1987.

Riessman, Frank. *The Culturally Deprived Child*. New York; Harper & Row, 1962.

Rossman, Martin L. "Imagery: Learning to Use the Mind's Eye," in Daniel Goleman and Joel Gurin (eds.), *Mind-Body Medicine: How to Use Your Mind for Better Health*. Yonkers, NY: Consumer Reports Books, 1993.

Rushbrook, Sara. "Messages of Video Games: Socialization Implications." Ph.D. Dissertation: University of California, Los Angeles, 1986.

Sagarin, Stephen. "Art in a Waldorf School." *Holistic Education Review*, Summer 1992.

Samples, Robert. *The Metaphoric Mind*. Reading, MA: Addison-Wesley, 1976.

Silverstein, Shel. *The Search: Where the Sidewalk Ends*. New York: Harper & Row, 1974.

Whittrock, M.C. "Education and the Cognitive Process of the Brain," in Jeanne Chall and Allan Mirsky (eds.), *Education and the Brain*. Chicago: University of Chicago Press, 1978.

Additional Resources

Armstrong, Thomas. *In Their Own Way: Discovering and Encouraging Your Child's Personal Learning Style*. Los Angeles: Jeremy P. Tarcher, 1987.

Barbe, Walter, and Raymond Swassing. *Teaching through Modality Strengths: Concepts and Practices*. Columbus, OH: ZanerBloser, 1979.

Bennett, Neville, et al. *Teaching Styles and Pupil Progress*. Cambridge, MA: Harvard University Press, 1976.

Davidman, Leonard. "Learning Style: The Myth, the Panacea, the Wisdom." *Phi Delta Kappan*, May 1981.

"Discover Your True Needs through Imagery." *Natural Health*, July/August 1993.

Entwistle, Noel. *Styles of Learning and Teaching*. New York: Wiley, 1981.

Fanning, Patrick. *Visualization for Change*. Oakland, CA: New Harbinger Publications, 1994.

Gendlin, Eugene T. *Focusing*. New York: Everest House, 1978.

Gregorc, Anthony F. "Learning and Teaching Styles: Potent Forces Behind Them." *Educational Leadership*, November 1979.

Kirby, Patricia. *Cognitive Style, Learning Style, and Transfer Skill Acquisition*. National Center for Research in Vocational Education, Ohio State University, 1979.

Miller, Ron (ed.). *New Directions in Education*. Brandon, VT: Holistic Education Press, 1990.

Murdock, Maureen. *Spinning Inward: Using Guided Imagery with Children for Learning, Creativity and Relaxation*. Boston: Shambala, 1987.

Ramirez, Manuel, and Alfredo Castaneda. *Cultural Democracy, Bicognitive Development, and Education*. New York: Academic Press, 1974.

Restak, Richard. "The Other Difference," in *Student Learning Styles*. Reston, VA: National Association of Secondary School Principals, 1979.

Rossman, Martin, M.D. *Healing Yourself with Mental Imagery*. Videocassette available from Thinking Allowed Productions, 2560 Ninth St., Suite 123, Berkeley, CA 94710.

Silverstein, Shel. *A Light in the Attic*. New York: Harper & Row, 1981.

Willis, George, and William H. Schubert (eds.). *Reflections from the Heart of Educational Inquiry: Understanding Curriculum and Teaching through the Arts*. Albany, NY: State University of New York Press, 1991.

Issues and Concerns

The Health Educator as Counselor

Controversy is the basis of change and, hopefully, improvement. Its lack signifies complacency, authoritarian limits on free expression, or the absence of realistic alternatives to existing circumstances. An articulate presentation of a point of view on a controversial matter breathes new life into abiding human and social concerns. Controversy prompts reexamination and, perhaps, renewal.

Health education, by its very nature and content, is controversial. Arguments exist over the most appropriate aims, most propitious means, and most effective teaching strategies to meet the issues and concerns faced in health education today.

H.G. Wells told us that human history becomes more and more a race between education and catastrophe. What is needed to win this race are new ideas regarding cultural change, human relationships, ethical norms, gender respect, the use of technology, and the quality of life. These new ideas, of course, may be "old" ones newly applied.

By whatever means, the remaining chapters will be directed toward confronting critical issues in health education that must be addressed if the educational experience is to be improved. The end result just might be a society in which people are not just filling space, time, or a social role but are capable of saying something worthwhile with their lives.

Additionally, it is impossible to work with people in health education without taking on the role of counselor, especially when dealing with such topics as sexuality, drug use, life-style, self-esteem, and behavioral change. As such, we in health education should understand at least the basic principles of the counseling process. Chapter 16 will integrate the work of Carl Rogers, Robert Carkhuff, and others into a cognitive-behavioral mode for counseling intervention.

As health educators and helpers, we need to understand our role in the counseling process, because there is a crying need for us to support those we are working with in ways that transcend our traditional professional boundaries. "Helping is not bound by the four walls of a therapist's office, nor by the minutes of a client hour. Helping occurs whenever there is a responsive and initiative interaction between people. Such interactions always result in a person's growth. We stop thinking in terms of therapist and client. Instead, we start thinking in terms of helper and helpee, members of the same team whose relationship is oriented entirely to a human being's growth" (Carkhuff, 1983).

Reference

Carkhuff, Robert R. *The Art of Helping.* Amherst, MA: Human Resource Development Press, 1983.

15 Identifying Concerns

There is a sixth-century Indian legend about a scorpion and a tortoise who were facing a swollen river. The scorpion begged the tortoise to carry it across. "I can't take you on my back," the tortoise replied. "You'd sting me."

"Why would I do that?" the scorpion wanted to know. "You'd be my life raft. If I stung you, we'd both drown."

"Well," said the tortoise, "since you put it that way, I guess it'll be all right. Hop on."

So, the scorpion climbed on the tortoise's back and they set out across the river. When they were almost to the shore, the scorpion stung the tortoise. As they were both going down, the tortoise turned to the scorpion and asked, "Just tell me this before we drown. Why did you do it? I have to know."

And the scorpion replied, looking perhaps a little regretful, "What can I tell you? I couldn't help myself. It's my nature."

Are there people who hate, have prejudices, or just don't like someone else because it is their nature? Or is it really that? More likely, they were raised that way, verbally and nonverbally inculcated with a whole list of hateful attitudes.

Closing ourselves off from our feelings frees us, at a price, from having to do anything about those feelings. Putting other people on a hate list often seems a safer bet than taking a chance on caring about them.

As a teacher, you need to help those who fall into this trap, understand that, by closing themselves off from their feelings about those who don't meet their standards, they pay a high price in terms of social and emotional health. Painting other people as bad or unacceptable puts the person who hates into a defensive mode all the time.

To fully relate to another, one must first relate to oneself. If we cannot embrace our own aloneness, we will simply use the other as a shield against isolation. Only when one can live like the eagle—with no audience whatsoever—can one turn to another in love; only then is one able to care about the enlargement of the other's being.

—Irvin D. Yalom

Self-Awareness

The objective of Gestalt therapy (Perls, 1969) is to help the client become fully aware of herself and her present experience. Awareness touches virtually every aspect of life: our ideas, feelings, and physiological actions as well as our appreciation for and relationship to the environment. Self-awareness gets us in touch with our own existence and reality, which leads to a greater responsibility for our attitudes, behaviors, and feelings and beliefs. Helping a person become aware of herself allows her to see her prejudices, what may be producing them, and what actions may be necessary to resolve them.

Time Out for Personal Thoughts
Even though there are plenty of reasons for us to behave in a purely selfish fashion, we are capable of amazingly selfless acts of altruism and sacrifice for others. Most of us, though we may be reluctant to claim we are the best exemplars of pure love for others, have given of ourselves in some ways. Can you list a few of the ways you feel you have given to others?

The Function of Health Education in Self-Awareness

The aim of cognitive-behavioral teaching is to assist learners in becoming more aware of themselves, their environments, and their personal needs. The effective health educator helps students come to grips with their emotions, feelings, and attitudes and helps them develop positive outlooks and behaviors toward those who are not like them.

The role of the educational process is to provide an atmosphere that is conducive to developing this self-awareness (Passons, 1975), helping those who are dealing with problems to recognize them and cope in positive ways. To be effective as a health educator and contribute to your own understanding, you must be open and aware of your role as an individual and a teacher. Ask yourself the following questions: Who am I? Where am I going? How can I help?

Cultural Diversity

Any teacher who does not consider cultural diversity a critical factor in the classroom is living in an environmental void. Personal beliefs, family, culture, gender, age, and socioeconomic background have a major effect on how students behave. Such factors have to be considered when making any judgments about class content or verbal and nonverbal behavior.

The larger issue, according to Ron Miller (1989), is whether education exists to enforce a conformity of language, behavior, value, thought, and experience for the sake of national economic goals, or to nurture the innate human possibilities of every living child. Cultural diversity, beliefs, and values should be respected and cultivated rather than buried under layers of rigid social discipline.

For education, cultural diversity is an opportunity to cultivate what Joanna Macy calls "The Greening of the Self" (1990): "We have to treat others as part of who we are, rather than as a *them* with whom we are in constant competition." This idea certainly falls in line with Glasser's contention that cooperation, not competition, in the classroom builds a sense of community and positive learning.

Cultural diversity is related to health issues as evidenced by the following questions:

- Which cultures have the highest longevity? Why?
- Which cultures have the lowest rate of cholesterol? Why?
- Which cultures have the lowest rate of infant mortality? Why?
- What cultural differences affect the use of condoms?
- What are the cultural differences concerning abortion?
- What are the unique eating habits of different cultures?

Corey et al. (1992) suggest these additional methods for identifying relevant dimensions of students' culture:

- Have students tell you something about their culture and how they think it influences their participation in the group.
- Ask students if they think many members of the group have a cultural perspective different from their own. If so, have them pick out those people and tell them what things they are likely to see differently.
- Have students pretend they are back home among members of their ethnic group. Then have them try to explain to this group what the class is all about. What would they say?
- Address the following request to a specific member: "I'm aware that many of us in this group are from a culture that is different from yours. Would it be okay with you if some of us expressed our assumptions or stereotypes about your culture? You can react to what you hear, which could help us reconsider some of our conclusions." (Be careful in this exercise, for it can be either powerful or hurtful.)

The important aspect of multiculturalism in health education is that each group adds a healthy aspect of their culture to the "melting pot" of good health. The teacher should research each group for the positive aspects of that culture's health contributions.

Gender Bias to Gender Respect

A recent study of gender bias in schools raised important questions about what teachers can do to equalize how teachers focus on females and males in the classroom. The study, sponsored by the American Association of University Women

(AAUW) and conducted by the Wellesley College Center for Research on Women (1991), contended that teachers pay more attention to boys than to girls, use teaching materials rife with harmful sex stereotypes, favor teaching methods more suited to male pupils, and stereotype girls in the curriculum. The researchers recommended evaluating teachers, administrators, and counselors on how well they promote gender-equitable education.

In health education, the purpose should be toward expanding girls' awareness of gender bias; it is still a male-dominated society in which girls and women are devalued and subjected to sexual and emotional abuse. Given women's complicated lives, health-education programs must be creative and understanding of gender issues and issue a strong message that women are qualified, talented, exceptional, and capable.

In his book *Shifting Worlds, Changing Minds* (1987), physicist Jeremy Hayward demonstrated how our fundamental (and largely unconscious) assumptions about reality—our *belief* contexts—profoundly shape our experience of the world. He used the following riddle to illustrate the effect of context on perception.

> *A father and his son are driving to a football game. They begin to cross a railroad crossing and, when they are halfway across, the car stalls. Hearing a train coming in the distance, the father desperately tries to get the engine started again. He is unsuccessful, and the train hits the car. The father is killed instantly, but the son survives and is rushed to the hospital for brain surgery. The surgeon, on entering the operating theater, turns white and says, "I cannot operate on this boy. He is my son." What is the relation between the boy and the surgeon?*

The answer? She is his mother. (The assumption most of us make is that surgeons are men.)

Attacking gender bias in the classroom begins with our language. The overuse of that pesky pronoun "he" is a good place to start, for women feel rightly that they are a separate entity, not a part of men. The current attempt to correct the bias is the alternate use of "he" and "she," which can be awkward. Another is the use of plural pronouns such as "their" and "we." Various jobs can be referred to in gender-neutral terms as well (police officer or mail carrier, for example).

Bias-free language is only one step in eliminating gender inequality. It also includes respecting the other sex's property, space, personal style, strengths, and preferences. The bottom line is, gender bias compromises women's self-esteem, their sense of ability, and their sense of identity. They are never given the complete opportunity to be who they are.

Dealing with gender issues is one way to get the sexes to confront their attitudes. Try this technique. Have the class respond in writing to the set of questions in the exercise, first individually and then in a group.

To end this topic without discussing men's issues would imply that men are totally at fault. This is not the position of the author. The important point here is that men are as much victims of their socialization as are women (Bly, 1990). Thus, we should not focus exclusively on men as the aggressors and women as the victims. While statistically correct, it does not tell the total story. As teachers, we must help men and women understand they are both casualties of the cultural-

Exercise: Gender Bias

Directions: Read each statement carefully and respond using the scale given. List your responses in the column provided.

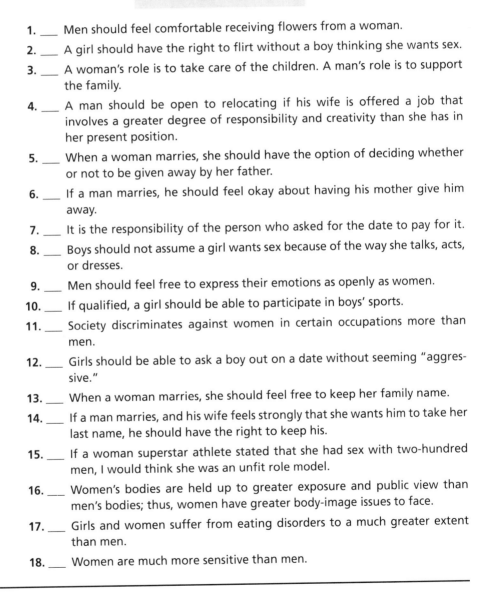

SCALE
1 = strongly agree
2 = agree
3 = neutral
4 = disagree
5 = strongly disagree

1. ___ Men should feel comfortable receiving flowers from a woman.

2. ___ A girl should have the right to flirt without a boy thinking she wants sex.

3. ___ A woman's role is to take care of the children. A man's role is to support the family.

4. ___ A man should be open to relocating if his wife is offered a job that involves a greater degree of responsibility and creativity than she has in her present position.

5. ___ When a woman marries, she should have the option of deciding whether or not to be given away by her father.

6. ___ If a man marries, he should feel okay about having his mother give him away.

7. ___ It is the responsibility of the person who asked for the date to pay for it.

8. ___ Boys should not assume a girl wants sex because of the way she talks, acts, or dresses.

9. ___ Men should feel free to express their emotions as openly as women.

10. ___ If qualified, a girl should be able to participate in boys' sports.

11. ___ Society discriminates against women in certain occupations more than men.

12. ___ Girls should be able to ask a boy out on a date without seeming "aggressive."

13. ___ When a woman marries, she should feel free to keep her family name.

14. ___ If a man marries, and his wife feels strongly that she wants him to take her last name, he should have the right to keep his.

15. ___ If a woman superstar athlete stated that she had sex with two-hundred men, I would think she was an unfit role model.

16. ___ Women's bodies are held up to greater exposure and public view than men's bodies; thus, women have greater body-image issues to face.

17. ___ Girls and women suffer from eating disorders to a much greater extent than men.

18. ___ Women are much more sensitive than men.

socialization process. We must discuss the issues of mythology, men's rights, and feminism in a life-affirming mix.

There is a change taking place in the feminist movement today. Some feminists feel strongly that male bashing is not the answer—that all heterosexual sex is *not* rape and that male oppression is a myth. Ricky Silberman, vice-chair of the U.S. Equal Employment and Opportunity Commission and member of both the Independent Women's Forum and the Women's Freedom Network, believes it is wrong to paint women as victims. She supports the concept that "new" feminists should distance themselves from the notion of women as the passive recipients of constant oppression, and instead promote women as individuals who do not need special protection but are on equal footing with men (*Boston Sunday Globe,* 1994).

Understanding and Dealing with Prejudice

Prejudice is a judgmental attitude flowing from blind or irrational beliefs that are often resistant to change. One kind of prejudice we all share is prejudice toward ourselves: "I'm stupid," "I just don't know how to do that," "I'm not accepted by others," and the like. The more prejudiced we are toward other people and events, the more prejudiced we are likely to be about ourselves.

Prejudice may take the form of hostility toward an entire group of people (e.g., gays or lesbians). It is a response to any person stereotyped as a group member rather than as a unique individual (Allport, 1958). Many people prejudge group members without ever having met them. Conversely, when someone is prejudiced *in favor* of a group, they often refuse to believe anything unfavorable about that group and even give them special considerations. (People's attitudes about the Reverend Jim Jones led them to their deaths in Jonestown, Guyana.)

Prejudice can be both the result and cause of misinformation about others. Knowing very little about a group they distrust can keep students from wanting to learn anything more, thus keeping themselves ignorant through the mechanism of *selective inattention.*

Exercise: Issues of Bias

Have students make a list of their prejudices. Have them be specific, and assure them that this list will not be shared with anyone. When they are done, have them draw a circle below their list. Have them look at their prejudices and divide them like slices of a pie, with their highest ranked prejudice the largest, and the size of each subsequent slice reflecting their prejudices in descending order. Then ask them to consider the following questions.

What was their largest prejudice?

What is this prejudice based on?

Would they like to reverse this prejudice?

What do they need to do to reverse this prejudice?

If you had a pleasant phone conversation with a blind date, would you feel uncomfortable to discover on meeting him that his ethnic background was not what you'd thought it was? Would you pursue the relationship?

How would you feel if your father remarried a woman of another race?

When describing your future stepmother to your friends, would you first refer to her ethnic background? Why?

Your best friend of years states that she is finally able to confide in you that she is gay. How would you respond?

If a friend recommended two tax attorneys—one male, one female—which one would you choose? Why?

You have been scheduled for major surgery. You have two choices, either a male surgeon or a female surgeon. Both have the same background and experience. Would you choose on the basis of gender? If so, why?

If two salespeople approached you at a car dealership—one obese, one not— whom would you ask for help? Why?

(continued)

If two salespeople approached you at a clothing store—one of color, one not—whom would you ask for help? Why?

A new coworker reveals that she spent two years receiving public assistance. Would you feel differently about her from the way you did before you knew this?

Sex Education: Abstinence versus Reality

An emotional debate about how to teach sexuality is raging across the country today. This debate is really between those who advocate either abstinence-based or reality-based sex education.

The supporters of the abstinence-based approach believe sex education should primarily promote sexual abstinence as the morally right choice. Its proponents feel that "pushing graphic sex" on children is pouring gas on an already burning fire.

The supporters of reality-based sex education seek a comprehensive, K–12 sex-education curriculum that presents basic information about human reproduction along with specific information on contraception, masturbation, homosexuality, and sexually transmitted diseases.

Educational Note

According to a recent study (Whitmire, 1994), the most effective sex-education classes combine abstinence training with traditional sex information. "School programs should teach youths how to say no to intercourse," said sex researcher Douglas Kirby in a paper sponsored by the Kaiser Family Foundation. But he also believed teachers should encourage students to use condoms if they choose to have intercourse.

Kirby looked at twenty-three school-based sex education programs and found

- *no indications that school-based sex education encourages fifteen- to nineteen-year-olds to experiment with sex. But evidence varied with age and gender: Classes leave fifteen- to seventeen-year-old girls more likely to initiate intercourse, while eighteen- and nineteen-year-old girls were less likely to do so. There was no impact on boys.*
- *the evidence that school-based clinics can reduce pregnancy rates is inconclusive.*
- *eighty-five percent of U.S. adults support school-based sex education.*

What's at Issue Here?

Figures from the Centers for Disease Control show that over half of the 70 percent of high-school seniors who report being sexually active say they don't practice safe sex. What this report shows is that young people are making choices on their own. Their study on teens, sex, and disease found that

- 72 percent of all high-school seniors have had sexual intercourse
- nearly one-fifth—19 percent—have had at least four partners
- among high-school students who are sexually active, only 45 percent report using a condom during their last sexual intercourse
- of 1,415 AIDS cases diagnosed in teenagers aged thirteen to nineteen and 12,712 in young people aged twenty to twenty-four, many were probably infected during adolescence
- 3 million teens have sexually transmitted diseases, including gonorrhea, chlamydia, herpes, and hepatitis B
- AIDS is the sixth leading cause of death among young people aged fifteen to twenty-four

The Reality of Teenage Sexual Behavior

As educators, parents, health professionals, and other community members vigorously debate the sex-education curricula in their public schools, more and more people are appearing before school boards requesting programs that provide students with accurate, unbiased information about reproduction, birth control, abstinence, and disease prevention. They know only too well that, as the debate lingers, more students will become sexually active and put themselves at risk for AIDS, other sexually transmitted diseases, emotional trauma, and unwanted pregnancies.

Few would disagree that something as basic as sexual behavior is the result of a chain of events so complex that we are often unaware of having made a choice about it. It is possible, however, that substantial numbers of youngsters do have the capacity to choose, in the same sense they choose the character that will mark them as adults—that is, through a sustained, lengthy process of considered and unconsidered behaviors. Although some influences—social and biological—are beyond our control, we should not accept the idea that people of "bad" character had no choice. To understand this is to also understand that we should establish a classroom climate that steers students into personal inquiry about what they need to feel and think based on the most accurate and comprehensive information we are capable of presenting. To provide a comprehensive, age-appropriate level of sexual knowledge that stresses responsibility and respect empowers students to make healthy sexual choices. This is the type of educational program young people want and need.

One of the most important goals of sex education should be teaching young people to act as they believe they should act based on *their* values while at the same time teaching them to respect the values of others. The teacher needs to help students develop well-defined values that will guide their sexual behavior.

In any discussion of sex and sexuality, the teacher can provide a creative classroom environment by allowing students to

- clarify and discuss issues of confusion about sex and sexuality
- examine their boundary issues (i.e., how far are they willing to go), and who determines these boundaries
- play a role reversal: let the girls become boys and the boys become girls, then have them discuss why they should not have sex
- brainstorm to come up with a sex-education program that would benefit lower level schoolchildren
- brainstorm how they could help lower the teen-pregnancy rate in their age group

Choosing a Sex-Education Curriculum

Consider some of the following viable suggestions from Planned Parenthood (1993) before investing time in the development of a curriculum for sex education:

- Are the goals and objectives of the curriculum clear and realistic?
- Does the curriculum contain accurate, reality-based information?
- Is the curriculum comprehensive?
- Does the curriculum meaningfully involve parents and other family members?
- What will it cost to implement the curriculum?
- Is the curriculum easy to use?
- Does the curriculum include lessons that help students to develop and practice effective communication skills?
- Does the curriculum support responsible behavior?
- Does the curriculum present clear messages about attitudes and values?
- Is the curriculum balanced?
- Is the curriculum inclusive and respectful of diversity?
- Is the curriculum appropriate to the developmental stage and learning needs of students?

Sex Information and Education Council of the United States (SIECUS)

Position Statement. Learning about sexuality goes from birth until death. Parents, peers, schools, religion, the media, friends, and partners all influence learning about sexuality for people at all stages of life. All too often, conflicting, incomplete, or inaccurate messages are received, and this frequently causes confusion.

SIECUS (1993) endorses the right of all people to comprehensive sexuality education. Comprehensive sexuality education addresses the biological, sociocultural, psychological, and spiritual dimensions of sexuality from (1) the cognitive domain (facts, data, and information); (2) the affective domain (feelings, values, and attitudes); and (3) the behavioral domain (the skills to communicate effectively and to make responsible decisions).

SIECUS affirms that parents are—and ought to be—the primary sexuality educators of their children. They support efforts to help parents fulfill this important role. In addition, they encourage religious leaders, youth and community-group leaders, and health and educational professionals to play an important role in complementing and augmenting the sexuality education received at home (Table 15–1).

Sex-education programs need to focus on *both* sexes, with an emphasis on social and moral issues. We must base our teaching on prevailing cultural and moral premises. To the question, Does sex education lead to more sex? Some research would indicate that the opposite is so. For example, Project SNAPP (developed by staffers at Children's Hospital, Los Angeles) conducted studies on its broad "abstinence-plus" approach, and results showed that the program worked (Griffin, 1995).

To support and conduct a sex-education program that is both equal and reality-based and that will *help* young people, start by

- accepting that they are sexual people
- giving behaviorally relevant information
- helping them gain the skills to prevent pregnancy and STDs

Table 15–1

SIECUS' Six Key Concepts to Include in a Comprehensive Sex-Education Program

Key Concept 1: Human Development

Reproductive anatomy and physiology

Reproduction

Puberty

Body image

Sexual identity and orientation

Key Concept 2: Relationships

Families

Friendship

Love

Dating

Marriage and lifetime commitments

Parenting

Key Concept 3: Personal Skills

Values

Decision making

Communication

Assertiveness

Negotiation

Finding help

(continued)

Table 15–1

Continued

Key Concept 4: Sexual Behavior

Sexuality throughout life

Masturbation

Shared sexual behavior

Abstinence

Human sexual response

Fantasy

Sexual dysfunction

Key Concept 5: Sexual Health

Contraception

Abortion

Sexually transmitted diseases and HIV infection

Sexual abuse

Reproductive health

Key Concept 6: Society and Culture

Sexuality and society

Gender roles

Sexuality and the law

Sexuality and religion

Diversity

Sexuality and the arts

Sexuality and the media

- teaching them negotiation skills to use with their partners
- helping them act publicly (i.e., go to a place to purchase contraceptives)
- consistently reinforcing all of these skills

Dealing with Gay and Lesbian Issues

School systems have a responsibility to recognize that they have many gay or lesbian students in their classes. They must not only provide a safe environment for them but also provide educational awareness about gay and lesbian issues. Most important, the unusually high suicide rates among young homosexuals due to the stigma attached to this sexual life-style begs our attention.

A learning session in gay/lesbian awareness should focus on homosexual identity, not sexual behavior. Gay and lesbian stereotypes should be discussed with an emphasis on understanding. Health educators should also incorporate gay and lesbian issues into their teaching (including civil rights, ending the ban in the military, adopting children, getting married, etc.). The educational focus should be toward erasing the stigma attached to homosexuality (Berne and Hamill, 1992):

> *Enhancing the students' level of moral reasoning through role-taking activities and discussions regarding moral dilemmas . . . can help eliminate homophobia. As children become less egocentric and more concerned with others, they become more altruistic, more empathic, and display more prosocial behaviors, such as cooperation, friendliness, kindness, generosity, and sharing.*

State School Board OKs Gay Guidelines

The Massachusetts Board of Education unanimously adopted guidelines for protecting and counseling gay students, the first state to do so. Schools are not obligated to adopt the guidelines, and proponents expect fights in every community. Jessica Byers, a seventeen-year-old lesbian who is a senior at Cambridge Latin School, said: "In most high schools, people are absolutely terrified to come out because they fear harassment and violence—not only by other students but by their teachers, too."

Also: Students at Bremerton High School in Washington state voted down an amendment to bar gay students from serving on the student council. Of the school's fifty-four homerooms, thirty-six voted against the measure.

Copyright © 1993, USA Today. Reprinted with permission.

Wright and Yates (1987) suggest asking ourselves the following questions to examine our own gay and lesbian attitudes:

1. "Do I make heterosexist assumptions?" Suggested approach: Use gender-free terminology in class discussions (such as *partners* or *persons* instead of *husband, wife, boyfriend,* or *girlfriend*).
2. "Do I ignore homophobic remarks?" Suggested approach: Consistently interrupt homophobic comments with interventions that encourage critical thinking. For example, if someone says "I think all queers should be locked up," ask her why she thinks that is a good idea. Get the class involved, if possible. Most important, don't let unacceptable terms like "queers" go unchallenged.
3. "Do I blame my audience for their misinformation?" Suggested approach: Remember that homophobia is learned. Use homophobic misinformation to reeducate the group by responding to questions truthfully and sufficiently. If the answer is unknown, you should research it or ask the group to do so.

4. "Do I use educational materials that assume all my students are heterosexuals?" Suggested approach? Be sure material is not purely heterosexual or homophobic.

Exercise: Checking Out Attitudes toward Gays and Lesbians

To check out learner attitudes and feelings about homosexuality, have them respond to the following set of questions using the key provided:

> **KEY**
> 1 = strongly agree
> 2 = agree
> 3 = neutral
> 4 = disagree
> 5 = strongly disagree

1. 1 2 3 4 5   Homosexuality is something I could never accept in another person or in myself.

2. 1 2 3 4 5   I would feel comfortable working with someone who is gay.

3. 1 2 3 4 5   If I found out that one of my friends was gay, I would not remain friends with him.

4. 1 2 3 4 5   I believe that gays should be allowed into the military.

5. 1 2 3 4 5   I believe that gays should not be allowed to teach, especially in elementary school.

6. 1 2 3 4 5   I would support gay and lesbian rights.

7. 1 2 3 4 5   I would feel that I had failed as a parent if I found out that my son or daughter was gay.

8. 1 2 3 4 5   I believe that gays, like heterosexual couples, have every right to get legally married.

9. 1 2 3 4 5   I would never support a law allowing gays to adopt a child.

10. 1 2 3 4 5   I have no problem with gay people, but they should not be allowed to work with children.

11. 1 2 3 4 5   I feel that homosexual behavior is abnormal.

12. 1 2 3 4 5   My feelings about gay and lesbian life-styles are mostly from what I have heard, not what I personally know.

13. 1 2 3 4 5   Personally, my feelings are that gays should be treated as equals.

14. 1 2 3 4 5   If a homosexual person made a pass at me, I would treat them as I would any heterosexual person doing the same thing.

15. 1 2 3 4 5   I would never shop at a store owned by a homosexual.

16. 1 2 3 4 5   I would vote for a homosexual political candidate.

17. 1 2 3 4 5   I would allow my child to watch a TV program with a homosexual in it.

18. 1 2 3 4 5   I would not attend a church or synagogue with a homosexual minister or rabbi.

19. 1 2 3 4 5   I would allow my child to attend a preschool that had gay and lesbian staff members.

20. 1 2 3 4 5   I would never see a homosexual doctor.

21. 1 2 3 4 5   I don't understand gay and lesbian life-styles; I would like to learn more, including:

Note: Have students share their responses to number 21 so you can include them in a lesson on gay and lesbian issues.

Are There Remedies for Prejudice?

Yes, according to some new research (Monteith et al., 1992, 1993). People who score high in prejudice on various widely recognized scales behave markedly different than people who score low in prejudice. People low in prejudice are much more likely to feel remorseful when they act in ways that violate their personal standards or beliefs, whereas highly prejudiced people are likely to become increasingly frustrated and angry. Unless that anger is defused by firm but nonjudgmental leadership, it can explode in the face of the people who are targeted.

Instead of feeling guilty about their behavior and saying "it's my fault," people who are high in prejudice are more likely to externalize blame—*"they're gay"* or *"they're* black," or "if *they* didn't hang around here, I wouldn't have to feel this way." They resent being forced to confront something they really don't like about themselves (Bass, 1993).

"It has to do with the nature of the 'should' standard," reports Monteith et al. (1993):

> In low-prejudiced people, the belief in not engaging in prejudicial behavior is a personally held moral standard and very much related to their self-concept. So when they violate that standard, they are angry at themselves. But for high-prejudiced people, that standard has been imposed by society at large or other people, and it isn't really based on a sense of moral obligation.

It is easier to change people's behavior when they are feeling remorseful than it is when they are angry and convinced they are right (Katz, 1960). But there are ways to defuse anger before it gets out of hand. Racial attitudes can be changed when community leaders continually reaffirm the need for acceptance of different groups and point out the inconsistency between the American ethos of egalitarianism and individual feelings of intolerance. When that inconsistency is exposed, even people who are highly prejudiced can bring their racial attitudes more in line with widely held democratic principles (Devine, 1989; Gaertner and Dovidio, 1986).

Cooperative-learning techniques (Glasser, 1990) are also designed to improve racial attitudes. Separate classes into small, racially mixed groups and assign a specific question, such as:

- What are the basic causes of racism?
- How would you deal with racism?
- How would you deal with racism in this class? In this school?

Researchers have found that, after working together in such teams, students are much more likely to say their friends are from other races or ethnic groups (Abrami et al., 1993).

When Students Argue for Unhealthy Values

If you get students into a discussion on cheating, some students will argue that it is acceptable under certain situations. These are called *situational values* and are based on a number of reasons that students may cite, including

- "Everybody else is cheating, so why shouldn't I?"
- "The teacher gives such unfair exams that I have to cheat to pass."
- "I have to work after school. I couldn't study, so if I don't cheat, I will flunk the exam."

Teachers who fall prey to this type of argument often don't know what else to say or do. They become victims of students who dominate the class discussion with poor or faulty thinking, much of which has been learned.

Time Out for Personal Thoughts

What short- and long-term consequences of cheating can you think of?

Short-term:

Long-term:

Hopefully, teachers who are skilled in leading the class are able to bring the discussion back to a rational moral foundation. The teacher who relies on the positive human qualities of students begins by challenging the idea that cheating is okay, pointing out the moral low in this country vis-à-vis white-collar crime, the Iran-Contra scandal, etc. A skilled teacher is able to get students to rethink their options by considering both the short- and long-term consequences of their choices. Most important, she first thinks about the particular student, not the particular issue under consideration.

Dealing with the Unpopular Student

If you ask schoolchildren to rank-order their classmates, you will almost always find the same names at the bottom of everybody's list. Several behaviors are likely to be the source of such unpopularity (Selman, 1987). Some children are so shy and withdrawn that they become isolated; others are disruptive, striking out physically or bullying others.

Children use relationships with peers to refine their abilities to share, to handle anger, and to sustain emotional closeness. "Our research shows very clearly," states Selman, "that the cutting edge of children's growth in reciprocity isn't with adults, it's with equals." If children go day after day without making friends, they become increasingly vulnerable to lifelong difficulties. Chronic peer rejection is linked with childhood depression, low self-esteem, early school-leaving, and delinquent behavior.

For teachers, the issue is not just how to help a rejected child, but how to handle the complex classroom dynamics as other children express their negative or ambivalent feelings. Peer relations are an important part of the climate of classrooms and schools, but it is not always clear whether, or how, to intervene. Many psychologists believe that the dynamics of early peer rejection are too complex for effective one-shot interventions.

Confronting Sexual Harassment

"Sexual harassment in schools is more than behavior of a molesting teacher or counselor. It includes actions long dismissed as adolescent pranks: harmful graffiti, pushing and touching in hallways, pep-rally skits that denigrate females, pornography passed in the classroom" (Lanpher, 1992).

A survey of sexual harassment in schools revealed the following statistics concerning teenage girls (LeBlanc, 1993):

Who reported being harassed?

- Girls nine to eleven years old: 2 percent
- Girls twelve to sixteen years old: 92 percent
- Girls seventeen to nineteen years old: 6 percent

What Constitutes Harassment?

Staff-to-Student Harassment

1. A male teacher placing his arms around middle-school girls and rubbing their backs as positive reinforcement for a job well done.
2. A teacher's inquiry into a student's personal, social, and sexual life.
3. Leering or staring at the intimate body parts of a student.
4. A bus driver playing a game with elementary students involving tickling and touching of the students by the bus driver.
5. A teacher showing favoritism toward students who welcome sexually suggestive comments or behavior.

Student-to-Student Harassment

1. Bra snapping, giving "snuggies" or "pantsing" (pulling down boys' or girls' pants or pulling up girls' skirts).
2. Students "rating" other students.
3. Students displaying or circulating centerfolds or other sexually explicit materials.
4. Name calling: "slut," "whore," "fag," "lesbian," "cow," or "dog."
5. Teasing students about their sexual activities or lack of sexual activity.
6. Students wearing sexually offensive t-shirts, hats, or pins.
7. Displays of affection between students (e.g., "making out" in the halls).
8. Suggestive comments about apparel.

Student-to-Staff Harassment

1. Students making sexually explicit and threatening comments to a staff member.
2. Students "hiding" sexually explicit materials in a classroom where a teacher will find them.
3. Students passing around sexually explicit, derogatory illustrations of the principal.
4. Students making obscene phone calls to a teacher at his or her home.

Source: *Shoop, Robert J., and Jack W. Hayhow. Sexual Harassment in Our Schools. Copyright © 1994, Allyn and Bacon. Used with permission.*

Who do they say is harassing them?

- Fellow students: 96 percent
- Teachers or counselors: 3 percent
- Administrators or other school staff: 1 percent

What form does the harassment take?

- Suggestive gestures, looks, or comments: 89 percent
- Touching, pinching, or grabbing: 83 percent
- Being leaned over or cornered: 47 percent
- Sexual notes or pictures: 28 percent
- Pressure to do something sexual: 27 percent
- Being forced to do something sexual: 10 percent

Where does it happen?

- In the classroom: 23 percent
- In the hall: 18 percent
- On a parking lot or playing field: 6 percent
- At a school activity away from school: 3 percent
- In the cafeteria: 1 percent
- Multiple locations: 44 percent

When does it happen?

- Every day: 39 percent
- Once a week: 29 percent
- Once a month: 21 percent
- Once a year: 11 percent
- In the presence of others: 92 percent
- Alone with the harasser: 8 percent

How do you respond?

- Tell harasser to stop: 74 percent
- Walk away: 46 percent
- Resist with physical force: 40 percent
- Do nothing: 13 percent
- Tell a friend: 66 percent
- Keep it to yourself: 24 percent
- Tell a parent: 18 percent
- Tell a teacher: 18 percent
- Tell a counselor: 2 percent

In the same vein, Dr. Nan Stein of the Massachusetts Department of Education states how she "really came to see that sexual harassment was this mundane occurrence that happened in stairwells, parking lots, cafeterias, classes, whatever. The girls had to work out incredible coping strategies. Ultimately, it was a denial of equal-education opportunity" (Lanpher, 1992). Stein developed the first sexual-harassment curriculum for high schools as well as a video for use by secondary schools and universities. She promotes a multipronged approach to dealing with sexual harassment in which the first step is training adults—school administrators, teachers, and other personnel—followed by working with students and getting them to thresh out for themselves what constitutes sexual harassment. "What one person may perceive as a compliment," says Stein, "another may feel demeaned by." She would also like to see trained personnel brought into schools so that students have someone to go to for advice without having to file a complaint.

In short, sexual harassment should be added to the repertoire of drug and alcohol discussions in school in an ongoing, systematic way—not addressed in one-shot assemblies (Lanpher, 1992).

Sexual harassment permeates the school environment . . . surveys show that it is pervasive, with four out of five students reporting that they have been the target of some form of sexual harassment during their school lives. Of those students, one in four report being targeted "often." And surprisingly, much of the problem

---

If You're Harassed . . .

Nan Stein's tips for students (and their parents) who feel they're the target of sexual harassment:

- *Tell someone and keep telling until you find someone who believes you. Find supporters and talk with them. The point is to find someone you can trust who will take the kinds of actions you want.*
- *Don't blame yourself. Harassment is unwanted and can make you feel trapped, confused, helpless, embarrassed, or scared. You certainly didn't ask for any of those feelings.*
- *Keep a written record of the incidents: what happened, when, where, who else was present, and how you reacted. Save any notes or pictures from the harasser.*
- *Find out who at your school is responsible for dealing with complaints about sexual harassment. If you feel uncomfortable talking to the designated people, go to an adult you like and trust. I'ts okay to bring a friend or parent with you to that meeting.*
- *Let the harasser know you don't like the behavior or comments. If you feel safe and comfortable doing so, tell the harasser his behavior bothers you and you want him to stop. Or write a letter that describes the behaviors you consider to be harassment, indicating that these bother you and that you want them to stop. Keep a copy. Write the letter with an adult advocate and have the adult hand-deliver the letter to the harasser so the harasser takes this letter seriously.*
- *You have the right to file a complaint with the U.S. Department of Education's Office for Civil Rights, with your state's department of education, or to bring a lawsuit under Title IX of the federal education laws.*

---

isn't initiated by adults; it's caused by student-to-student harassment in high school, junior high and middle schools, and even in elementary schools.

Clearly, something needs to be done to confront sexual harassment, and health education has the most appropriate curriculum options to deal with it. To start the classroom thinking about sexual harassment, separate the girls and boys and have each group work out a list of what they consider sexual harassment. Have each group present their lists to the class, followed by a discussion. Finally, see if the class can agree on a single list.

The following questions can be asked to increase student awareness of sexual harassment (Strauss, 1992):

Exercise: Sexual-Harassment Awareness

Circle "T" if you think the statement *usually* true. Circle "F" if you think the statement *usually* false.

T F **1.** Sexual harassment has been a problem for me.

T F **2.** Sexual harassment is a problem in the schools.

T F **3.** Boys can be victims of sexual harassment.

T F **4.** If a girl dresses or behaves in a sexy way, she is asking to be sexually harassed.

T F **5.** Sexual harassment can occur between people of the same sex.

T F **6.** Women in professional jobs (teachers, lawyers, engineers, doctors, etc.) are not as likely to be sexually harassed as women in blue-collar jobs (factory workers, waitresses, truck drivers, etc.).

T F **7.** Women rarely file false charges of sexual harassment.

T F **8.** Saying no is usually enough to stop sexual harassment.

T F **9.** If sexual harassment occurs between students in the school, it is illegal, and the school is responsible.

T F **10.** Women who work in jobs that are usually held by men (construction workers, accountants, surgeons, etc.) are more likely to be sexually harassed.

T F **11.** Most women enjoy getting sexual attention at work and at school.

T F **12.** Most men enjoy getting sexual attention at work and at school.

T F **13.** The only people who can harass women are those in positions of authority (employers, teachers, administrators).

T F **14.** Women use their sex appeal to get what they want at work and at school.

T F **15.** One of the best ways to deal with sexual harassment is to ignore it.

T F **16.** Women of color are sexually harassed more often than white women.

(continued)

T F 17. Most victims of sexual harassment report it to their employer or school principal.

T F 18. If *he* didn't like the sexual attention but *she* meant it only as flirting, then it was not sexual harassment.

T F 19. Teasing and flirting are not a big deal. They make school and work fun.

T F 20. Schools and workplaces should know if sexual harassment is occurring among their students or employees.

A survey sponsored by the NOW Legal Defense Fund and Wellesley College's Center for Research on Women (LeBlanc, 1993), found that girls are not passive victims of harassment. Nearly two-thirds of the respondents said they had told their harassers to stop; one-third had resisted with physical force. The survey also showed that in spite of—or perhaps as a result of—adult inaction, girls are learning that harassment is something they don't have to take. Health educators must teach boys—and men—that they must act accordingly.

Teachers and Harassment

The scheme dreamed up by a Chicago fourth grader to falsely accuse a teacher she disliked of sexual abuse should be a wake-up call for all teachers. Here is an explosive example of how teachers are vulnerable in the 1990s with regard to the whole issue of teacher-student relationships. In this age of political correctness, all teachers must be aware that their professional lives are on the line. This is most true for male teachers. Male teachers must be aware that teaching sex education is like walking in a mine field; they cannot be perceived as having personal involvement with students, particularly female students. Even innocent, casual touching can be totally misconstrued.

This does not in any way deny that harassment of students by teachers is a real problem. But, the no-touch policy has forced a great many teachers to rethink their personal approaches to teaching. As we all know, touching is a very important and encouraging part of teaching; it conveys the message that we care and understand, on a personal level. But it can inadvertently send a double message.

A compromise may be forming. Shoop and Hayhow (1994), recommend a "continuum of contact": more physical expressions of support in the early grades, where it's acceptable for a teacher to hold a hand or wipe a tear, and less in middle school and high school, where even innocent hugs can confuse students who are forging their sexual identities. Such a policy, clearly defined and understood by students and teachers, is vital to making schools physically and emotionally safer.

Understanding the Other Sex

Health educators need to follow up the unit on sexual harassment with a discussion about mutual understanding. Understanding the other sex (a term I feel is much more appropriate than "opposite sex") is the best road to more positive relations.

One area to focus on deals with men—their fear of sexual rejection and the powerlessness it engenders. Allow the men to express their feelings about sexual rejection while the women listen. Next, allow the women in the group to express what, if any, role they play in men's feelings of rejection. Male students have to be fully involved in this exercise, and the emphasis has to be on male empowerment and female empowerment equally.

Resolving Conflict in the Learning Environment

As violence becomes more prevalent on city streets, on television, and at home, some educators say children are acting out more violently in schools. Add to this racism, sexism, and anti-gay behavior and we are not talking about isolated incidents anymore. "Violence is not usually isolated from other aspects of a damaging way of life," wrote David Hamburg, president of the Carnegie Corporation, in a report on violence-prevention programs (Hamburg, 1992):

> Violence and related problems have to be, to some extent, thought of together in terms of generic interventions to make differences in the lives of kids. How do kids grow up, particularly in poverty-concentration areas? Can you improve the life chances in substantial ways that would diminish the risk of their becoming involved in violence and other risks as well?

The program proposed by Hamburg uses a technique called *conflict resolution* (or cooperative rule setting) in which conflicting students are brought together with a neutral third party, usually a peer, who leads the students in a discussion to resolve their problems. This process works well in a classroom setting (see Chapter 6).

To take this process a step further, a teacher can ask students to establish cooperative rules of behavior at the beginning of a new school year. Have students establish simple, positive classroom guidelines that describe their ideal learning environment and include words like safe, happy, supportive, and understanding. The students in this collaborative venture "own" these rules; thus, they own a share of the responsible behavior that leads to meeting these rules.

In addition, these rules should be phrased as something to *do* versus something to *stop doing*. By saying "don't do that" we violate a vital tenet of reality therapy: that someone is more receptive to concrete representation than to negative command (Glasser, 1965). For example, probably every teacher has said to a student, "Don't do that again or I will send you to the principal," the result of which is that the student repeats the previous action. In simple terms, "don'ts" often fail to get a desired behavior. They are negative, and perhaps a particular student has had an overload of negatives throughout her life. Thus, she tunes out anything that follows the word (Berne, 1961).

Five elements that contribute to an atmosphere in which people can act nonviolently to resolve conflict are as follows (Judson, 1984):

- *Affirmation.* People need to feel empowered so that they feel confidence in themselves and in taking creative action.
- *Sharing of feelings.* Through a sharing of feelings, people are able to hear and empathize with others in conflict situations.
- *Establishing a supportive community.* Create an atmosphere in which each student is (and feels) a part of the whole.
- *Problem-solving.* Learning ways of solving problems is the most viable way of diffusing a problem before it escalates.
- *Enjoying life.* Teaching young people to enjoy life is at the very core of a nonviolent learning environment.

Eight Steps to Good Discipline

Schools (or any other learning environments) can be good places to be given certain educational concepts. These concepts are as follows (Glasser, 1977):

- *Be personal.* Use personal pronouns, e.g., "I care enough about you to be involved, to be your friend."

- *Refer to present behavior.* Awareness of behavior is the first step. Avoid references to the past. Emphasize positive attitudes and behavior.
- *Stress value judgments.* Ask students to evaluate their own attitudes and behaviors.
- *Plan.* Work with students to formulate alternatives. Keep the plan simple. Build success into the plan. The decision to improve their behavior must be theirs.
- *Be committed.* Build in a way to check back and follow up. Give positive reinforcement.
- *Do not accept excuses.* Eliminate excuses to show you know students can succeed. Work with them. Don't give up.
- *Do not punish.* Punishment not only lifts responsibility from students but sends a message that you have reached the end. Set rules and sanctions with them. They have to understand that they are responsible for their actions.
- *Never give up.* Each of us must define "never," but hang in there longer than the student thinks you will.

Synthesis

There is a personal element in every task that health educators and students do together, whether it be teaching and learning, designing a curriculum, or discussing health issues. How people think and feel about each other and what they are doing influences the inhibition or release of talent, effort, and most important, cooperative achievement. Young people can be effectively disabled by uncertainty about their relation to the people around them. Such uncertainty is partly the fear of expressing deeply felt opinions, of trying to do difficult or previously untried things (some people would call that being creative), or of doing anything that others will see and judge.

Supplementing class discussions with indirect counseling techniques can trigger developmental processes. For example, role playing and role reversal can be used to deal with gender issues, sexual harassment, and prejudice. Similarly, there are exercises that can enhance a student's capacity for empathy, his listening skills, and his communication skills, all of which reduce misunderstanding.

Directing the learning experience in ways that confront conflicts brings a process whereby issues of race, sex, sexual preference, etc. can be discussed and, hopefully, creatively resolved by the class.

References

Abrami, Philip C., et al. *Using Cooperative Learning.* Montreal, Quebec: Centre for the Study of Classroom Process, Concordia University, 1993.

Allport, Gordon. *The Nature of Prejudice.* Garden City, NJ: Doubleday, 1958.

Bass, Alison. "New Studies on Prejudice Point to Possible Remedies." *Boston Globe,* 17 May 1993.

Berne, Eric. *Transactional Analysis in Psychotherapy.* New York: Grove Press, 1961.

Berne, Linda A., and Shelley Hamill. "Homosexuality: Exploring Your Feelings." *Journal of School Health,* September/October 1992.

Bly, Robert. *Iron John: A Book about Men.* Reading, MA: Addison Wesley, 1990.

Centers for Disease Control. "Trends in Sexual Risk Behavior among High-School Students: United States, 1990, 1991, 1993." *Morbidity and Mortality Weekly Report* 44:7, 24 February 1995.

Corey, Gerald, et al. *Group Techniques.* Pacific Grove, CA: Brooks/Cole, 1992.

Devine, P.G. "Stereotypes and Prejudice: Their Automatic and Controlled Components." *Journal of Personality and Social Psychology,* January 1989.

Gaertner, S.L., and J.F. Dovidio. "The Aversive Form of Racism," in J.F. Dovidio and S.L. Gaertner (eds.), *Prejudice, Discrimination, and Racism.* San Diego, CA: Academic Press, 1986.

Glasser, William. *Reality Therapy: A New Approach to Psychiatry.* New York: Harper & Row, 1965.

___. "10 Steps to Good Discipline." *Today's Education,* November/December 1977.

___. *The Quality School: Managing Students without Coercion.* New York: Harper Perennial, 1990.

Griffin, Katherine. "Sex Education that Works." *Health,* May/June 1995.

Hamburg, David, quoted in Amy Mednick, "Resolving Youthful Conflict." *Boston Globe,* 21 June 1992.

Hayward, Jeremy. *Shifting Worlds, Changing Minds.* Berkeley, CA: Shambhala, 1987.

Judson, Stephanie (ed.). *A Manual on Nonviolence and Children.* Philadelphia, PA: New Society, 1984.

Katz, D. "The Functional Approach to the Study of Attitudes." *Public Opinion Quarterly,* Summer 1960.

Lanpher, Katherine. "Reading, 'Riting, and 'Rassment." *Ms.,* May/June 1992.

LeBlanc, Adrian Nicole. "Harassment at School: The Truth Is Out." *Seventeen,* May 1993.

Macy, Joanna. "The Greening of the Self." *Common Boundary,* July/August 1990.

Miller, Ron. "American Education and Cultural Conformity." *Holistic Education Review,* Winter 1989.

Monteith, Margo J. *Self-Regulation of Stereotypic Responses: Implications for Prejudice Reduction Efforts.* Unpublished doctoral dissertation, University of Wisconsin, Madison; 1992.

___, et al. "Self-Directed versus Other-Directed Affect as a Consequence of Prejudice-Related Discrepancies." *Journal of Personality and Social Psychology,* February 1993.

Passons, W.R. *Gestalt Approaches to Counseling.* New York: Holt, Rinehart & Winston, 1975.

Perls, Fritz. *Gestalt Therapy Verbatim.* Moab, UT: Real People Press, 1969.

Planned Parenthood. *Choosing a Sexuality-Education Curriculum.* Planned Parenthood Federation of America, 1993.

Selman, R.L., and M. Glidden. "Negotiation Strategies for Youth." *School Safety,* Fall 1987.

Sex Information and Education Council of the United States. *SIECUS Position Statement.* New York: SIECUS, 1993.

Shoop, Robert, and Jack W. Hayhow, Jr. *Sexual Harassment in Our Schools: What Parents and Students Need to Know to Spot It and Stop It.* Boston: Allyn and Bacon, 1994.

Silberman, Ricky, quoted in "New Breed of Feminist Challenges Old Guard." *Boston Sunday Globe,* 29 May 1994.

Stein, Nan, quoted in "If You're Harassed . . . " *USA Today,* 18 May 1993.

Strauss, Susan. *Sexual Harassment and Teens.* Minneapolis, MN: Free Spirit, 1992.

Wellesley College Center for Research on Women. *How Schools Shortchange Girls.* American Association of University Women, 1991.

Whitmire, Richard. "School-Based Sex Education." *USA Today,* 24 January 1994.

Wright, B., and R. Yates. "AIDS and Homophobia: A Perspective for AIDS Educators." *Feminist Teacher,* Fall 1987.

Yalom, Irvin D. *When Nietzsche Wept.* New York: Basic Books, 1992.

Additional Resources

Berne, Linda A., and Shelley Hamill. "Homosexuality: Exploring Your Feelings." *Journal of Health Education,* September/October 1992.

Butler, Karen L., and T. Jean Byrne. "Homophobia among Preservice Elementary Teachers." *Journal of Health Education,* September/October 1992.

Comer, James P., and Alvin F. Poussaint. *Raising Black Children.* New York: Plume, 1992.

Creative Conflict Resolution. Pamphlet available from the Boston Area Educators for Social Responsibility, 19 Garden Street, Cambridge, MA, 1993.

Education that Works: An Action Plan for the Education of Minorities. Contains descriptions of dozens of individual projects specifically targeted at minority students. Write to: Project Director, Quality Education for Minorities Project, 1818 N Street NW, Suite 350, Washington, DC 20036. Phone: (202) 659–1818.

Galvin, Maryanne, and Donald A. Read. "Combating Racism and Sexism in Health Education: Some Issues, Responsibilities, and Possibilities." *Health Education,* March/April 1983.

Konner, Melvin. *Childhood: A Multicultural View.* Boston: Little, Brown, 1991.

Lacey, Ella P. "U.S. Census Procedures: A Backdrop for Consideration of Ethnic and Racial Issues in Health Education Programming." *Journal of Health Education,* January/February 1992.

Massachusetts Department of Education. "No Laughing Matter: High School Students and Sexual Harassment." 25-minute videotape. Call (617) 388–3300.

Massachusetts Department of Education. "Who's Hurt and Who's Liable: Sexual Harassment in Massachusetts Schools." Free pamphlet. Call (617) 388–3300.

Page, Randy M., et al. "Interpersonal Violence: A Priority Issue for Health Education." *Journal of Health Education,* July/August 1992.

Safe Schools Coalition, 5351 Gulf Drive, P.O. Box 1338, Holmes Beach, FL 34218. Phone (813) 778–9140.

Teaching Tolerance, a new tool for combating racism, is now available from the Southern Poverty Law Center. The program offers a curriculum package, "America's Civil Rights Movement," that includes a video and magazine focusing on teaching strategies and exercises for increasing racial and religious sensitivity. Write to: Southern Poverty Law Center, 400 Washington Avenue, Montgomery, AL 36104. Phone: (205) 264–0286.

"Tune In to Your Rights: A Guide for Teenagers about Turning Off Sexual Harassment," pamphlet available from the University of Michigan. Call (313) 763–9910.

Wichert, Susanne. *Keeping the Peace: Practicing Cooperation and Conflict Resolution with Preschoolers.* Philadelphia, PA: New Society, 1989.

16 The Health Educator as Counselor

Trying something new might seem only a small step in your life. If you feel discouraged, remember the words of the ancient Chinese sage, Lao-tzu. We typically notice and applaud the "nine-story tower" and forget that there was *ever* only a "heap of earth." We learn to distrust our ability to accomplish anything when we let our eyes rest only on the finished product.

A Humanistic Approach to Counseling

In the 1950s, humanistic psychology, the core of the human-potential movement whose leading spokesperson was Abraham Maslow (1954), emerged as a third force—an alternative to Freudian psychoanalysis on the one hand and to behavioral psychology on the other.

Humanistic psychology, more philosophic than scientific, objected to the psychoanalytic view that the individual's personality and behavior are determined by his or her life experiences, especially those of childhood, and also to the behaviorist view that individual actions are a set of conditioned responses to stimuli. Humanistic psychology stressed the individual's power to choose how to behave and right to self-fulfillment. It held that behavior should be judged not in terms of supposedly objective scientific standards but in terms of the individual's own frame of reference. If a person considered a non-competitive, laid-back life, that was a valid goal for him or her, not a symptom of a character flaw; so, too, was a gay life-style, sexual freedom, and other departures from social norms. Humanistic psychology, therefore, had great appeal, especially for the young during the individualistic 1960s.

> *Big things of the world can only be achieved by attending to their small beginnings. . . . A tree as big as a man's embrace springs from a tiny sprout. A tower nine stories high begins with a heap of earth.*
>
> —LAO-TZU

Out of this psychology emerged a crop of new therapies. Though widely disparate, they are all based on the doctrine that everyone possesses inner resources for growth and self-healing, and that the goal of counseling is not to change the person but to remove obstacles, such as poor self-esteem or the denial of feelings, to the person's use of these inner resources. As a health educator, your role is not to guide the individual toward some scientific ideal of mental or physical health but to help her grow toward her own best self.

The Crucial Ingredient in Counseling: You

Imagine that a student you have been working with in a group session on sexuality comes to you one day and asks if she can talk with you privately. After some preliminaries, she says,

> *I feel like I am living a lie with my family, with my friends, with everyone. . . . I know that I am gay, but I have told no one, not even my best friend. I feel very self-conscious, even though my friends say nothing to me. Although all of them have boyfriends, I don't because it would be a lie for me to have one. I don't even like boys. I knew a long time ago that I liked girls better, that it is a girl I want to be with, to love. What should I do?*

It is important that you take a moment and think through what you consider the central issues troubling this girl. Write down what you would say to her:

After this exercise, you may have glanced ahead to find the "correct" answer. Well, you won't find it; nor do I believe there is one appropriate thing to say to a person who has a concern or is coping with conflict. Chances are that you *have* a correct response—something that you offered of yourself that helps clarify the reality of this student's position. The objective of this chapter is to help you understand and expand your typical response and enhance your ability to generate new possibilities for your students. You will find those whom you help will also generate new ways to manage their lives more effectively.

Return to your response and read what you wrote. Before you go any further, have several other people respond to the question, and record what they say. Are their responses helpful? Would they lead the girl in a different direction than yours did? Is one response necessarily better than another? Remember, *what you say to a person in a helping relationship says as much about you, or more, than it does about the person.*

Person-Centered Counseling

One approach to counseling that takes into consideration the quality of the counselor/client relationship is that of Carl Rogers. He published *Client-Centered Therapy* in 1951, and its widespread effect subsequently made him one of the chief spokespersons in the field of humanistic psychology.

According to Rogers, humans are organic creatures who are capable of growth but who may, on occasion, need to be reminded of how to go about releasing their potential. This total acceptance of the individual provided the orientation for Rogers' subsequent therapeutic developments. The person who wanted advice was no longer to be categorized as a patient but looked upon as a client. This eliminated the earlier medical model because, since the person was no longer seen as "sick," there was no need to delve into his past experiences to determine the cause of his "illness." Client-centered therapy focused on the present. Additionally, the person, not the "problem," was discussion, and feelings were more important than the intellect.

The Focus of Person-Centered Counseling

Person-centered counseling focuses on an individual's inherent tendency toward self-actualization, that is, the essential forces within a person working toward self-maintenance and self-enhancement (Maslow, 1954). This process is thwarted in early life when *conditions of worth* (usually parental standards of right and wrong) are placed on experiences. A person begins to value her own experiences by the criteria of these externally imposed conditions instead of by her own inherent response.

This creates a discrepancy between a person's self-esteem and her experience. Those experiences not in line with the self-image are distorted or completely shut off from conscious awareness. The work of the health educator is not only to heal these divisions but also to heal all mind-body separations (see Chapter 2).

There are three significant characteristics of a successful teacher-centered therapist: genuineness, empathic understanding, and unconditional positive regard. Of these characteristics, genuineness, or *congruence,* is the most basic. Genuineness signifies that the therapist is in touch with his own feelings and can be fully present in the relationship with the client. He can express himself freely with no attempts at role playing. Genuineness leads to an openness in the client's feelings and empathic understanding. Essential to empathic understanding, in turn, is nonpossessive caring and acceptance—i.e., unconditional positive regard.

According to Rogers, these qualities will be perceived and positively responded to, and the client will develop greater awareness and gradual acceptance and trust in her own inner processes. The helper should not attempt to advise or direct the person in this growth process. He trusts the person's ability to provide her own direction; that is, he trusts the constantly evolving self-actualization process. Because person-centered therapy relies so heavily on the human qualities of the individuals involved and the genuineness of the relationship, it can be easily applied in a wide variety of situations where the aim is to increase understanding and enhance personal growth.

Most important for us in health education, the individual must gain a sense of herself as a valuable person in more than just one aspect of her being. She needs a belief in her own intrinsic worth. Humanistic counseling says that we are valuable simply because we are human beings. If we can cultivate that sense of worth, reinforcing it both by our treatment of others and by our attitudes toward ourselves, we will help create healthier, more productive, more contributing human beings.

Some Important Ethical Considerations

Students often seek out a person they trust. They have established a sense of trust prior to actually sharing with that person. Confidentiality is a basic factor in this relationship. According to Rogers (1957), we must create an empathic, warm, and respectful climate conducive to client openness and self-disclosure.

The core of ethical responsibility is *to do nothing to harm the client*. Health educators are not trained in the area of counseling (unless they receive such on their own); thus, they should review the guidelines for ethical responsibility of the American Psychological Association and those suggested by Ivey and Simek-Downing (1980):

- *Maintain confidentiality.* Respect your client's personal privacy. Do not discuss what is said during an interview with others. If you are unable to maintain confidence, the client must be told *before* you begin talking. The client can then decide whether or not the data should be shared. If a definite danger to the client or society is shared, ethical guidelines suggest that confidence be broken to protect the safety of the client or others. You must always be aware, however, that the prime responsibility of the therapist is to the individual client.
- *Recognize your limitations.* There is a certain intoxication that comes when you first learn some techniques of counseling. Beginning counselors are tempted to delve deeply into their friends' or clients' inner selves. This is potentially dangerous. A beginning counselor should work under a professional's supervision and seek advice and suggestions for improvement. Professionalism is knowing one's own limitations.
- *Avoid asking for irrelevant details.* Beginning counselors are often fascinated with the "war stories" of clients' lives. They will sometimes ask extremely personal questions about the client's sex life, travel experiences, etc. A sure sign of a poor counselor is giving prime attention to the details of a client's life while missing how he feels and thinks. Counseling is for the client's gain, not for expansion of information.

- Treat the client as you would like to be treated. Put yourself in his place. Every person desires to be treated with respect, dignity, kindness, and honesty. The building of good rapport begins by making the client feel accepted. This is achieved by respecting the client's thoughts and feelings and by treating the client as a person. A trusting relationship develops from the abilities of both client and counselor to be honest.

Looking at our own professional code of ethics (AAHE, 1994), we should most certainly add the following:

- Health educators should accurately communicate the potential benefits and consequences of services.
- Health educators should be truthful about their qualifications and the limitations of their expertise and provide services consistent with these qualifications and limitations.
- Health educators should be committed to providing professional services equitably to all people.
- Health educators should respect the rights of others to hold diverse values, attitudes, and opinions.
- Health educators should protect individuals' privacy and dignity.

It must be recognized that, despite confidentiality guidelines, individual schools, school districts, communities, and states require that child abuse, spousal abuse, drug abuse, etc. be reported to specific authorities. In these cases, you *must* advise the person with whom you are dealing that the information they are providing you with may be subject to state, local, community, or school-district disclosure regulations. It would be wise to check out the specifics prior to participating in a counseling session where these issues seem likely to crop up.

Response Theory

How you initially respond to someone may determine whether or not that person discusses a conflict situation in more depth or stops talking completely. The manner in which you respond can also have a great influence on how a student will think and act in the future. Regardless of what a helper does, the client is influenced in one direction or another. Fortunately, most of us are interested in helping people achieve their own goals rather than the goals and objectives of the helper.

Some effective listening skills are suggested by David Hutchins and Claire Cole in their book *Helping Relationships and Strategies* (1992):

- Listen carefully to what the client says and how it is said.
- Avoid interrupting, and allow the client to complete sentences and ideas.
- Use silence to encourage the client to continue talking, thus giving the client time and space to verbalize feelings that may be difficult to talk about (especially if the client has never expressed them before).

- Use reflection to clarify the client's meaning. Reflection is mirroring the essence of the client's communication in concise terms.
- Ask questions to ascertain important details: what, where, when, how, under what circumstances, how often, etc.
- Help the client systematically explore relevant content.
- Reflect similarities and discrepancies between what the client says (thinking), how the client says it (feeling), and what the client does (acting).
- Elicit feedback from the client to ensure the accuracy of the helper's perceptions.

Introspection, the rapport of our thoughts, ideas, reactions, moods, and feelings, is very important here. *Don't ever judge a person until you have heard them out. Don't ever let another teacher or counselor intrude on your judgments.*

Knowing how individuals function is essential to the entire counseling process. When establishing a working relationship, attempt to explore and understand the factors that underlie the person's behaviors and decide on a particular strategy. Know when to get involved and when not to.

How to Proceed

Between knowing, caring, and helping are some critical elements. Let's look at nine steps to helping students eliminate or decrease unhealthy behavior:

1. Help the student clearly identify the target behavior. If the behavior is complicated, break it down into individual parts. Help the student be as specific as possible.
2. Analyze the various individual aspects of the behavior to determine what contingencies exist against change. Note all the positive and negative reinforcers for the current behavior. How strong are these reinforcers?
3. Identify ways to eliminate or decrease the target behavior. What natural and logical approaches are available to help in this process? Determine what adverse consequences or positive gains can be achieved by changing the behavior. The student himself is most important in this process; let him know it. Put the responsibility totally on his shoulders. Have him write up just what he is going to do to achieve this goal.
4. Look into ways of initiating or strengthening the desired behavior. It is often wise to increase one of the student's positive behaviors when you decrease a negative one. For example, a student who is into after-school activities such as sports should increase this activity to decrease a negative behavior such as smoking.
5. Discuss the important elements for change: desire, persistence, attainability, and supportive contact.
6. Implement the behavioral change. Start with a target date, a working-through period and a change date. Specific dates must be secured from the student to head off procrastination.

7. Provide positive feedback, and evaluate the student's progress as they go along.

8. Continue supportive contact until the target behavior has been decreased or eliminated for a reasonable period of time.

9. Follow up with the student periodically to see if the desired behavioral change has been maintained.

Truly believing that your students are unique is really all you need to feel to help. The helper's objective is to gain an understanding of the client's concern in the problem situation. In exploring the problem, you must try and determine the following specifics (Hutchins and Cole, 1992):

- Who is involved in the situation? Are others (individuals or groups) consistently present when the problem occurs?
- Where do the events occur? At home or work, or in recreational settings?
- When do the incidents happen? Early in the day, at mealtime, late at night?
- What is the immediacy, frequency, and severity of the problem? Does the situation recur every day, once a week, each month, or every few months? Is it a crisis or a relatively harmless situation?
- What are the unique circumstances associated with the problem?

The Aim of Helping

In helping, there must be an overall goal. You don't go about encouraging positive change in someone unless you know where you are going. The most important goal of this book is to promote healthier behavior, which requires us to use cognitive-behavioral skills. We must help those we are working with know where they are in the present before they can develop new patterns of behavior.

Robert Carkhuff and Richard Pierce (1976) suggest three goals for helping students:

1. **Self-exploration.** To find out where they are, students must be taught to explore their own image of self, their physical environment, and the people around them.

2. **Understanding.** A sign of a successful explorer is discovery. The history books remember Leif Erikson and Columbus but say nothing about Horatio Nonentitti, an unhappy man who set out on a great quest, got lost in a fog bank, and ended up back in his home port with nothing of significance to report. But discovery itself is often not enough. Columbus eventually realized that he had not found a new route to the Indies, but a new land entirely. In other words, what the explorer finds is not always what she set out for. She must struggle to *understand* what she finds. A student who initially says "I am angry" may eventually understand she really means "I am disappointed in my inability to do something." Self-exploration is only meaningful if it leads to a greater degree of understanding.

3. **Constructive action.** To reach a goal, an individual must *act*. It is at this stage that the teacher helps initiate new behavior. Constructive action, based

on self-exploration and clear understanding, helps the student move toward a desired goal.

To help another, you have to know what he needs. The only way to find that out is to ask him.

Synthesis

The challenge in health education and personal counseling is that we often face students who choose to avoid issues of unhealthy behavior. Instead of making courageous, autonomous, and healthy choices, they limit themselves by responding in noncommittal ways and developing patterns of conforming, controlling, withdrawing, and self-destructive behaviors.

Those who conform often do so at the expense of their own identities. They often ignore their own preferences, relinquish their freedom, and give up the privilege to be self-determined. Personal health counseling can help those you are working with realize that *their* lives should be about *their* choices.

References

Association for the Advancement of Health Education. "Code of Ethics for Health Educators." *Journal of Health Education,* July/August 1994.

Carkhuff, Robert R., and Richard M. Pierce. *Teacher as Person.* Washington, DC: National Education Association, 1976.

Hutchins, David E., and Claire G. Cole. *Helping Relationships and Strategies.* Pacific Grove, CA: Brooks/Cole, 1992.

Ivey, Allen E., and Lynn Simek-Downing. *Counseling and Psychotherapy: Skills, Theories, and Practice.* Englewood Cliffs, NJ: Prentice-Hall, 1980.

Lao-tzu, *Tao the Ching.* John C.H. Wu (trans.); Paul K.T. Sih (ed.). New York: St. John's University Press, 1961.

Maslow, Abraham H. *Motivation and Personality.* New York: Harper and Row, 1954.

Rogers, Carl. *Client-Centered Therapy.* Boston: Houghton Mifflin, 1951.

____. "The Necessary and Sufficient Conditions of Therapeutic Personality Change." *Journal of Consulting Psychology* 21, 1957.

Additional Resources

American Journal of Health Behavior. PNG Publications, P.O. Box 4593, Star City, WV 26504-4593.

Brimmer, Lawrence M., and Ginger MacDonald. *The Helping Relationship: Process and Skills.* Needham Heights, MA: Allyn and Bacon, 1996.

Corey, Marianne Schneider, and Gerald Corey. *Group Process and Practice.* Pacific Grove, CA: Brooks/Cole, 1992.

Dass, Ram, and Paul Gorman. *How Can I Help?* New York: Knopf, 1985.

Havens, Leston. *Learning to Be Human.* Reading, MA: William Patrick, 1994.

Klingman, Avigdor. "Health-Related School Guidance: Practical Applications in Primary Prevention." *Personnel and Guidance Journal,* June 1984.

McMahon, Susanna. *The Portable Therapist: Wise and Inspiring Answers to the Questions People in Therapy Ask Most.* New York: Dell, 1992.

Neimark, Jill, Clare Conway, and Peter Doskoch. "Back from the Drink." *Psychology Today,* September/October 1994.

Page, Randy M., and Tana S. Page. *Fostering Emotional Well-Being in the Classroom.* Boston: Jones and Bartlett, 1992.

Peck, M. Scott. "The Importance of Being Civil." *Common Boundary,* March/April 1993.

Rowan, John. *The Reality Game: A Guide to Humanistic Counseling and Therapy.* New York: Routledge, 1991.

Sloman, Jim. *When You're Troubled: The Healing Heart.* Tiburon, CA: Ocean Blue Publishing, 1993.

Stensrud, Robert, and Kay Stensrud. "Counseling for Health Empowerment." *Personnel and Guidance Journal,* February 1982.

___. "Holistic Health through Holistic Counseling: Toward a Unified Theory." *Personnel and Guidance Journal,* March 1984.

Three Approaches to Counseling by Allen E. Ivey. Available on videocassette from Microtraining and Multicultural Development, P.O. Box 9641, North Amherst, MA 01059-9641. Video shows students how to engage in and integrate three different types of helping relationships: psychodynamic-dream analysis, humanistic positive reframing, and behavioral assertiveness training.

Three Approaches to Psychotherapy. Three-part series available on videocassette from Psychological and Educational Films (An Everett L. Shostrom Company), 3334 E. Coast Hwy., #252, Corona Del Mar, CA 92625. The famous "Gloria" series, this video is a pioneer in educational film-making in the field of psychology. Includes the work of Rogers, Perls, and Ellis in actual counseling sessions with Gloria.

Appendix A: Report of the 1990 Joint Committee on Health Education Terminology

One of the essential underpinnings of any profession is a body of well-defined terms used to enable members to communicate easily and with the clarity necessary for understanding among themselves and with others. The field of health education has changed dramatically in the past two decades. The definitions in this report provide a common interpretation of terms frequently used by health educators in a variety of settings. Therefore, the terms presented here are defined for use by the professional health educator as well as by other individuals and groups.

The Committee recognized that other health professionals (e.g., physicians, nurses, etc.) are concerned with and involved in health education as a part of their professional role and that they may have a different orientation. Consequently, they may use different terminology from that contained in this report. It is hoped, however, that the terms defined will be of help to these groups to clarify terminology used by health education professionals.

Words referring to health service and related personnel (e.g., patient educator, health counselor) or words which are in general use and understood by a variety of professionals (e.g., mass communication, objectives, self-help, self-care, evaluation) are not included. The Committee chose to define community and school health education and associated terminology, because degrees are offered in these areas. Other areas (e.g., patient and worksite health education) were omitted because they tend to be areas of emphasis rather than degrees.

There may be other interpretations of the words defined; however, those presented in this report are as many health educators view them today. The terms included reflect trends, concepts and practices. They help to explain what the profession is, who its practitioners are and how they function. Additional uses might include the following:

- articulating the health education professional preparation program to other units on college and university campuses
- assisting governmental agencies in planning effective health education policies and programs
- assisting educational boards in determining appropriate health education word usage
- guiding accrediting and credentialing agencies
- explaining the field of practice to other professionals

Source: Report of the 1990 Joint Committee on Health Education Terminology. 1991. *Journal of Health Education* 22 (2):97–108. Reprinted with permission.

- establishing a basis for consistency of language use in the professional litera-ture and in research endeavors and grantsmanship

Historically, the Public Health Education Section of the American Public Health Association (APHA) developed a statement of terminology about 1927. The first committee report on terminology was published by the American Phys-ical Education Association in 1934. The American Association for Health, Physi-cal Education, and Recreation (AAHPER) presented a report on health and physical education terminology in 1950–51. Another AAHPER joint committee was appointed in 1962 to foster and improve understanding on the part of school and public health educators. After nine years, AAHPER again took the lead which resulted in a 1973 joint committee terminology report. In 1990, the Association for the Advancement of Health Education (AAHE), an Association of the Ameri-can Alliance for Health, Physical Education, Recreation and Dance (AAHPERD), continued this leadership by convening a joint committee of delegates of the Coalition of National Health Education Organizations (CNHEO)* and a represen-tative from the American Academy of Pediatrics to update the earlier terms and to add relevant new definitions.

The Association for the Advancement of Health Education provided staff sup-port as well as funding for the Terminology Committee meeting. Additional finan-cial support for dissemination of the report was contributed by the majority of organizations represented. The meeting was convened at the AAHE/AAHPERD headquarters in Reston, Virginia, August 2–5, 1990.

Process of Formulating the Definitions

The charge to the Committee was to review the 1973 Report of the Joint Com-mittee on Health Education Terminology, to determine which terms are still rele-vant, to delete those considered outdated, to revise as deemed appropriate, and to add new terms currently used in the health education field. Individual mem-

---

*The Coalition was established in 1973 to provide a vehicle for collaboration of all major national health education organizations. Its primary mission is to mobilize the resources of the Health Educa-tion profession in order to expand and improve health education, regardless of the setting. Each mem-ber organization appoints one delegate and one alternate. The following organizations are members: American Public Health Association, School Health Education and Services Section and the Public Health Education and Health Promotion Section; American College Health Association; American School Health Association; Association for the Advancement of Health Education, American Alliance for Health, Physical Education, Recreation and Dance; Association of State and Territorial Directors of Public Health Education; Society for Public Health Education, Inc.; and the Society of State Direc-tors of Health, Physical Education and Recreation.

The Coalition facilitates national level communication, collaboration and coordination among the member organizations; provides a forum for the identification and discussion of health education issues; formulates recommendations and takes appropriate action on issues affecting member inter-ests; serves as a communication and advisory resource for agencies, organizations and persons in the public and private sectors on health education issues; and serves as a focus for the exploration and resolution of issues pertinent to professional health educators.

bers came with reference documents to be used in the process. AAHE library materials also were available. The committee was cochaired by the coordinator of the Coalition and the AAHE delegate to the Coalition.

A draft document was completed during the meeting and subsequently circulated to a select number of outside reviewers for comment. The final document was presented as a Committee Report to the AAHE Board of Directors.

After acceptance by the AAHE Board of Directors, the Report was published in the *Journal of Health Education* and copies were provided to organizations whose delegates served on the Joint Committee. Each organization was encouraged to disseminate the final report to a wide audience.

Criteria

The 1973 report was reviewed carefully. Some terms from this report were excluded, some repeated verbatim, some revised, and new terms were added based upon the criteria listed below.

Essentialness—is basic to the field of health education and necessary for communication.

Authoritativeness—is recognized or accepted by the profession as official language.

Significance—is so important in communication within and among groups that its use requires common interpretation.

Encompassment—is sufficiently broad and inclusive to eliminate unnecessary additional definitions but is restrictive enough to have clear meaning.

Usage—occurs frequently enough to affect and effect communication.

Adaptability—can be used effectively by various health professions and other individuals and groups.

Clarity—definition is necessary to maintain consistency of use among disciplines.

Contextual Definitions

Health education takes place within the broad context of health. Certain health terms are defined to clarify how health education functions. These are:

Health

There are many definitions written for the word *health*. Three examples are provided.

- "A state of complete physical, mental, and social well-being, and not merely the absence of disease and infirmity" (World Health Organization, 1946).

- "A quality of life involving dynamic interaction and independence among the individual's physical well-being, his (sic) mental and emotional reactions, and the social complex in which he (sic) exists" (Health Education).
- "An integrated method of functioning which is oriented toward maximizing the potential of which the individual is capable. It requires that the individual maintain a continuum of balance and purposeful direction with the environment where he (sic) is functioning" (Dunn, 1967).

Health Promotion and Disease Prevention

Health promotion and disease prevention is the aggregate of all purposeful activities designed to improve personal and public health through a combination of strategies, including the competent implementation of behavioral change strategies, health education, health protection measures, risk factor detection, health enhancement and health maintenance.

Healthy Life-style

A healthy life-style is a set of health-enhancing behaviors, shaped by internally consistent values, attitudes, beliefs and external social and cultural forces.

Official Health Agency

An official health agency is a publicly supported governmental organization mandated by law and/or regulation for the protection and improvement of the health of the public.

Voluntary Health Organization

A voluntary health organization is a nonprofit association supported by contributions dedicated to conducting research and providing education and/or services related to particular health problems or concerns.

(Note: Private voluntary organization—PVO—is the term used outside the U.S.A. to denote a voluntary health organization; in some countries and in connection with the United Nations, the term nongovernmental organization—NGO—is used.)

Private Health Agency

A private health agency is a profit or nonprofit organization devoted to providing primary, secondary and/or tertiary health services, which may include health education.

Primary Health-Education Definitions

Certain health-education terms are generic and are defined here, as follows.

Health-Education Field

The health education field is that multidisciplinary practice which is concerned with designing, implementing and evaluating educational programs that enable individuals, families, groups, organizations and communities to play active roles in achieving, protecting and sustaining health.

Health-Education Process

The health-education process is that continuum of learning which enables people, as individuals and as members of social structures, to voluntarily make decisions, modify behaviors and change social conditions in ways which are health enhancing.

Health-Education Program

A health-education program is a planned combination of activities developed with the involvement of specific populations and based on a needs assessment, sound principles of education and periodic evaluation using a clear set of goals and objectives.

Health-Educator

A health-educator is a practitioner who is professionally prepared in the field of health education, who demonstrates competence in both theory and practice and who accepts responsibility to advance the aims of the health-education profession.

Examples of settings for health educators and the application of health education include, but are not limited to, the following:

- schools
- communities
- post-secondary educational institutions
- medical-care institutions
- voluntary health organizations
- worksites (business and industry)
- rehabilitation centers
- professional associations
- governmental agencies
- public-health agencies
- environmental agencies
- mental-health agencies

Certified Health-Education Specialist (CHES)

A certified health-education specialist (CHES) is an individual who is credentialed as a result of demonstrating competency based on criteria established by the National Commission for Health Education Credentialing, Inc. (NCHEC).

Health-Education Coordinator

A health-education coordinator is a professional health educator who is responsible for the management and coordination of all health-education policies, activities and resources within a particular setting or circumstance.

Health-Education Administrator

A health-education administrator is a professional health educator who has the authority and responsibility for the management and coordination of all health-education policies, activities and resources within a particular setting or circumstance.

Health Information

Health information is the content of communications based on data derived from systematic and scientific methods as they relate to health issues, policies, programs, services and other aspects of individual and public health, which can be used for informing various populations and in planning health education activities.

Health Literacy

Health literacy is the capacity of an individual to obtain, interpret and understand basic health information and services and the competence to use such information and services in ways which are health enhancing.

Health Advising*

Health advising is a process of informing and assisting individuals or groups in making decisions and solving problems related to health.

---

*The Committee believes that Health Counseling is a term that should be defined by the health counseling profession.

Definitions Related to Community Settings

The terms that relate more specifically to community or public health education are defined here, as follows.

Community Health Education

Community health education is the application of a variety of methods that result in the education and mobilization of community members in actions for resolving health issues and problems which affect the community. These methods include, but are not limited to, group process, mass media communication, community organization, organization development, strategic planning, skills training, legislation, policy making and advocacy.

Community-Health Educator

A community health educator is a practitioner who is professionally prepared in the field of community/public health education who demonstrates competence in the planning, implementation and evaluation of a broad range of health promoting or health enhancing programs for community groups.

Definitions Related to Educational Settings

The terms that relate more specifically to school health education are defined here, as follows.

Comprehensive School Health Program

A comprehensive school health program is an organized set of policies, procedures and activities designed to protect and promote the health and well-being of students and staff which has traditionally included health services, healthful school environment and health education. It should also include, but not be limited to, guidance and counseling, physical education, food service, social work, psychological services and employee health promotion.

School Health Education

School health education is one component of the comprehensive school health program which includes the development, delivery and evaluation of a planned instructional program and other activities for students preschool through grade twelve, for parents and for school staff, and is designed to positively influence the health knowledge, attitudes and skills of individuals.

School Health Services

School health services are that part of the school health program provided by physicians, nurses, dentists, health educators, other allied health personnel, social workers, teachers and others to appraise, protect and promote the health of students and school personnel. These services are designed to insure access to and the appropriate use of primary health care services, prevent and control communicable disease, provide emergency care for injury or sudden illness, promote and provide optimum sanitary conditions in a safe school facility and environment and provide concurrent learning opportunities which are conducive to the maintenance and promotion of individual and community health.

School Health Educator

A school health educator is a practitioner who is professionally prepared in the field of school health education, meets state teaching requirements and demonstrates competence in the development, delivery and evaluation of curricula for students and adults in the school setting that enhance health knowledge, attitudes and problem-solving skills.

Comprehensive School Health Instruction

Comprehensive school health instruction refers to the development, delivery and evaluation of a planned curriculum, preschool through twelve, with goals, objectives, content sequence and specific classroom lessons which includes, but is not limited to, the following major content areas:

- community health
- consumer health
- environmental health
- family life
- mental and emotional health
- injury prevention and safety
- nutrition
- personal health
- prevention and control of disease
- substance use and abuse

References

Dunn, H. *High Level Wellness.* Virginia: R.W. Beatty, 1967, pp. 4–5.

Health Education: A Conceptual Approach to Curriculum Design, School Health Education Study. Washington, DC: 3M Education Press, p. 10.

Johns, E.B., Chair. Joint Committee on Health Education Terminology. Report of the Joint Committee on Health Education Terminology. *Health Education* 4:6 (1973), p. 25.

Moss, B., Chair. Joint Committee on Health Education Terminology. *Journal of Health and Physical Education* 21:41 (1950).

Rugen, M. *A Fifty-Year History of the Public Health Section of the American Public Health Association, 1922–1972.* Washington, DC: American Public Health Association, 1972, p. 9.

Williams, J.F., Chair. Report of the Health Education Section of the American Physical Education Association. Definitions of terms in health education. *Journal of Health and Physical Education* 5:16–17 (1934), pp. 50–51.

World Health Organization. *Constitution of the World Health Organization.* Geneva: World Health Organization, 1946.

Yoho, R., Chair. Joint Committee on Health Education Terminology. Health education terminology. *Journal of Health, Physical Education, Recreation* 33:27–28 (1962).

Appendix B: Terminology and Names

Terms and names often have several conceptual definitions. The following are the definitions that apply in the context of this book.

Accommodation. In Piaget's theory of cognitive development, accommodation is adaptation as a result of outside pressures: "Mental life is accommodation to the environment." However, adaptation is also viewed as an equilibrium between assimilation and accommodation" (Piaget, 1952).

Applied behavior analysis. A strategy used to modify behavior. The behavior is carefully specified and observations are made of the antecedents and consequences of the behavior. After the observations are made, attempts are made to alter the conditions that control the behavior.

Assimilation. In Piaget's theory of cognitive development, assimilation is the process by which the child reduces the universe to his own terms (Piaget, 1952). Assimilation is always associated with accommodation, since attempts to assimilate objects or events into established schemes of action or thought lead to adjustments of the schemes.

Behavioral control. The belief that an individual has the ability to influence the aversiveness of a situation.

Behavioral goal. The results we seek to achieve using a behavioral approach to teaching. Behavioral goals typically include the process (e.g., *thinking, feeling,* and *behaving*) as well as the results (e.g., practicing safe sex). Behavioral goals may involve changing covert behavior, such as feelings or thoughts, overt behavior, such as speaking before groups, or both.

Behavior medicine. An interdisciplinary field that applies theories and techniques from the behavioral sciences to the treatment and prevention of illness.

Behavior modification. A generic term referring to the applied use of behavioral psychology to bring about change in human behavior. Based on Skinner's operant-conditioning paradigm, its central tenet is that all behavior is primarily learned and maintained as a result of an individual's interaction with her environment (including other individuals). As such, behavior is susceptible to change by control over features of the environment. Per the three-term analysis of behavior (or ABC model), behavior change may be achieved by manipulating either the conditions for or the consequences of behavior, in line with the law of effect (Kessen, 1983). Simply stated, this means that rewarded behavior will tend to increase in frequency, while behavior followed by punishing consequences will tend to decline.

Behavior therapy. A form of behavior modification that includes techniques such as aversion therapy and systematic desensitization.

Bonding. The affection and recognition between a mother and a child that is supposedly established by physical contact soon after birth. Klaus and Kennell (1976) reported that mothers who had such contact showed more physical affection for their newborn babies and were more positive toward their children when they were a year old. Attempts to replicate these results have not had great success (Svejda et al., 1982); in general, mechanisms and possible critical periods for bonding have not been established (Myers, 1984). Nevertheless, there is plenty of evidence that failure to form *any* secure emotional bonds in infancy causes deviance and psychopathology.

Concept learning. Learning to categorize different experiences. This process has been much studied using the concept-identification method: A person is presented with a series of stimuli, some of which have been designated as new categories. Success in identifying the new category is demonstrated by the ability to classify it correctly.

Dewey, John. Professor at the University of Michigan and Columbia University who criticized the atomistic conception of psychic functions and the separate study of stimuli and responses. He stressed instead the adaptive meaning and unity for the individual in his or her interaction with the environment. He is most famous as a proponent of child-centered teaching techniques that stress cooperation between pupil and teacher in the classroom.

Educational attainment and locus of control. Locus of control refers to an individual's perception of reinforcement contingencies. The more a person sees a connection between her own behavior and what happens to her, the more "internal" she is considered to be. Conversely, the less she perceives this connection, seeing instead the consequences as due to luck, chance, or the influence of others, the more "external" the person is considered to be. Originating in Rotter's social-learning theory (1966), locus of control has been related to an impressive array of significant behavior ranging from academic achievement to psychological adjustment. There are multiple measures of locus of control available.

Ellis, Albert. Born in Pittsburgh, Dr. Ellis grew up in New York City, where he studied at the College of New York and at Columbia University. In his work as a marriage and family counselor, Ellis observed that people were gaining much insight by means of traditional psychotherapeutic methods but were not making enough headway in actually solving their problems. With this dilemma in mind, he formulated a therapy based on the premise that emotional problems are primarily caused by irrational attitudes and beliefs about oneself, others, and the world at large. Rational-emotive therapy (RET) is an attempt to focus on specific irrational patterns of thought and subsequent disturbing behavior. Clients are taught to become aware of their irrationalities and discard them, in order to confront difficulties in a logical way and increase the chance of living a productive and pleasurable life.

Empathy. The understanding and sharing of another person's emotional experience in a particular situation.

Empowerment. Empowering education is defined by Ira Shor (1992) as "a critical democratic pedagogy for self- and social change." It is a student-centered program for multicultural democracy in school and society. It approaches individual growth as an active, cooperative, and social process, because the self and society create each other. Human beings do not invent themselves in a vacuum, and society cannot be made unless people create it together. The goals of this pedagogy are to relate personal growth to public life by developing strong academic knowledge, habits of inquiry, and critical curiosity about society, power, inequality, and change.

Glasser, William. A practicing psychiatrist who heads the Institute for Reality Therapy in Canoga Park, California. Essentially, Glasser's reality therapy is aimed toward helping individuals become more in touch with the world about them. It provides persons with assistance in learning new ways of fulfilling their needs in real-life situations. We depend primarily on involvement with other people to fulfill our needs, yet our associations with them are complicated on varying levels. To the reality therapist, all behavior is designed to accomplish the fulfillment of these human needs for belonging, love, power, fun, and freedom. Glasser claims that we all have similar needs, but we vary in our ability to fulfill them. To be worthwhile, we must maintain a satisfactory standard of behavior, and for this reason reality therapy includes teaching morals, values, and right-and-wrong behavior. Responsibility is another basic tenet of reality therapy, defined as the ability to fulfill one's needs in a way that does not deprive others of the ability to fulfill theirs. This is accomplished by personal involvement of the therapist (teacher) with the client. A variety of techniques and skills from other theories may be employed in the process.

Humanistic education. An approach toward educating the whole person that originated from humanistic psychology and is due, in large measure, to the pioneering work of Carl Rogers (1983). Roger's work as a psychotherapist in the 1950s led him to the view that human beings have an innate potential for growth and learning, and that this potential could be released by the companionship of a teacher if the latter possessed the essential qualities of genuineness, warmth, and empathy. Genuineness refers to the ability to reveal oneself and one's true feelings. Warmth refers to the ability to accept and value another person unconditionally. Empathy refers to the ability to see someone else's situation through one's own eyes and to communicate that understanding with a gentle, nonauthoritarian clarity. Rogers preferred the word "facilitator" to that of "teacher" and came to extend his ideas from the psychotherapeutic to the school context, arguing that these same personal qualities were invaluable in an educator of whatever sort.

Identification. A core concept in psychoanalytic theory. The process through which a subject assimilates aspects of others (objects) and constitutes his own personality from the results.

Imagery. Mental visualization used in conjunction with strategies such as covert reinforcement and covert sensitization. The mental image of a behavior or situation should include all the sensations of the actual behavior or situation.

Internalization. In social-psychological terms, the adoption of attitudes or behavior patterns by an individual. Much of socialization and education is involved with encouraging the individual to internalize behavioral norms—the morals and values of his group. Full internalization is when a behavior takes place not just because it is rewarded or punished but because it is seen as correct or appropriate.

Learning strategies. Activities with the goal of increasing learning that are executed intentionally. Such strategies in the learner are either internal cognitive strategies (e.g., imagery) or external strategies (e.g., note taking).

Locus of control. The degree to which an individual perceives the events in his life to be under his control.

Maslow, Abraham. Maslow was born in Brooklyn and studied Gestalt psychology at the New School for Social Research, although most of his study was done at the University of Wisconsin. He was an articulate spokesperson for humanistic psychology, a school that has had a profound influence on the concept of humanistic education. Humanistic psychology opposes the Freudians and behaviorists, centering instead on the individual and her personal experience. Its tenets are defined as

> the focus on experience as the primary phenomenon in the study of human behavior.

> emphasis on such distinct human qualities as choice, creativity, valuation, and self-realization as opposed to thinking about human beings in mechanistic and reductionist terms.

> choosing meaningful problems for study, rather than emphasizing objectivity at the expense of significance.

> valuing the dignity and worth of each person and developing his inherent potential.

Modeling. Providing a person with a visual, verbal, or manual representation of the behavior you want her to engage in. This is also known as *imitation learning* (Bandura, 1969).

Peer group. The term is used in two different senses: first, it is defined as a group of friends or associates who share common values, interests, and activities; second, it refers to virtually all persons of the same age, reflecting the fact that schools tend to be age-graded. Peer-group influence, therefore, can be the influence that friends exercise on one another or the influence exerted by a much wider category of age-mates. The term *peer-group influence* is generally restricted to discussions of adolescents despite the fact that there is little evidence that such influence is either highly distinctive or greater among adolescents than among other age groups.

Piaget, Jean. A Swiss biologist concerned not only with the extent of children's intellectual capacities at different ages but also with the kind of experiences that lead to intellectual growth. It was mainly because of the latter interest that Piaget's ideas have played so large a part in recent debates about education.

Rogers, Carl. The late Carl Rogers wrote extensively about his experience and research in psychotherapy. His book *On Becoming a Person* (1961) is a classic. He has written also what, in the author's opinion, is the best book in the field of humanistic education. This book, *Freedom to Learn for the Eighties* (1983), is Carl Rogers' attempt to give educators his pertinent thoughts about learning that have been so popular and rewarding to those in psychology. His theme is that learning can be enjoyable when the teacher becomes a "learning facilitator" and deals with feelings as well as with the intellect. The book shows how three educators—a sixth-grade teacher, a professor of college freshmen, and a graduate faculty member—provide in different ways an exciting facilitated-learning environment in which their students thrive. He also presents the attitudes that he feels the successful learning facilitator must have and suggests ways for achieving them.

Self-esteem. An evaluation of the self that individuals make and customarily maintain. It expresses an attitude of approval or disapproval and indicates the extent to which individuals believe themselves to be capable, significant, successful, and worthy.

Sexual bias. Behavior and attitudes resulting from belief in sex stereotypes or adherence to restrictively defined sex roles.

Sexual harassment. Unwelcome sexual advances, requests for sexual favors, and other inappropriate verbal or physical conduct of a sexual nature.

Social-learning theory. An explanation of various aspects of human behavior and personality with reference to principles derived from experiments on learning.

Socialization. A technical term that gained currency in anthropology, psychology, and sociology during the late 1930s, which describes the process wherein an individual becomes a competent member of society.

Spirituality. The word "spirit," which comes from the Latin for "breathing," connotes both a sense of vital force and of something invisible. By extension, spirituality can refer to the notion of an invisible realm that functions in human life not merely alongside the visible but also inextricably bound to it. Other planes of being occur alongside the visible plane. For my purposes, the word spirit is preferable to "religious" self because it is not limited to an organized communal practice (Occhiogrosso, 1991).

Target behavior. The behavior an individual aspires to alter with a behavior-management plan.

Teacher-pupil interactions. The encounters between teachers and students is at the heart of the process of schooling, so they have been a major research topic in educational psychology. All theories of learning and cognitive development revolve around their implications for teacher strategies and techniques (especially the work of Piaget and Bruner).

References

Bandura, A. *Principles of Behavior Modification*. New York: Holt, Rinehart & Winston, 1969.

Boden, M.A. *Piaget*. New York: Viking, 1980.

Klaus, Marshall H., and John H. Kennell. *Maternal-Infant Bonding*. St. Louis: Mosby, 1976.

Maslow, Abraham. *The Farther Reaches of Human Nature*. New York: Viking, 1971.

Myers, B.J. "Mother-Infant Bonding: The Status of the Critical Period Hypothesis." *Developmental Review*, 1984.

Occhiogrosso, Peter. *Through the Labyrinth: Stories of the Search for Spiritual Transformation in Everyday Life*. New York: Viking Penguin, 1991.

Piaget, J. *The Origins of Intelligence in Children*. New York: International Universities Press, 1936.

___. "Piaget's Theory," in W. Kessen (ed.), *Handbook of Child Psychology*. New York: Wiley, 1983.

Rogers, Carl. *On Becoming a Person*. Boston: Houghton Mifflin, 1961.

___. *Freedom to Learn for the Eighties*. Columbus, OH: Charles Merrill, 1983.

Rotter, J.B. "Generalized Expectancies for Internal versus External Control of Reinforcements." *Psychological Monographs*, 1966.

Shor, Ira. *Empowering Education: Critical Teaching for Social Change*. Chicago: University of Chicago Press, 1992.

Svedja, M.J., B.J. Pannabecker, and R.N. Emde. "Parent-to-Infant Attachment: A Critique of the Early 'Bonding' Model," in *The Development of Attachment and Affiliative Systems*. New York: Plenum, 1982.

Appendix C: Additional Readings

One of the problems in compiling a list of books is that there are so many good ones to choose from. What I have listed is far from being comprehensive.

Armstrong, Thomas. *In Their Own Way*. Los Angeles: Jeremy P. Tarcher, 1987.

This book speaks to millions of parents and teachers with children experiencing less than desirable success in school. The author shows that, in most cases, these children are individuals with distinct personal learning styles (linguistic, spatial, interpersonal, etc.) and explains how to help them acquire knowledge according to these aptitudes. With chapters on attitude, imagination, attention, self-esteem, and nutrition.

Bennett, William J. *The Book of Virtues*. New York: Simon & Schuster, 1993.

The author has collected hundreds of stories in an instructive and inspiring anthology that will help children understand and develop character—and help adults teach them.

Borysenko, Joan. *Fire in the Soul: A New Psychology of Spiritual Optimism*. New York: Warner Books, 1993.

In this enlightening book, Dr. Borysenko goes beyond psychology as currently practiced and taps a deeper vein of healing. She reveals the power of spiritual optimism, a philosophy that views life crises as opportunities for personal growth and spiritual homecoming.

Branden, Nathaniel. *The Power of Self-Esteem*. Deerfield Beach, FL: Health Communications, 1992.

If you wish to know what self-esteem depends on and how to nurture it in your students, support it in your schools, and encourage it in the classroom, this is the book for you. It offers a clear message of hope. Nathaniel Brandon shows why self-esteem is basic to psychological health, achievement, and positive relationships. He introduces six basic practices for daily living that can help establish and maintain self-esteem in one's life and personal relationships, and provides guidelines for teachers, parents, managers, and therapists to help support the self-esteem of others.

___. *The Six Pillars of Self-Esteem*. New York: Bantam, 1994.

The author reveals the pathways to actualizing and celebrating our remarkable selves and offers a foundation on which to build our families, our schools, and self-esteem in young and old.

Burns, David D. *Ten Days to Self-Esteem*. New York: Quill, 1993.

In this book, the author presents an innovative approach to mood problems. Written in a remarkably clear and understanding style, this book will help you identify the causes of mood slumps and develop a more positive outlook on life.

Chopra, Deepak. *Unconditional Life: Mastering the Forces that Shape Personal Reality*. New York: Bantam Books, 1991.

Filled with dramatic case histories, *Unconditional Life* brings together disciplines ranging from modern physics and neuroscience to the ancient traditions of Indian wisdom. Dr. Chopra's thesis is that our perception creates our experience—we live inside the boundaries of our conditioning, and yet boundless freedom lies outside them.

Currie, Elliott. *Reckoning: Drugs, the Cities, and the American Future*. New York: Hill and Wang, 1993.

The author offers an incisive, original argument about the social roots of the drug crisis and the steps we must take to solve it. Drawing on a vast body of research, he examines the uses and limits of traditional strategies—law enforcement, treatment, and legalization, arguing that our only hope to reverse the crisis lies in a more profound reckoning with its underlying causes: the growing disintegration of our cities' economic and social structures.

Fanning, Patrick. *Visualization for Change*. Oakland, CA: New Harbinger Publications, 1994.

The author gives a very clear, concise, and accurate picture of the workings of the immune system. Patrick Fanning's detailed visualizations for fighting cancer, arthritis, and allergies are fascinating. He also provides applications for self-improvement, stress reduction, and self-esteem.

Fervis, Kathe, and Carol Montag (eds.). *Progressive Education for the 1990s: Transforming Practice*. Brandon, VT: Holistic Education Press, 1991.

This volume brings together thirty-three essays from the early years (1988–90) of the pioneering journal *Holistic Education Review*. The authors are teachers and principals in public and alternative schools, educational scholars, and independent writers and consultants who are developing (and in many cases implementing) truly progressive solutions to the challenges of education today. Their writings demonstrate how a holistic perspective, broadly defined, offers alternatives to the conventional, narrowly technical, and managerial solutions generally proposed in education reform.

Garrett, Laurie. *The Coming Plague: Newly Emerging Diseases in a World out of Balance*. New York: Farrar, Straus and Giroux, 1994.

The author plunges into an exhaustive history of the AIDS-genesis question and virtually everything known about it through mid-1994. Along the way, she disposes of arguments that HIV represents a U.S. germ-warfare experiment gone wrong, a monstrous genocidal plot against the black race, or a colossal distraction from the real cause of AIDS—a "self-destructive" gay life-style. Garrett's AIDS chapter—only about 15 percent of her panoramic examination of the recent relationship between humans and pathogens—contains dozens of informative surprises, even for those who think themselves reasonably up-to-date about AIDS.

Gerstner, Louis V. Jr. *Reinventing Education: Entrepreneurship in American Public Schools.* New York: Dutton, 1994.

The Next Century Schools program is based on a simple, yet radical idea: to make public school educators think like entrepreneurs! No idea or innovation is off limits. *Reinventing Education* is the first report on the program's amazing success.

Glasser, William. *The Quality School.* New York: Harper & Row, 1990.

In this book, Glasser claims that we must stop settling for minimal goals, such as reducing dropout rates and dealing with discipline problems, and start convincing students to work hard because there is quality both in what they are asked to do and how they are asked to do it.

Halberstam, Joshua. *Everyday Ethics: Inspired Solutions to Real-Life Dilemmas.* New York: Penguin, 1994.

The perfect handbook for understanding what constitutes moral relationships with friends, enemies, and one's own self in common situations.

Hazelton, Deborah M. *Solving the Self-Esteem Puzzle.* Deerfield Beach, FL: Health Communications, 1991.

The author shows us how to build our self-confidence, resolve lingering shame issues, and reclaim the self-worth we deserve.

James, Muriel, and John James. *Passion for Life: Psychology and the Human Spirit.* New York: Penguin Books, 1991.

This extraordinary and imaginative guide identifies the seven basic urges that are expressions of the spiritual self in all of us, showing us exactly how we learn to fulfill these fundamental needs.

Judson, Stephanie (ed.). *A Manual on Nonviolence and Children.* Philadelphia, PA: New Society Publications, 1984.

This resource contains over one-hundred exercises, games, and agendas developed, tested, or used by the Friends Committee on Nonviolence and Children in Philadelphia. It helps children gain a concrete understanding of how values extend to the world.

Kilpatrick, William. *Why Johnny Can't Tell Right from Wrong: Moral Illiteracy and the Case for Character Education.* New York: Simon & Schuster, 1992.

The best way to encourage moral growth, says Kilpatrick, is to return to the proven model of character education, with its emphasis on setting good examples and good habits of behavior. Kilpatrick explains why this approach works and gives examples of school systems that have switched to character education with impressive results.

Kreidley, William J. *Creative Conflict Resolution*. Glenview, IL: Scott, Foresman and Company, 1984.

Creative Conflict Resolution will help you respond constructively to the conflicts that occur in every K–6 classroom. This resource book offers over twenty conflict-resolution techniques along with fourteen reproducible worksheets and over two-hundred class-tested activities and cooperative games.

Lawson, Annette, and Deborah L. Rhode. *The Politics of Pregnancy: Adolescent Sexuality and Public Policy*. New Haven: Yale University Press, 1993.

This collection of articles provides an excellent sustained treatment of the adolescent pregnancy crisis while also challenging the assumption that it *is* a crisis. Bringing together truly talented scholars with diverse perspectives, this book provides a model of interdisciplinary dialogue.

Lewis, Hunter. *A Question of Values: Six Ways We Make the Personal Choices that Shape Our Lives*. New York: Harper & Row, 1990.

Not only does Lewis illuminate our own values and those of others, he also helps us sort through a variety of social issues—for example, whether values should or should not be taught in the classroom or the general problem of moral education in American schools and colleges. He makes brilliant sense of the moral and ethical confusion of our times.

Lickona, Thomas. *Education for Character: How Our Schools Teach Respect and Responsibility*. New York: Bantam Books, 1992.

Masterfully interweaving the findings of our fifty years of psychological and educational research with examples drawn from his own extensive experience in schools, Lickona provides a sorely needed approach to character education in a pluralistic society.

Martz, Larry. *Making Schools Better*. New York: Times Books, 1992.

An upbeat look at innovative programs in a dozen schools that are boosting academic performance and helping troubled students at the same time. Full of human interest, the book is designed to inspire more teachers and parents to take small steps with children that could lead to a giant step for American education.

Naylor, Thomas H., William H. Willimon, and Magdalena R. Naylor. *The Search for Meaning*. Nashville, TN: Abingdon Press, 1994.

The authors present a seven-step process for coming to grips with what it means to be a human being who lives, loves, works, plays, and confronts the concept of death. A guide to coming to terms with life and its meaning.

Orenstein, Peggy. *School Girls: Young Women, Self-Esteem, and the Confidence Gap.* New York: Doubleday, 1994.

Orenstein takes us behind the scenes—into the classroom, schoolyard, and family home—and, with her natural gift for listening to young women, powerfully illuminates the forces that shape and so often break the precarious confidence of American girls. *School Girls* is provocative and deeply troubling, and it should be read by anyone who cares about education, the rights of women, and the future of the next generation.

Pearce, Joseph Chilton. *Evolution's End: Claiming the Potential of Our Intelligence.* New York: Harper & Row, 1992.

Staggering and inspirational insights, discoveries, and teachings on the nature of reality. Teachers will gain greatly by reading this book.

Peck, M. Scott. *The Difference Drum: Community Making and Peace.* New York: Touchstone, 1987.

A very practical and optimistic book about community. For those teachers who would like to establish a "just community" in their classroom, begin with this.

Peele, Stanton. *Diseasing of America: Addiction Treatment out of Control.* Boston: Lexington Books, 1989.

This book documents the scientific fallacies of the addiction-as-disease movement. It points the way to positive personal and social change and shows how society can support people in outgrowing or avoiding addiction altogether.

Rodin, Judith. *Body Traps: Breaking the Binds that Keep You from Feeling Good about Your Body.* New York: Morrow, 1992.

The author examines why we fall into self-defeating, health-damaging obsessions and what we can do to escape them. Making use of her ground-breaking research, the author illustrates the most common traps people fall into in pursuit of the elusive beauty ideal: self-image distortion, competition, and food and exercise abuse.

Sontag, Susan. *Illness as Metaphor and AIDS and Its Metaphors.* New York: Doubleday, 1989.

An exemplary demonstration of the power of the intellect in the face of the lethal metaphors of fear in both illness and AIDS.

Strauss, Susan. *Sexual Harassment and Teens: A Program for Positive Change.* Minneapolis, MN: Free Spirit Publishing, 1992.

Provides a complete course in sexual harassment you can start using today. This book helps you identify and solve sexual-harassment problems that may exist in the teaching/learning environment and prevent future problems.

Warter, Carlos. *Recovery of the Sacred: Lessons in Soul Awareness.* Deerfield Beach, FL: Health Communications, 1994.

Whether looking for a deeper understanding of human potential, the meaning of life, or an escape from the material world in which we live, more and more people are seeking ways to connect with their spiritual identity. Warter says that "when we understand that we *are* soul—we don't *have* a soul— we *are* soul, we enter into the big story wherein love, light, timelessness, and wholeness is our destiny."

Wichet, Susanne. *Keeping the Peace: Practicing Cooperation and Conflict Resolution with Preschoolers.* Philadelphia, PA: New Society Publishers, 1989.

Keeping the Peace helps parents, teachers, and other caregivers create an environment in which the level of conflict is low enough that the adults can guide the resolution process in such a way that it works for the child and can be used again by the child.

Appendix D: Code of Ethics for Health Educators

Preamble

Health education is a process concerned with designing, implementing, and evaluating educational programs that enable individuals, families, groups, organizations, and communities to play active roles in achieving, protecting, and sustaining health. Its purpose is to contribute to health and well-being by promoting lifestyles, community actions, and conditions that make it possible to live healthful lives. Health educators have professional responsibilities to the community and society in which they work and live. They apply and make public their knowledge of health with integrity and dedication to the truth. Health education is not the answer to every health problem and should not be positioned as a stand-alone, independent strategy. However, carefully planned and implemented programs are an essential component of effective health promotion, disease prevention, treatment, and care.

Health education is based on humanitarian and democratic ideals. Health educators are dedicated to improving the health of individuals and groups through educational intervention and other strategies that are characterized by respect for competing value systems, an overriding commitment to self-determination, justice, and the right of individuals to make informed choices. Health educators employ a recognized body of knowledge about human health and disease in order to promote well-being. They liberate people through the honest exchange of accurate and valid information, with appropriate consideration and respect for human diversity and the right of individuals and communities to determine their own ways of living.

Effective health education is planned with input from representatives of target populations and is influenced by the nature of the health problem and setting (e.g., school, community, workplace, or health care organizations). Health education methodologies and strategies are uniquely tailored to address the circumstances of a given population, person, or situation, and are consistent with empirically supported health education and learning theories.

Health educators have knowledge of scientific, behavioral, cultural, and philosophical foundations of health and health behavior. As a result of their professional preparation, health educators are able to apply this knowledge in planning, implementing, and evaluating health education programs.

This Code of Ethics provides a common set of values designed to guide health educators in resolving many of the ethical dilemmas experienced in professional life. These guidelines regarding professional conduct of health educators require a commitment to behave ethically and to encourage and support the ethical behavior of others.

Article 1: Responsibility to the Public

Health educators' ultimate responsibility is to educate people about health in order to promote wellness and quality of life. Health educators recognize that decisions about health are made at individual, family, peer, community, societal, and global levels. When there is a conflict of interest among individuals, groups, agencies, or institutions, health educators consider all issues and give priority to the principles of responsibility and freedom of choice.

Section 1

Health educators support the right of individuals to make informed decisions regarding their own health.

Section 2

Health educators encourage actions and social policies which support the best balance of benefits over harm for all affected parties.

Section 3

Health educators accurately communicate the potential benefits and consequences of services.

Section 4

Health educators act on conditions that can adversely affect the health of individuals and communities.

Section 5

Health educators are truthful about their qualifications and the limitations of their expertise and provide services consistent with these qualifications and limitations.

Section 6

Health educators are committed to providing professional services equitably to all people.

Section 7

Health educators respect the rights of others to hold diverse values, attitudes, and opinions.

Section 8

Health educators protect individuals' privacy and dignity.

Article II: Responsibility to the Profession

Health educators are responsible for the reputation of their profession. Their professional behavior is consistent with the Code of Ethics. When appropriate, they consult with colleagues in order to promote ethical conduct.

Section 1

Health educators maintain their professional competence through continued study and education.

Section 2

Health educators treat all individuals equitably in professional actions (e.g., hiring, promotion, retention, work assignments, and admission policies) regardless of age, gender, race, ethnicity, national origin, religion, sexual orientation, disability, socioeconomic status, or any basis prescribed by law.

Section 3

Health educators encourage and accept critical discourse in order to improve the profession.

Section 4

Health educators contribute to the development of the profession by sharing program components they have found to be effective.

Section 5

Health educators to not manipulate or violate others' rights in sexual, emotional, financial, or other ways.

Section 6

Health educators are aware of possible conflicts of interest and exercise integrity in these situations.

Section 7

Health educators give appropriate recognition to students and colleagues for their professional contributions.

Article III: Responsibility to Employers

Health educators recognize the boundaries of their professional competence. They provide services and programs for which they are qualified by education and experience and they are accountable for their professional activities.

Section 1

Health educators accurately represent their own qualifications and the qualifications of others they recommend.

Section 2

Health educators use current professional standards, theory, and guidelines as criteria when accepting consultations, when delegating health education activities, and when making referrals.

Section 3

Health educators accurately represent potential program outcomes to employers.

Section 4

Health educators make known competing commitments, conflicts of interest, and endorsement of products when the quality of health education delivered could be adversely affected by these activities.

Section 5

Health educators openly communicate to employers when expectations or job-related assignments conflict with professional ethics.

Article IV: Responsibility in the Delivery of Health Education

Health educators promote integrity in the delivery of health education and respect the fundamental rights, dignity, confidentiality, and worth of all people by adapting strategies and methods to the needs of different populations.

Section 1

Health educators are sensitive to the variety of cultural and social norms.

Section 2

Health educators promote the right of individuals and groups to be actively involved in all aspects of the educational process.

Section 3

Health educators use educational strategies and methods that reflect the Code of Ethics and applicable laws. If neither law nor the Code of Ethics provides guidance in resolving an issue, health educators consider other professional standards as well as their own personal standards of ethical behavior, and consult other health educators.

Section 4

Health educators implement strategies and methods that enable individuals to adopt healthy lifestyles through choice rather than by coercion.

Section 5

Health educators conduct regular evaluations of program effectiveness.

Section 6

Health educators provide educational interventions that are grounded in a theoretical framework and supported by empirical evidence.

Article V: Responsibility in Research and Evaluation

Health educators contribute to the health of the population and to the profession through research and evaluation activities. When planning and conducting research or evaluation, health educators do so in accordance with federal and state laws and regulations, organizational and institutional policies, and professional standards.

Section 1

Health educators conduct research in accordance with recognized scientific and ethical standards.

Section 2

Health educators ensure that the consent of participants in research is voluntary and informed.

Section 3

Health educators implement standards to protect the rights, health, safety, and welfare of human research participants.

Section 4

Health educators maintain confidentiality and protect the privacy of research participants in accordance with law and professional standards.

Section 5

Health educators take credit, including authorship, only for work they have actually performed and give credit to the contributions of others.

Section 6

Health educators who serve as research or evaluation consultants discuss their results only with those to whom they are providing service, unless maintaining such confidentiality would jeopardize the health or safety of others.

Section 7

Health educators honor commitments they have made to research participants.

Section 8

Health educators report the results of their research and evaluation accurately and in a timely fashion.

The AAHE Code of Ethics was developed over a two year period of time by a committee appointed by the AAHE president. Over 500 health educators working in a variety of settings participated in providing opinions on the various drafts of the document. Credit is given to SOPHE's Code of Ethics which served as a basis for the development of this document. The preface includes information adopted from the report of the 1990 joint committee on health education terminology and a joint document of WHO and IUHE published in 1991, titled "Meeting Global Challenges: A Position Paper on Health Education." (Association for the Advancement of Health Education, 1900 Association Drive, Reston, VA 22091, 703/476-3437.)

Appendix E: Interactive Video

Interactive video, as used in this context, is a process of getting students involved in what they are viewing. This requires the health educator to preview the video numerous times in order to highlight important ideas and direct questions that require specific answers and that elicit the students' thoughts and feelings.

After showing a video, have students get into small groups to share feelings and specific responses or get into one large group to do the same. In either case, your role should be specific in terms of what you want from the group.

In the samples provided here, the films *Philadelphia* and *Forrest Gump*, the questions revolve around such relevant health issues as personal morals and values, gay/lesbian life-styles, AIDS, and drug abuse. Questions are presented and specific cognitive answers are provided to help your students get the most out of the exercise.

Questions for the film *Philadelphia*

1. After the first courtroom scene, Andy and Joe get on the elevator. What does the writing on the elevator door say?
2. There is a scene in the clinic where Andy observes a man with AIDS having his blood drawn. The phlebotomist says, "We're going to have to start looking for veins in your feet, sweetheart." Why do you think Andy is affected by this scenario?
3. When Andy is called to the conference room to discuss the *Highline v. Sanders Systems* case, Charles asks, "Who would you like to see win this case?" Andy responds, "Highline." When asked why, he says, "If Sanders Systems wins, an energetic young company is destroyed." At this point, do you think Andy's answer is representative of his values?
4. When asked by a law partner what the lesion on his forehead was caused by, Andy says he was hit by a racquetball. Why do you think he chose to conceal his disease from the firm?
5. In the emergency room, the doctor tells Miguel that he is "not a member of [Andy's] immediate family," and he could have him "removed from the ER." Do you think he was being discriminatory because they are homosexuals? Explain.
6. In Joe's office, Joe notices everything Andy touches—where he puts his hat down, his cigar, and the picture of the baby he holds. Joe is apparently uncom-

---

Source: Patricia A. Houston, MEd., CHES.

fortable. Do you think this attitude is representative of society's attitude toward people with AIDS? Can you cite a specific example?

7. In Joe's office, Andy flashes back to the day he was fired. What, if anything, was peculiar to you about this scene?

8. Joe asks, "Didn't you have an obligation to tell your employer you had this dreaded, deadly, infectious disease?" How do you feel about someone purposefully concealing his or her HIV status?

9. When Andy leaves Joe's office, he stands in front of the door and cries. The door has the name of the law firm on it. What is the name of the law firm and what is it in reference to?

10. Why did Joe leave the doctor's office without getting his blood drawn?

11. In Joe's kitchen, he says, "You can call me old-fashioned; you can call me conservative; just call me a man." What do you feel Joe was insinuating by this comment?

12. Joe says to his baby, Clarise, "Stay away from your Aunt Teresa." Why do you think he said that?

13. Why did the director of the film show us the scenes of Joe holding the door open for a woman in the delicatessen and giving Santa Claus money, as they appear to have no bearing on the plot?

14. In the library, the librarian tells Andrew that he found the information on HIV discrimination. He then states, "We do have a private research room available." Andy says, "I'm fine right here, thank you." The librarian then asks, "Wouldn't you be more comfortable in a research room?" How does Andy respond?

15. How was discrimination defined in the law book?

16. The director chose to have the summons delivered during the basketball game. Why do you suppose he chose basketball rather than another sport?

17. In the corridor after the basketball game, Charles says, "Andy brought AIDS into our offices, into our men's room. He brought AIDS into our annual cocktail family picnic." What is your reaction to this remark?

18. How does Andy's family treat him? Would you and your family respond the same way if someone in your family had AIDS?

19. What did Andy's mother say when he asked her about going to court?

20. What does the first picket sign shown say?

21. In the bar scene, a man began teasing Joe about his sexuality. Do you think Joe responded appropriately?

22. In the drug store, a law student tries to "pick up" Joe. He becomes offended that the law student thought he was gay. How do you think Joe can represent a gay man when he has such strong feelings about being identified as a gay?

23. In court, Joe attacks his own witness by asking him if he is gay using a multitude of slang terms. Why do you think Joe burst out like that? Could it have been dealt with another way?

24. One law partner says, "I felt and still feel nothing but the deepest sympathy and compassion for people like Melissa who contracted this terrible disease through no fault of their own." What was the underlying statement here?

25. When Andy and Miguel argue about Andy's "time left," they decide to throw a party instead of planning his memorial service. Why?

26. How is the aria from the opera related to Andy?

I bring sorrow to those who love me. It was during this sorrow that love came to me. Live still. I am life. Heaven is in your eyes. I am divine. I am oblivion. I am God who comes down to the earth and makes the earth a Heaven. I am love, I am life.

27. After the party, Joe goes home and holds his daughter, then his wife. Why do you think he did this?

28. When Andy is on the stand and unbuttoning his shirt to reveal his lesions, what did two of the defense lawyers say to each other?

   a. "My God, what a nightmare."
   b. "He asked for it."

29. When Charles is on the stand, he says, "Read your bible, Mr. Miller." Why does he say this?

30. When Mr. Seidman was on the stand, he said he would probably regret not talking to Andy about his health for as long as he lived. Why do you think he feels this way?

31. How do *you* feel about people who have AIDS?

32. Does your attitude about people who have AIDS differ depending on their sexual orientation as well as their being male or female?

33. Do you think justice was served by the jury's verdict?

34. If you worked in a medical setting, would you want a law passed mandating HIV testing for staff and patients alike?

35. Did this film have any impact on your attitude toward people who are infected with AIDS?

Answers to Specific Questions

1. "No justice, no peace."
7. They placed his chair at the far end of the room, away from everyone else.
9. ___ & Shilts's Legal Services. Randy Shilts is author of *And the Band Played On.*
14. "No. Would it make you more comfortable?"
15. "Formulating opinions about others not based on their individual merits but rather on their membership in a group with the same characteristics."
19. "I didn't raise my kids to sit on the back of the bus. Get in there and fight for your rights."
20. "AIDS cures homosexuality."

Questions for the Film Forrest Gump

1. When you first see Forrest, how do you feel about him? How is this reflective of your value of people?

2. On the bench, he says to the nurse, "Mamma says life is like a box of chocolates; you never know what you're gonna get." What does this mean?

3. We find out that Forrest is named after General Nathan Bedford Forrest of the Ku Klux Klan. What are the different values associated with the KKK?

4. After getting his foot caught in the street drain, Forrest's mother says to him, "Don't ever let anybody tell you they're better than you, Forrest. If God had intended everybody to be the same, he would have given us all braces on our legs." What value does this statement promote?

5. When the principal doesn't want to let Forrest attend a "normal" school, Forrest's mother sleeps with him to get her son into it. How do you feel about this?

6. Forrest's mother lies to him when he asks what a vacation is. Why do you think she did this? Should she have done this?

7. On the bus to school, when nobody will let Forrest sit with them, Jenny says, "you can sit here if you want." What value does this represent?

8. On the bus, Forrest tells Jenny that his Mamma says "stupid is as stupid does." What does this phrase mean to you?

9. When Forrest goes to visit Jenny at her house, they run into the field and hide from her father. Why are they running?

10. While running away from the local boys, Forrest runs through the football game. In the next scene, we find out that Forrest attended the University of Alabama on a football scholarship. How do you feel about this?

11. On the University of Alabama campus, a rally is being held to protest black students attending classes. What are the different values represented at this rally?

12. While in the army, Forrest sees a picture of Jenny in *Playboy* magazine. She was thrown out of school for this. What values are presented here, and should they have affected her school status?

13. After Forrest carries Jenny off the stage, they walk down the street. Jenny asks Forrest if he thinks she can fly off the bridge. What is she alluding to?

14. After Jenny leaves Forrest on the bridge, he goes to Vietnam. What are the different values here?

15. In Vietnam, Forrest's platoon is attacked. Forrest carries out everybody he could find, including Lieutenant Dan, who wanted to be left to die. How do you feel about this? Should Forrest have left Dan to die?

16. After Forrest carried Bubba out of the woods, Bubba asks, "Why did this happen, Forrest?" What is he asking?

17. After receiving the Medal of Honor, Forrest walks to the mall in Washington where he speaks to the crowd. What are the different views expressed here?

18. What does the phrase "like peas and carrots" mean?

19. At the Black Panther party, a man hits Jenny. What value does he hold about women? How does Jenny respond?

20. How did Jenny learn to expand her mind in California?

21. When Forrest meets Lieutenant Dan again, he asks him if he met Jesus. What does religion have to do with values?

22. On New Year's Eve in Lieutenant Dan's apartment, one of the women asks Forrest if he is "stupid or something," and Dan gets angry. Why?

23. When Forrest goes to the White House with the ping-pong team, he sees people searching an office building with flashlights. What is he seeing?

24. After being discharged from the army, Forrest endorses a ping-pong paddle even though he doesn't like it. What value is represented here?

25. One day while Forrest is shrimping, Lieutenant Dan shows up to work with him. Why did he do this?

26. Why did the man on the bench laugh when he found out that Forrest was the owner of the Bubba-Gump Shrimp Company?

27. When Jenny comes home to see Forrest and they see the house she grew up in, Jenny gets angry and throws rocks at the house. What does Forrest say?

28. When Forrest asks Jenny to marry him, she says, "You don't want to marry me, Forrest." Why does she say this?

29. The morning after Forrest and Jenny make love, Jenny leaves. Why?

30. While running across the United States, Forrest picks up a group of followers. Why were they upset when he stopped running?

31. Forrest visits Jenny in her apartment and finds out that they have a child together. Why didn't Jenny tell Forrest long ago that he parented her child?

32. In the park, we find out that Jenny has an unknown virus. What do you think this is?

33. Why does Jenny ask Forrest to marry her when she didn't want to marry him before?

34. When Jenny dies, what does Forrest tell Jenny his Momma says about dying?

35. Throughout the movie, we see the assassinations of John Kennedy, Robert Kennedy, and John Lennon and the attempted assassinations of Wallace and Reagan. What is the commonality among all these killings, and how do you feel about it?

36. What was the purpose of this movie?

37. What kind of values does Forrest have?

38. Whom can you identify with best in the movie, and why?

Answers to Specific Questions

9. Jenny's father was abusive to her. She was trying to get away from him.
13. Suicide
20. Using drugs
23. Watergate
27. "Sometimes there just aren't enough rocks."
34. "Dying is a part of life."

Index